9 X

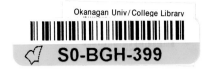
DATE DUE

Weeding June 2015

This title was selected for retention in the library because of the circulation stats indicated higher use: **9X**

BRODART

The Concept of Defense Mechanisms in Contemporary Psychology

Uwe Hentschel   Gudmund J.W. Smith
Wolfram Ehlers   Juris G. Draguns
Editors

The Concept of Defense Mechanisms in Contemporary Psychology

Theoretical, Research, and Clinical Perspectives

With 51 Illustrations

Springer-Verlag
New York Berlin Heidelberg London Paris
Tokyo Hong Kong Barcelona Budapest

Uwe Hentschel, Ph.D., Department of Personality Psychology, University of Leiden, 2300 RB Leiden, The Netherlands

Gudmund J.W. Smith, Ph.D., Department of Psychology, University of Lund, S-22350 Lund, Sweden

Wolfram Ehlers, M.D., Center for Psychotherapy Research, D-70597 Stuttgart 70, Germany

Juris G. Draguns, Ph.D., Department of Psychology, The Pennsylvania State University, University Park, PA 16802, USA

Library of Congress Cataloging-in-Publication Data
The Concept of defense mechanisms in contemporary psychology:
  theoretical, research, and clinical perspectives / Uwe Hentschel . . .
  [et al.], editors.
      p.   cm.
  Includes bibliographical references.
  ISBN 0-387-94003-0.—ISBN 3-540-94003-0
  1. Defense mechanisms (Psychology)   I. Hentschel, Uwe.
  [DNLM: 1. Defense Mechanisms.   WM 193 C744]
  BF175.5.D44C66   1993
  155.2—dc20   92-48254

Printed on acid-free paper.

Production coordinated by Chernow Editorial Services, Inc., and managed by
   Christin R. Ciresi; manufacturing supervised by Jacqui Ashri.
Typeset by Best-set Typesetter Ltd., Hong Kong.
Printed and bound by Edwards Brothers, Inc., Ann Arbor, MI.
Printed in the United States of America.

9 8 7 6 5 4 3 2 1

ISBN 0-387-94003-0 Springer-Verlag New York Berlin Heidelberg
ISBN 3-540-94003-0 Springer-Verlag Berlin Heidelberg New York

Preface

What is the scientific status and the "truth value" of the concept of defense mechanisms? Among contemporary psychologists, three types of answers to this question may be expected. Some would wholeheartedly endorse the theoretical, clinical, and research value of this notion; others would reject it outright. Between these two extremes, a large number of observers, perhaps the majority, would suspend their judgment. Their attitude, compounded of hope and doubt, would capitalize on defense as an interesting and promising concept. At the same time, these psychologists would express skepticism and disappointment over its clinical limitations, theoretical ambiguity, and research failures.

The present volume is primarily addressed to the audience of hopeful skeptics—those who have not given up on the notion of defense, yet have been frustrated by the difficulties of incorporating it into the modern, streamlined structure of psychology. To this end, we have brought together theoretical and empirical contributions germane to defense together with reports about their applications to clinical and personality assessment, especially in relation to psychopathology, psychosomatics, and psychotherapeutic intervention.

The idea for this volume originated at the 24th International Congress of Psychology in Sydney, where the four editors found themselves at the Symposium on Experimental Psychodynamic Research. Members of the audience asked about the availability of a systematic and up-to-date overview of this topic, and it became apparent that there was no such resource in the current or recent literature. As we immersed ourselves in this topic, we became aware of the magnitude and difficulty of the task. Above all, decisions about inclusion and exclusion had to be faced and the recurrent question about where to draw the line had to be answered. Our response was to concentrate on percept-genetic techniques, clinical ratings, personality questionnaires, and projective tests. We also allocated some space to speech samples and psychophysiological indicators in relation to defenses. In this manner, we ended up with 28 contributions. Their collective and principal objective is to highlight the advantages and the potentials of the currently active approaches to empirical research on defense mechanisms. At the same time, we have endeavored not to hide the unsolved problems and the inherent difficulties and limitations of this research area.

The results of these studies are varied. The method specificity of a great many findings is evident. To overcome these limitations, we have included nine theoretically oriented chapters, which we hope will be helpful in articulating the theoretical issues and the conceptual assumptions that are shared by the contributors to the volume. Although the chapters can be read separately, in any order, we recommend that the reader new to this field turn to Chapter 7, especially if he or she desires an introduction to the percept-genetic approaches. In any case, the chapters are extensively cross-referenced so that the readers can easily turn their sights from theory to research and vice versa.

Conceived at an international congress, the present volume has retained a cosmopolitan outlook. Contributions from the United States, Great Britain, Sweden, Germany, Israel, Chile, and the Netherlands are included. Inevitably, a high proportion of the chapters are written by authors who are not native speakers of English. As editors, we have tried to keep in mind the problems that have resulted from this circumstance and to improve the clarity and usage of the text whenever we could. We can only hope that these efforts have been reasonably successful, and we apologize to our readers for any avoidable peculiarities and idiosyncrasies that we have failed to spot.

The boundaries of the concept of defense are fuzzy, and unsolved problems and unanswered questions abound. The four editors, however, share the conviction that there is enough validated and applicable information to sustain the interest of both basic researchers and practitioners and to justify the pursuit of the theoretical and empirical objectives posited in this book. What fascinates us—and we hope to transmit our enthusiasm to some of our readers—is the possibility of merging the psychodynamic and the experimental traditions of investigation. Our belief is that this merger is one of the waves of the future in psychology. If so, we hope that this book will serve as an invitation to develop new avenues of experimental psychodynamic investigation and to refine and extend the existing approaches.

We are grateful to all the contributors who have complied with the difficult conditions inherent in delivering an electronically stored manuscript. Our thanks go to the editors and employees at Springer-Verlag, especially for allowing us more pages than originally allocated, and to the Swedish Council for Humanistic and Social Science Research for the financial support extended to this project. Last but not least, we thank several people who have helped us in the production process: M. Weijand for coordinating and correcting work, G. Veltema and A. Wentzel for retyping parts of the text and the tables, and M. Echteld for preparing some of the figures in Harvard Graphics.

Uwe Hentschel
Gudmund J.W. Smith
Wolfram Ehlers
Juris G. Draguns

Contents

Part III Personality and Applied Psychology

Part V Psychosomatics

Contributors

Daniela Aeschelmann, Department of Psychotherapy, University of Ulm, D-7900 Ulm, Germany

Renate Arnold, M.D., University Hospital, D-7900 Ulm, Germany

Frits J. Bekker, Ph.D., Department of Personality Psychology, University of Leiden, 2300 Leiden, The Netherlands

Sidney J. Blatt, Ph.D., Department of Psychiatry, Yale University, New Haven, CT 06520, USA

Nicola Ciani, M.D., Department of Psychiatry, Torvergata University, 00100 Rome, Italy

Hope R. Conte, Ph.D., Albert Einstein College of Medicine of Yeshiva University, Bronx, NY 10461, USA

Phebe Cramer, Ph.D., Department of Psychology, Williams College, Williamstown, MA 01267, USA

Juris G. Draguns, Ph.D., Department of Psychology, The Pennsylvania State University, University Park, PA 16802, USA

Herbert Dreier, Department of Psychology, University of Mainz, D-6500 Mainz, Germany

Wolfram Ehlers, M.D., Center for Psychotherapy Research, D-70597 Stuttgart 70, Germany

Roland Fellhauer, Gelderland Clinic, D-4170 Geldern, Germany

Janny Fronczek, Department of Psychonomics, University of Amsterdam, 1018 WB Amsterdam, The Netherlands

Inez Gitzinger, Ph.D., Werner Schwidder Clinic for Psychosomatic Medicine, 7812-Bad Krozingen, Germany

Louis A. Gottschalk, M.D., Ph.D., Department of Psychiatry and Human Behavior, College of Medicine, University of California, Irvine, CA 92717, USA

Uwe Hentschel, Ph.D., Department of Personality Psychology, University of Leiden, 2300 RB Leiden, The Netherlands

Arn Hosemann, Ph.D., Daimler Benz Research Institute, D-1000 Berlin, Germany

Per Johnsson, Department of Psychiatry, University of Lund, S-22185, Lund, Sweden

Horst Kächele, M.D., Department of Psychotherapy, University of Ulm, D-7900 Ulm, Germany

Marianne E. Kardos, The Cambridge Hospital, Cambridge, MA 02139, USA

Manfred Kießling, Gesellschaft zur Förderung Persönlichkeits- und Sozialpyschologisches-Forschung, University of Mainz, D-6500 Mainz, Germany

Paul Kline, Ph.D., D.Sc., Washington Singer Laboratories, Department of Psychology, University of Exeter, Exeter EX44QG, England

Carl-Walter Kohlmann, Ph.D., Institute of Psychology, University of Mainz, D-6500 Mainz, Germany

Hans Kreitler, Ph.D., Department of Psychology, Tel Aviv University, 69978 Tel Aviv, Israel (deceased)

Shulamith Kreitler, Ph.D., Department of Psychology, Tel Aviv University, 69978 Tel Aviv, Israel

Joachim Küchenhoff, Ph.D., Psychosomatic Clinic, University of Heidelberg, D-6900 Heidelberg 1, Germany

Falk Leichsenring, Ph.D., Department of Clinical Group Psychotherapy, University of Göttingen, D-3400 Göttingen, Germany

Fernando Lolas, M.D., Psychiatric Clinic, University of Chile, Santiago 7, Chile

Rolf Manz, Department of Psychotherapy, University of Heidelberg, D-6900 Heidelberg, Germany

Christopher J. Pagano, Ph.D., The Cambridge Hospital, Cambridge, MA 02139, USA

J. Christopher Perry, Ph.D., Institute of Community and Family Psychiatry, Sir Mortimer B. Davis-Jewish General Hospital, Montréal, Québec H3T 1E4, Canada

Rainer Peter, Center for Psychotherapy Research, D-7000 Stuttgart 70, Germany

Robert Plutchik, Ph.D., Albert Einstein College of Medicine of Yeshiva University, Bronx, NY 10461, USA

Marion Reinsch, Department of Personality Psychology, University of Leiden, 2300 Leiden, The Netherlands

Gerhard Reister, M.D., Department of Psychosomatic Medicine and Psychotherapy, Heinrich Heine University, D-4000 Düsseldorf 12, Germany

I. Alex Rubino, M.D., Percept-Genetic Laboratory, Torvergata University, 00141 Rome, Italy

Barbara E. Saitner, Ph.D., University of Cologne, 5000 Köln 41, Germany

Christina Schwilk, M.D., Department of Psychotherapy, University of Ulm, D-7900 Ulm, Germany

Claudia Simons., Department of Psychotherapy, University of Ulm, D-7900 Ulm, Germany

Hans Sjöbäck, Ph.D., Department of Psychology, University of Lund, S-22350 Lund, Sweden (deceased)

Gudmund J.W. Smith, Ph.D., Department of Psychology, University of Lund, S-22350 Lund, Sweden

Heidi Teubner-Berg, Gesellschaft zur Förderung Persönlichkeits- und Sozialpyschologisches-Forschung, University of Mainz, D-6500 Mainz, Germany

Wolfgang Tress, M.D., Ph.D., Department of Psychosomatic Medicine and Psychotherapy, Heinrich Heine University Düsseldorf, D-4000 Düsseldorf 12, Germany

Gunilla van der Meer, Department of Psychology, University of Lund, S-22350 Lund, Sweden

Bert Westerlundh, Ph.D., Department of Psychology, University of Lund, S-22350 Lund, Sweden

Introduction: Defense Mechanisms in Clinical Practice, Theoretical Explanation, and Experimental Investigation

UWE HENTSCHEL, GUDMUND J.W. SMITH, WOLFRAM EHLERS, and
JURIS G. DRAGUNS

Over the last few years, the concept of defense mechanism has increasingly come into focus both in theory and in empirical investigation. No longer the virtually exclusive concern of psychoanalytically oriented clinicians, defense mechanisms are demonstrating their usefulness over a wide spectrum of areas of interest to both theoreticians and practitioners in the behavioral sciences. Such popularity has brought with it problems and difficulties. The defense enterprise runs the risk of becoming unwieldy and amorphous. Defenses have come to mean very different things to different people, and the concept may become so vague as to be nonfalsifiable—retroactively invoked with impunity, yet of little use in formulating specific and differential predictions. The number of designated defense mechanisms has been increasing exponentially, and their applications have been expanding in all directions, from the consulting rooms of psychoanalysts to the training programs of fighter pilots.

What then is the justification for yet another book about defense mechanisms? Certainly, there has been no paucity of such publications. Like many other concepts, mechanisms of defense have gone through a lengthy process of gestation and maturation. Originally a cornerstone of psychoanalytic conceptualization, they have entered everyday speech, as exemplified by such common phrases in several Western languages as "I must have simply repressed it." Academic psychologists have variously ignored the concept of defense, scrutinized it skeptically, or accepted it with reservations. The related concept of coping has enjoyed more success, less burdened as it is by the assumption of the unconscious. Since the two concepts are closely, perhaps even inextricably connected, their somewhat diverging fortunes exercise pressure upon the field to decide between acceptance and rejection. As already suggested, in the last few years the scale has been tipped toward an ever more general, though as yet not universal, acceptance. The formulations within the DSM-IV, currently in the prefinal stages of its development, testify to the trend of incorporating the notion of defense into diagnostic formulations and criteria. Numerous attempts have been undertaken to capture general defensiveness or specific defenses by means of paper-and-pencil scales. Interdisciplinary connections have been forged, on the conceptual and empirical levels, between differences across persons and stimuli in adaptive performance, implicit in the notion of defense, and trends and concepts in biology and medicine that are focused on the subject. Hentschel, Smith, and Draguns (1986) have noted the parallels between percept-genetic assumptions, prominent in the current investigation of defense mechanisms, and the notions of functional region discussed by von Uexküll (1921) and the *Gestaltkreis* as treated by von Weizsäcker (1947). A noteworthy trend in contemporary biology is focused on the personal history of the subject or its epigenesis in the constant interplay of personal experience, behavior, and environment. Thus Maturana and Varela (1988) speak of drift in the course of the simultaneous and bilateral interchange which affects the subject and the environment alike.

As Hernandez Peón, Scherrer, and Velasco (1956) have demonstrated, the afferent conduction from the peripheral parts of the nervous system can be dependent on central influences that comprise the subjective emotional experiences. These observations, once again, highlight the importance of the subject, in both theory and experimentation. And yet, the notion of the subject remains too global and holistic to be conveniently incorporated into empirical research. The challenge is to delimit more specific variables of predictive value. Defense mechanisms hold promise in this respect, for several reasons. For one, they constitute a psychodynamic concept that encompasses the naturally occurring unconscious and affective contents of human information processing, so often artificially excluded in the interest of "neat and tidy" experimentation. Moreover, inferences can be made from the momentary manifestation of defense to the more abiding, structural characteristics of the individual. Defenses span the range of maladaptive to adaptive behavior, and at the same time they represent an empirically observable and measurable concept. The potential attractiveness of the concept of defense then lies in its scope: from the neuronal substrate to complex real-life events. Defense mechanisms are embedded in the social representation of various actions and conceptions, and they are crucial in coping with reality. To be sure, they could be more "neatly" classified and arranged; there are too many similar labels and diverging operational definitions.

In this volume, we grouped the chapters into five major sections, corresponding to, besides general issues, four areas of empirical research and application, namely methodological considerations, personality and applied psychology, clinical assessment and psychotherapeutic intervention, and psychosomatic research. These four sections are preceded by a set of chapters that provide a general introduction and, above all, present the theoretical underpinning for the understanding of the concept of the defense as well as the rationale for the several styles and modes of its current investigation.

Of necessity, we have started at the source; defense mechanisms were discovered and described in the psychotherapeutic setting. From there they traveled to the experimental laboratory and came to be observed, assessed, and manipulated in a variety of practical contexts. And yet the progression has never been unidirectional: experimental observations have informed clinical practice, and practical findings have been brought to bear upon theoretical formulations. At this point, we are witnessing an especially lively interchange among theoreticians, researchers, and practitioners. The present volume is testimony to the vitality of this interaction. Our hope is that it may not only document it, but foster and promote its growth and cultivation.

The variety of the current research methods and tools makes an exhaustive categorization difficult. Nonetheless, the several types of investigation can be organized under the following headings: clinical observations, self-report inventories, projective techniques, and percept-genetic methods. Cutting across this fourfold scheme is the contrast between observational and correlational studies on the one hand and of those based on experimental control and manipulation on the other. Research on defense mechanisms has gone beyond observation and recording, and its present state testifies to the feasibility of predicting the occurrence of defense, under experimental or naturalistic conditions.

So far, this preview of the volume's content has been grounded in general considerations, within psychology and beyond it. We should not, however, forget that the concept of defense originated and developed within a specific theoretical context, that of psychoanalysis. It therefore behooves us to bridge the gap between the origins of the concept and its current differentiated state in contemporary psychoanalysis.

The shift from the id to the ego has paved the way for psychoanalysis to come into contact with the concepts of contemporary psychology and other related sciences that deal with human experience. In the late writings of S. Freud the far-reaching effects of psychoanalysis are found by applications of psychoanalysis in all social sciences: "Strictly speaking there are only two sciences: psychology, pure and applied, and natural science" (Freud, 1933, p. 1).

From 1945 to 1970 Hartmann, the leading theoretician in the post-Freudian days, emphatically asserted that psychoanalysis must become a general psychology (Hartmann, 1964). Murphy (1960) was also emphatic in asserting that psychoanalysis should provide a unified theory of behavior without literal adherence to Freud's formulations. The structure of contemporary psychoanalytic theory can be described by some relevant perspectives in psychology.

The interpersonal perspective in psychoanalysis focuses attention on a larger transactional field by including cultural, societal components in the developmental, operationally oriented scheme. Empirical psychoanalytic research includes interpersonally defined mechanisms of defense like archaic or early defense mechanisms (see Chapters 17 and 28 in this book). Projective identification is a good example of the expanding concept of defense in interpersonal communication. Sandler (1987) described three stages for the development of this defense concept. In the first stage Klein's (1946) original definition of projective identification focused on the person's fantasy life: "Much of the hatred against parts of the self is now directed towards the mother. This leads to a particular form of identification which establishes the prototype of an aggressive object-relation. I suggest for these processes the term 'projective identification.' When projection is mainly derived from the infant's impulse to harm or to control the mother, he feels her to be a persecutor" (Klein, 1946, p. 102). In the second stage Heimann (1950), Racker (1968), and Grinberg (1962) substantially extended projective identification by bringing it into conjunction with the analyst's identification with the self- or object representation in the patient's unconscious fantasies, and with its effect on countertransference. The countertransference reaction could then be a possible source of information for the analyst about what was occurring in the patient. The central contribution of the third stage of development is the container model of Wilfred Bion (1962, 1963), which describes the capacity of the caretaking mother to be attentive to and tolerant of the needs, distress, and anger as well as the love of the infant, and to convey reassurance that she can both contain these feelings and respond to them in a considered and appropriate way. Through this the infant learns that his or her distress is not catastrophic. In the analytic situation the patient, in a similar way, can learn that those parts that he or she had considered to be dangerous can be accepted as aspects of the self that are not harmful.

The structural system of 1923 replaced the topographic system of Freud from 1900. Gill (1963) and Arlow and Brenner (1964) devoted extensive work to this point. Peterfreund (1971) argued that the traditional formulations of ego psychology and structural hypotheses lack explanatory power. Their replacement by information processing and systems models must restore consistency with neurophysiology. Moser (1968) with his cognitive model of defense gave an example for the conceptual integration of defense into contemporary cognitive psychology. In the present volume, Gottschalk and Fronczek (Chapter 23), Lolas (Chapter 13), and Kohlmann (Chapter 12) have made contributions toward integrating psychophysiological methods and findings into the study of defense.

The replacement of the drive concept by modern formulation of emotion theory (Dahl, 1991) makes new research designs possible in the realm of general and clinical psychology, as exemplified by Krause and Lütolf (1988) in their study on affect regulation in psychoanalytic treatment.

Models of the mind (Gedo & Goldberg, 1973) show that different concepts of metapsychology are relevant for developmental stages in the process of psychotherapy. The developmental perspectives of defense should stimulate a reconceptualization of defense mechanisms as they occur in psychotherapy. Perry, Kardos, and Pagano have initiated this effort in Chapter 8. The assumption of a hierarchical order of defense mechanisms constructed on a continuum from very pathological to mature, which by the empirical studies of Vaillant (1974) so strongly has improved the validity of the concept in general, does not make redundant the continued need for elaborated definitions of specific mechanisms and efforts to reach a widely accepted consensus on these (cf. Vaillant, 1992).

Once again, we return then to a fundamental theme: how the concept of defense has radiated from its origins in psychotherapy to be brought to bear upon the elucidation of the therapy situation. Without neglecting the psychotherapeutic focus, however, we have deliberately cast the net as widely as possible, in conceptualizations, approaches, methods, and topics. In the process, we have become aware of the limits of the present state of knowledge about defenses.

As yet, there is no way of comparing the manifestations of defense mechanisms across the various methods used for their observation. Conversely, with methods held constant, the several mechanisms cannot be conclusively and objectively compared. In light of these limitations, what is the incremental information that the book is able to provide? We think that the specific applications underscore the potentialities and the limits of the various methods and thereby delimit the frontiers of knowledge. For example, it is not necessary to have a constant standard of comparison to be able to determine which defense mechanisms promote the healing process in bone marrow transplant patients or what defenses enhance attention deployment.

The focus of the book is on the content of the various problems investigated. We have not, however, neglected methodological considerations, but we have not reached the point of being able to recommend one model research design for the study of defense mechanisms. The time is not yet ripe for a definitive evaluation of defense-oriented research. This situation is not that different from natural sciences (e.g., biomedicine, in which customarily the method of data gathering and evaluation is incorporated into the report of the results). In psychology, this problem is exacerbated by the linguistic dependence of its constructs. In any case, the empirical study of defense appears to us to be such an exciting and significant enterprise that we felt compelled to emphasize the multitude of the current research approaches. As editors, we have adopted the role of reporters in limiting ourselves to the communication of a complex pattern in as realistic a manner as we could.

References

Arlow, J.A. & Brenner, C. (1964) *Psychoanalytic concepts and the structural theory*. Madison, CT: International Universities Press.

Bion, W.R. (1962) *Learning from experience*. London: Heinemann.

Bion, W.R. (1963) *Elements of psychoanalysis*. London: Heinemann.

Dahl, H. (1991) The key to understanding change: Emotions as appetitive wishes and beliefs about their fulfillment. In J.G. Safran L. (Ed.), *Emotion, psychotherapy and change* (pp. 130–165). New York: Guilford Press.

Freud, S. (1933) The new introductory lectures. In *The standard edition of the complete psychological works of Sigmund Freud: Vol. 22*. London: Hogarth Press.

Gedo, J.E. & Goldberg, A. (1973) *Models of the mind*. Chicago: University of Chicago Press.

Gill, M.M. (1963) Topography and systems in psychoanalytic theory. *Psychological Issues: Monogra. 10*. Madison, CT: International Universities Press.

Grinberg, L. (1962) On a specific aspect of countertransference due to the patients projective identification. *International Journal of Psychoanalysis, 43*, 436–440.

Hartmann, H. (1964) *Essays in ego psychology*. Madison, CT: International Universities Press.

Heimann, P. (1950) On countertransference. *International Journal of Psychoanalysis, 31*, 81–84.

Hentschel, U., Smith, G., & Draguns, J.G. (1986) Subliminal perception, microgenesis, and personality. In U. Hentschel, G. Smith, & J.G. Draguns (Eds.), *The roots of perception: Individual differences in information processing within and beyond awareness* (pp. 3–36). Amsterdam: Elsevier.

Hernández Peón, R., Scherrer, H., & Velasco, M. (1956) Central influences on afferent conduction in the somatic and visual pathways. *Acta Neurologica Latina Americana, 2*, 8–22.

Klein, M. (1946) Notes on some schizoid mechanisms. *International Journal of Psychoanalysis, 27*, 99–110.

Krause, R. & Lütolf, P. (1988) Facial indicators of transference processes within psychoanalytic treatment. In H. Dahl, H. Kächele, & H. Thomä (Eds.), *Psychoanalytic process research strategies* (pp. 241–256). Berlin: Springer.

Maturana, H.R. & Varela, F.J. (1988) *The tree of knowledge. The biological roots of human understanding*. Boston: New Science Library.

Moser, U., Zeppelin, I. von, & Schneider, W. (1968) *Computersimulation eines Modells neurotischer Abwehrmechanismen. Ein Versuch zur Formalisierung der psychoanalytischen Theorie* [Computer simulation of a model of neurotic defense mechanisms. An attempt at formalizing psychoanalytic theory] (Bulletin 2). Department of Psychology, University of Zürich.

Murphy, G. (1960) Psychoanalysis as a unified theory of social behavior. *Science and Psychoanalysis, 3*, 140–149.

Peterfreund, E. (1971) *Information, systems and psychoanalysis. An evolutionary biological approach to psychoanalytic theory*. Madison, CT: International Universities Press.

Racker, H. (1968) *Transference and countertransference*. Madison, CT: International Universities Press.

Sandler, J. (1987) The concept of projective identification. In J. Sandler (Ed.), *Projection, identification, projective identification* (pp. 13–26). London: Karnac.

Uexküll, J. von (1921) *Umwelt und Innenwelt der Tiere* [The environment and inner world of animals]. Berlin: Springer.

Vaillant, G.E. (1974) *Adaptation to life*. Boston: Little, Brown.

Vaillant, G.E. (1992) The historical origin and future potential of Sigmund Freud's concept of the mechanisms of defense. *International Review of Psychoanalysis*, *19*, 35–50.

Weizsäcker, V. von (1947) *Der Gestaltkreis* [The gestalt region]. Stuttgart: Thieme.

Part I
General Issues

1
A Critical Perspective on Defense Mechanisms

PAUL KLINE

In this brief introductory chapter I shall describe the psychoanalytic notion of defense and show that as it has been elaborated and developed in psychology, it has undergone various changes such that what is now described as defenses or coping bears little resemblance to the original psychoanalytic propositions. These developments, it will be argued, are of considerably less psychological interest than the originals, since they have largely abandoned the unconscious aspects of defenses. However, it will be shown that it is possible to support a concept of defense that is in accord with the essence of psychoanalysis and with recent information theoretic accounts in psychology. The implications of this for the scientific study and measurement of defenses are also discussed.

Freudian Psychoanalytic Defense Mechanisms

Freud (1923) makes clear the nature of defense mechanisms. The neurotic conflict takes place between the ego and the id, the ego seeking to bar the expression of certain instinctual impulses by using defense mechanisms. In psychoanalysis these defense mechanisms have been carefully delineated and described, and Fenichel (1945) and Anna Freud (1946) contain excellent summaries of them. Before I briefly list the Freudian defense mechanisms, two further points should be made. These defenses are unconscious and can be categorized (Fenichel, 1945) as successful (where expression of the instinctual drive is allowed) and unsuccessful (where, because the instinct is not expressed, continuous repetition of the defense is required).

Sublimation

Sublimation refers to successful defenses and is not, in itself, a defense. Freud (1916), indeed, argued that sublimation consists in abandoning the sexual aim for another, which is no longer sexual. Indeed this deflection of aims is the most common definition of sublimation in psychoanalytic theory. There are various defenses within this category.

Reversal into Opposites (Freud, 1915). There are two processes involved in defense by reversal into opposites:

1. Change from active into passive: for example, sadism becomes masochism.
2. Reversal of content: for example, love becomes hate.

Turning Against Subject. Exhibitionism is voyeurism turned on the self.

Repression

Erdelyi (1990) has pointed out the ambiguity and diffuseness of Freud's terminology concerning repression and defense. He identifies in the writings of Freud 32 different phrases. However there is a general consensus, and I shall adopt here the definition in which Freud (1915) states that the essence of repression lies in the function of rejecting and keeping something out of consciousness. There are two types of repression.

1. Primal repression. This is the first phase of repression and refers to the denial of entry into consciousness of the mental presentation of the instinct.
2. Repression proper. This concerns the mental derivatives and associations of the repressed presentation, which are also denied entry into consciousness. The mental energy that belongs to repressed instincts is transformed into affects, especially anxiety, which renders repression an unsuccessful defense.

Denial

In denial the ego wards off by literally denying them some perceptions from the external world that would be painful. Freud (1925a) cites a patient who denied that a figure in his dream was his mother. Freud says that we amend it: it was his mother.

Projection

The attribution of one's own unacceptable impulses and ideas to others is called projection. This defense, together with reaction formation, is involved in the delusional persecutions of paranoia (Freud, 1911).

Reaction Formation

Reaction formation is a defense that results in the creation of an attitude opposite to the instinct that is defended against. Freud (1908) claims that the cleanliness of the anal character is a reaction formation against anal erotism.

Undoing

Undoing is a defense characteristic of obsessional neurosis (Freud, 1909b). This is described as negative magic, which endeavors to "blow away" the consequences of some event and the event itself. Something is done that actually or magically is the opposite of something that actually or in the imagination was done (Fenichel, 1945).

Isolation

According to Freud (1925b), isolation is peculiar, to obsessional neurosis. Experiences are isolated from their associations and emotions. The isolation of sexuality from the rest of life, which allows men to express their sexuality without guilt, is an example of this defense (Fenichel, 1945).

Regression

Freud (1925b) argues that the process by which the ego regresses to an earlier stage can be used as a defense. Thus the obsessional frequently regresses to the anal-sadistic level.

These are the main defenses described in Freudian theory, As can be seen, they are all means of protecting the ego from pain, caused by instinctual impulses. However, in addition to defenses against instincts, the ego attempts to defend itself against affect. The same mechanisms are used, but there are a few other examples in psychoanalysis of defenses against affect.

Defenses Against Affect

Postponement of Affect. Freud (1918) cites a common example in which a man's grief at the death of a sister received no expression until he was inexplicably overwhelmed by grief at Pushkin's grave a few months later.

Displacement of Affect. Another example was a special case of displacement. Often there is displacement of object, as in fear of father displaced to animals (Freud, 1909a). Displacement can be seen when sexual excitement is displaced to irregularities of breathing or heart rhythm or indeed in the claim that anxiety is displaced sexual energy (Freud, 1906).

Identification with the Aggressor. Anna Freud (1946) regarded identification with the aggressor as the introjection of the object against which the affect was directed. The anti-Semitism of Jews is an example of this defense.

This brief description of the main defenses in psychoanalytic theory makes it clear that they are unconscious ego mechanisms aimed at preventing pain mainly from internal sources but also from the external world. Their psychological interest and importance springs from the fact that defenses help to explain and give insight into behaviors and feelings that otherwise would remain incomprehensible. The whole of human history suggests that we do not live in a rational world without defenses. It is also clear that the distinctions are to some extent arbitrary. Thus displacement and postponement of affects are hardly different, and reversal into opposites and turning against the subject are highly similar. Thus it would be expected that as the study of defenses continued, on a clinical and subjective basis, other new categories would be used. This is indeed the case and while, in a chapter of this length it is impossible to list them all, I shall briefly describe some of the more influential modern accounts.

The Work of Vaillant and Horowitz

Vaillant (e.g., 1977) has devoted considerable effort to the study of defenses, basing his work on that of Anna Freud. In his 50-year investigation of college men and in his studies of control groups, 18 defenses were assessed. These were classified according to developmental level, primitive to mature. Mature defenses were more adaptive and led to better mental health. In these studies the deliberate conscious effort to put out of mind unpleasant and insoluble problems was adaptive. Note the use of the words "conscious" and "deliberate". Vaillant's notion of defense is far more broad than that of Freud since it includes also unconscious defenses. Vaillant defines the following defenses:

Primitive, pathological defenses: delusional projection, psychotic denial, projection.

Immature defenses: projection, schizoid fantasy, hypochondriasis, passive–aggressive behavior, acting out.

Neurotic defenses: intellectualization, repression, reaction formation, association.

Mature defenses: altruism, humor suppression, humor, anticipation, sublimation.

I shall now list the defenses described in Horowitz (1989), a book that includes all the defenses of Vaillant and other classifications. It should again be noted that these defenses are in some cases very different from those of Freud, in that they are conscious and, rather than being mental mechanisms of any kind, are simply overt behaviors. This implies that the concept of defense, despite the use of the old psychoanalytic terminology, has changed. After the defenses have been defined, we discuss Horowitz's conceptualizations.

Acting out. Impulsive action, which may involve displacement, without thought of consequences (e.g., delinquent acts rather than expressing hostility directly to parents).

Altruism. Needs are met by fulfilling the needs of others rather than one's own.

Conversion of Passive to Active. Person becomes active as defense against weakness—identification with the aggressor.

Denial. Defined as in psychoanalysis.

Devaluation. Stress and conflicts are dealt with by attributing exaggerated negative qualities to self and others.

Disavowal. To avoid stress, person claims the matter is trivial or that emotions are not important. This is highly similar to denial.

Displacement. Defined as in psychoanalysis.

Dissociation. Conflicts and stress are dealt with by temporary failure of consciousness to integrate the dangerous material.

Distortion. Meanings of stressful topics are altered. Devaluation, disavowal, exaggeration, and minimization are forms of distortion.

Exaggeration. Certain meanings can be given exaggerated value—personal ability to argue can be overestimated to avoid fear during an oral examination.

Humor. Humor can be used to deal with problems, as Freud (1905) discusses in some detail.

Idealization. Exaggerated positive qualities are attributed to self or others. It is difficult to see how this defense differs from exaggeration.

Intellectualization. Emotional implications of a topic are avoided by treating it on a purely intellectual level. This chapter might be seen as an example of this defense.

Isolation. As in psychoanalytic theory.

Minimization. Topic is undervalued to avoid stress—highly similar to disavowal.

Omnipotent Control. For fear of being abandoned or failed by others, the person acts as if in total control of the object.

Passive Aggression. Stress and conflict are dealt with by indirectly expressing aggression toward others.

Projection. As in psychoanalytic theory.

Projective Identification. Hateful aspects of self are attributed to a person to whom one is close, thus enabling one to be angry with this other person and provoking hostility in him or her.

Rationalization. Finding good reasons for what one wants to do.

Reaction Formation. As defined in psychoanalytic theory.

Regression. As in psychoanalytic theory.

Repression. As in psychoanalytic theory.

Somatization. Conflicts and stress are dealt with by preoccupation with physical symptoms.

Splitting. Oneself and others are viewed as all good or all bad, there being no integration of positive and negative qualities.

Sublimation. As in psychoanalytic theory.

Suppression. Intentionally avoiding thinking about the source of pain.

Turning Against Self. Aggression, or any impulse is redirected to self.

Undoing. Defined by Horowitz somewhat differently from psychoanalysis: here it is the expression of an impulse followed almost immediately by its opposite.

From these definitions of defenses as they are used in the modern psychological literature, a number of points should be noted. The term is far more broad than the original psychoanalytic concept. Thus it embraces Freudian unconscious defenses, conscious acts such as suppression, and actions such as acting out. Similarly, altruism would not be seen as a defense in psychoanalytic theory but as the result of a defense—sublimation. Exaggeration and disavowal are entirely conscious and would seem to fit better the notion of coping mechanism as defined by Lazarus and his colleagues (Lazarus & Folkman, 1984). Thus the list groups together terms that are categorically different. The psychological significance of the original defenses was precisely that they were unconscious and thus influenced the behavior and feelings of the individual in ways that were inexplicable to him or her and by no means obvious to an observer. Conscious defenses, however, seem to have relatively less interest in affording insight into behavior simply because they are so obvious, at least to the observer and to the subject if pointed out. This is particularly true of the coping mechanisms, discussed by Lazarus and Folkman (1984). Folkman and Lazarus (1980, p. 233) define coping as "the cognitive and behavioral efforts made to master, tolerate or reduce, external and internal demands and conflicts among them. Such coping efforts serve two main functions: the management or alteration of the person–environment relationship that is the source of stress (problem-focused coping) and the regulation of stressful emotions (emotion-focused coping)." Furthermore, there are two aspects to coping that are intertwined: primary appraisal, in which the significance of an event or experience is evaluated in terms of the well-being of the subject, and secondary appraisal, in which the coping resources (behavior and responses designed to deal with the problems) are evaluated. This recent and influential viewpoint on coping is notable because coping has become such an umbrella term that it actually includes social behavior such as calling on friends or relatives for help. This conceptualization, although it includes psychoanalytic notions of defenses, is so broad as to become, in this writer's view, of little value. Thus if faced with conflict, whatever a person does is conceptualized as the individual's way of coping. In other words, if a conflict occurs, with this definition a person copes. This conceptualization of coping is an example of what Smedslund (1984) has referred to as a noncontingent proposition, and I shall not consider it further.

These linguistic difficulties surrounding the work of Lazarus and colleagues lead us on to the information theoretic approaches to the notion of defenses, which have been well expounded by Marcel (1983) and Erdelyi (1985, 1988). Thus, in discussing perceptual defense, which is an experimental analogue of repression (Kline, 1981), Erdelyi (1988) points out the linguistic confusion in some of the experimental psychological conceptualizations of the problem. For example, if perception is seen as an all-or-nothing event, perceptual defense is impossible, since for perceptual defense to take place it is necessary to perceive the stimulus, the event which the perceptual defense is supposed to prevent. However, if perception is reformulated in information theoretic terms this problem disappears. Thus it is a subset of computed perceptions that become conscious. Others remain below the level of awareness, although still affecting our conscious perceptions (Dixon, 1981). Similarly, as Erdelyi (1988) argues, if terms such as force, cathexis, and anticathexis, terms all implicated in the psychoanalytic concept of defenses, are conceived in the classical tradition of physics, that force = mass × acceleration, then Freudian theory is absurd. However, if the notion of forces is reformulated as interaction and counteractions (as is done by Fenichel, 1945), Erdelyi argues that there is little scientific or philosophical objection. Psychodynamic theory is no different from modern cognitive theories, although, of course, it is an empirical matter whether it is correct. Indeed Erdelyi (1990) is absolutely explicit on this point. He reanalyzes some of the early work on remembering by Bartlett (1932) to show that the Bartlettian descriptions of schemas have considerable overlap with the Freudian concepts of defenses and concludes that the only difference is that Freud's mechanisms are, rightly or wrongly, assumed to play a defensive role. Thus he suggests that the defense mechanisms provide the neglected defensive side of the pervasive operation of schemas in our lives. Clearly there is no antithesis between cognitive psychology and defenses, in this formulation.

I shall now examine the work of Horowitz, who has made extensive studies of defenses and attempted to synthesize cognition and defense (e.g., Horowitz, 1988, 1989). His work is neatly summarized in Horowitz, Markham, Stinson, Fridhandler, and Ghannam (1990). As these authors point out, Haan (1977) had attempted to link defenses to certain cognitive processes by arguing that these led to certain outcomes such as defenses or coping. However the problem with this work is that the cognitive processes discussed are idiosyncratic and not in accord with recent cognitive theory. Horowitz, however, has tried to avoid this pitfall. In his work (Horowitz et al., 1990), defense mechanisms are regarded as defensive outcomes of regulation, efforts that might, in different circumstances, also have outcomes that would be labeled either adaptive regulation or dysregulation, defined as succumbing to stress. In this account there are three kinds of regulatory process, whose aim is to control the conscious experience of emotions and ideas, although the former also affect the expression and communication of the latter. These are the regulation of mental set, the regulation of person schemas and role models, and the regulation of conscious representation and sequencing. It is as a result of the outcome of these processes that defenses occur. Some examples will clarify the point. Thus altering the schema of another person can result in projection while sequencing ideas by seeking information can result in intellectualization.

Although this work of Horowitz is a determined attempt to link cognition and defense I am not convinced of its success. The choice of cognitive processes is somewhat arbitrary and would not be undisputed in cognitive psychology. The classifications do not appear to be at all mutually exclusive. Consider the example, given earlier, of intellectualization. This is claimed to be the outcome of the regulatory control process, sequencing ideas by seeking information. However intellectualization is not the outcome of this process. It is the process itself. Similarly rationalization is arranging information into decision trees rather than the outcome of it. The adaptive counterpart of rationalization, in this analysis, is problem solving. However the distinction between these two seems quite arbitrary. The notion of maladaptive and adaptive, which is surely cultural and subjective, is not useful in a truly scientific account. Since, however, there are undoubtedly cultural evaluative aspects of Freudian theory, the notion of defenses is not at risk. Thus problem solving would not necessarily be regarded as different from rationalization, or, indeed, intellectualization, with which it seems better juxtaposed. Certainly the brilliant work of some scientists could be seen as defensive, as indeed are the great literary creations of the world. This notion of adaptive and maladaptive stands no scrutiny, as a psychological phenomenon. However it is not my intention to subject the work of Horowitz to particular, detailed criticism. It is sufficient to see that it is an attempt to weld together cognition and defense, in a way that regards defenses as a maladaptive outcome of certain cognitive processes, even though, as was argued earlier in this discussion, this claim cannot always be maintained. However it suffers, compared to the work of Erdelyi, for example, from the choice of the cognitive processes based on the clinical research of Horowitz and his colleagues and would not fit easily into the cognitive approaches of experimental psychology, as described by Marcel (1983).

Conclusions

In 80 years there have been changes in the notion of defense, although, perhaps surprisingly, not as many as might have been expected—evidence that the concept, however difficult to formulate with precision, is still useful, in some guise or other, to understand emotional experiences. I think one clear conclusion may be drawn. Over these years the concept of defense has become far more broad. It began, in psychoanalytic theory, as a general term for an unconscious mechanism of ego protection. This became more precisely delineated into a number of unconscious defense mechanisms. These have been studied by clinical psychologists, and the concept of defenses has merged into a larger one of coping mechanisms, some unconscious, some conscious, and some actual behaviors designed to deal with stress. The term, indeed, embraces concepts that bear in some cases little psychological similarity. More recently attempts have been made to tic in the notion of defense to cognitive psychological concepts, thus bringing defenses into the orbit of experimental psychology. It appears from these studies that the original Freudian defense mechanisms, as unconscious processes to avoid pain, even if differently described, are still useful concepts in that they appear in most lists and descriptions. However one distinction seems essential—that between the defenses or coping mechanisms that are unconscious (the group in which the psychoanalytic defenses fall) and those that are not. This distinction is important because it profoundly affects the measurement of defenses, and precise valid measurement is critical for the scientific investigation of defenses. As has been argued (Kline, 1987), the measurement of unconscious processes by questionnaire is virtually impossible. This rules out many purported measures of defenses. What is needed, as the work in percept-genetics (Kragh and Smith, 1970) shows, as does research by Dixon (1981) and Erdelyi (1985) just for example, are subliminal stimuli. Silverman (1983), with his subliminal approach to the study of motivation and conflict, also supports this case.

In conclusion, therefore, it can be argued that the psychoanalytic notion of defense, even if it has to be conceptualized within a different framework, has stood the test of time. Care must be taken, in its objective investigation, that our measures are not so simplistic as to lose the essential unconscious nature of the concept, a danger particularly acute since the term "defense" has been widened to include a large variety of coping mechanisms.

References

Bartlett, F.C. (1932) *Remembering*. Cambridge: Cambridge University Press.
Dixon, N.F. (1981) *Preconscious processing*. Chichester: Wiley.

Erdelyi, M.H. (1985) *Psychoanalysis: Freud's cognitive psychology*. New York: Freeman.

Erdelyi, M.H. (1988) Some issues in the study of defense processes: Discussion of Horowitz's comments with some elaborations. In M.J. Horowitz (Ed.), *Psychodynamics and cognition*. Chicago: University of Chicago Press.

Erdelyi, M.H. (1990) Repression, reconstruction and defense: History and integration of the psychoanalytic and experimental frameworks. In J.L. Singer (Ed.), *Repression and dissociation* (pp.1–31). Chicago: University of Chicago Press.

Fenichel, O. (1945) *The psychoanalytic theory of neurosis*. New York: Norton.

Folkman, S. & Lazarus, R.S. (1980) An analysis of coping in a middle-aged community sample. *Journal of Health and Community Behavior*, *21*, 219–230.

Freud, A. (1946) *The ego and the mechanisms of defence*. London: Hogarth Press and The Institute of Psychoanalysis.

Freud, S. (1966) *The standard edition of the complete psychological works of Sigmund Freud*. London: Hogarth Press and The Institute of Psychoanalysis.

Freud, S. (1905) *Jokes and their relation to the unconscious: Vol. 8*.

Freud, S. (1906) *My views on the part played by sexuality in the aetiology of the neuroses: Vol. 7*, p. 271.

Freud, S. (1908) *Character and anal erotism: Vol. 9*, p. 169.

Freud, S. (1909a) *Analysis of a phobia in a five-year-old boy: Vol. 10*, p. 3.

Freud, S. (1909b) *Notes upon a case of obsessional neurosis: Vol. 10*, p. 153.

Freud, S. (1911) *Psychoanalytic notes on an autobiographical account of a case of paranoia (dementia paranoides): Vol. 12*, p. 3.

Freud, S. (1915) *Repression: Vol. 14*, p. 143.

Freud, S. (1916) *Introductory lectures on psychoanalysis: Vol. 15*.

Freud, S. (1918) *From the history of an infantile neurosis: Vol. 17*, p. 3.

Freud, S. (1923) *The ego and the id: Vol. 19*, p. 3.

Freud, S. (1925a) *Negation: Vol. 19*, p. 235.

Freud, S. (1925b) *Inhibition, symptoms and anxiety: Vol. 20*, p. 77.

Haan, N. (1977) *Coping and defending*. New York: Academic Press.

Horowitz, M.J. (Ed.) (1988) *Psychodynamics and cognition*. Chicago: University of Chicago Press.

Horowitz, M.J. (1989) *Introduction to psychodynamics*. London: Routledge.

Horowitz, M.J., Markman, H.C., Stinson, C.H., Fridhandler, B., & Ghannam, J.H. (1990) A classification theory of defense. In J.L. Singer (Ed.), *Repression and dissociation* (pp. 61–84). Chicago: University of Chicago Press.

Kline, P. (1981) *Fact and fantasy in Freudian theory* (2nd ed.). London: Methuen.

Kline, P. (1987) The scientific status of the DMT. *British Journal of Medical Psychology*, *60*, 53–59.

Kragh, U. & Smith, G. (1970) *Percept-genetic analysis*. Lund: Gleerup.

Lazarus, R.S. & Folkman, S. (1984) *Stress, appraisal and coping*. New York: Springer.

Marcel, A.J. (1983) Conscious and unconscious perception: An approach to the relations between phenomenal experience and perceptual processes. *Cognitive Psychology*, *15*, 238–300.

Silverman, L.H. (1983) The subliminal psychodynamic activation method: Overview and comprehensive listing of studies. In J. Masling (Ed.), *Empirical studies of psychoanalytic theories* (pp. 69–100). Hillsdale NJ: Analytic Press.

Smedslund, J. (1984) What is necessarily true in psychology. *Annals of Theoretical Psychology*, 2, 241–272.

Vaillant, G.E. (1977) *Adaptation to life*. Boston: Little, Brown.

2
Defense Mechanisms in the Clinic and in the Laboratory: An Attempt at Bridging the Gap

JURIS G. DRAGUNS

Defense mechanisms were discovered in the clinic, tested in the experimental laboratory, and applied to the explanation of human conduct in all its ramifications. As yet, the three strands of clinical observation, research investigation, and conceptual formulation have not merged into an integrated whole. Hence the need for this volume. The contributors aspire to fill the gaps between these three reference points of exploration and discovery. The present chapter attempts to take stock of the present state of knowledge in these areas and to offer a personal, and perhaps subjective, view of the needs for future investigation. Emphasis is placed on controlled experimentation as the method of choice of scientific inquiry into the phenomena of defense and most other variables in psychology. In the ideal case, a continuous interplay is envisaged among clinicians, experimenters, and theoreticians. This uninterrupted dialogue is, again in the optimal scenario, expected to produce the development of clinically observed and experimentally verified phenomena, linked by means of testable and heuristically fruitful concepts. As yet, close to a century after the formulation of the concept of defense by Freud (1894/1964; 1896/1964), we are miles removed from this ambitious goal. Let us therefore briefly and cursorily assess the state of the notion of defense, with a particular emphasis on the links between the three facets of this inquiry. As mentioned, one component of the proposed enterprise is taking stock of what is known and what has been accomplished; the other aspect of this undertaking is pointed toward the unknown and the future. What remains to be done to close the gap between the clinicians, the experimenters, and the theoreticians?

Early Formulations and Conceptual Developments

The concept of defense was first invoked by Freud (1894/1964; cf., Madison, 1961) to explain the origin of psychogenic symptoms and their peculiar persistence in the face of concerted attempts to remove them.

To this end, Freud (1894/1964) described how a threatening impulse is banished from awareness. The consciousness of its existence is obliterated, but its capacity to impel the person's behavior remains intact. What Freud had identified was, of course, repression, and over two decades the term was used interchangeably with defense. Gradually, Freud and his associates described other expressions of defense that appeared to differ qualitatively from repression. In 1926 Freud (1926/1963) undertook to differentiate these two terms sharply. Defense was to be the supraordinate, inclusive concept; repression was destined to remain one of the categories of defense, albeit perhaps the most important, even the prototypical one. Most of the psychoanalysts accepted this distinction, even though the debate has not died down to this day on the respective advantages and disadvantages of equating or differentiating these two concepts and on the status of repression as one defense mechanism among many or as a special, pivotal component of the defense structure (cf. Fenichel, 1945; Madison, 1961; Matte Blanco, 1955; Sjöbäck, 1973). Of greater importance was the four-stage sequence proposed by Freud and consisting of the activation of an *impulse*, the experience of on intrapsychic *conflict* over its expression, the mobilization of *anxiety*, and its eventual reduction by the imposition of a *defense* (cf. Freud, 1894/1964, 1926/1963). In the psychoanalytic situation, this sequence can be observed, albeit rarely in its entirety. What is obstructed from view is filled in on the basis of plausible, first-order inference. In a less readily observable manner, this progression occurs in a variety of real-life settings; as such it constitutes an important manifestation of "psychopathology of everyday life" (S. Freud, 1901/1948; Jones, 1911). Several decades later, toward the end of Freud's career, a number of defense mechanisms had been described. Their names were well known to the practicing analysts, and their operations were routinely noted and interpreted in the course of psychoanalysis. Yet Freud never undertook the task of systematically sifting and integrating the accumulated observations and formulations on defense mechanisms. It remained for his daughter to do so. Her classical monograph (A. Freud, 1946) stands at the boundary between the classical period of psychoanalysis and the emergence of ego psychology. As such, it deserves to be considered separately.

Contributions of Ego Analysts: Anna Freud and Others

Anna Freud (1946) described the 10 prominent defense mechanisms that had emerged from the psychoanalytic literature by that time: regression, repression, reaction formation, isolation, undoing, projection, introjection, turning against the self, reversal, and sublimation. However, Anna Freud did a lot more than that. She specified the purposes of the defense mechanisms, their role in guiding behavior in psychopathology and health, and their positive and negative consequences. In S. Freud's original formulation, the concept of defense was anchored in clinical observation, especially in relation to symptom formation and psychopathology. A. Freud shifted the focus from psychopathology to adaptation. Defenses, she recognized, reduce or silence inner turmoil, but they also help persons cope with the demands and challenges of reality. Even though the most conspicuous and dramatic illustrations of defense come from the clinic, defenses are an integral point of functioning of psychologically unimpaired and undistressed human beings. To be sure, a price is paid for overcoming anxiety by means of defense mechanisms. It is exacted in the form of a reduced awareness of both self and environment. Perception, memory, and judgment may experience impairment or distortion as a result. At the same time, as more recent contributors have recognized, defenses may help bring about socially valued achievements. Vaillant (1977, p. 7) likened them to "an oyster [which], confronted with a grain of sand, creates a pearl." This recognition has stimulated the search for a chronological, developmental or adaptive hierarchy of defenses. One such scheme was proposed by Vaillant (1977), who grouped defense mechanisms at four levels: I, psychotic mechanisms (delusional projection, denial, and distortion); II, immature mechanisms (projection, schizoid fantasy, hypochondriasis, passive–aggressive behavior, and acting out); III, "neurotic" defenses (intellectualization, repression, displacement, reaction formation, and dissociation); and IV, mature mechanisms (altruism, suppression, anticipation, and sublimation). At the lowest level, the mechanisms distort reality; at the highest, they bring about its integration with interpersonal relations and private feelings. At intermediate points, defenses alter distress and modify the experience of feelings, even though they may appear odd, inappropriate, or socially undesirable to the outside observer. It may be noticed that Vaillant placed most of the "classical" defense mechanisms on A. Freud's list at level III. Not coincidentally, they were observed while psychoanalyzing neurotic patients. Vaillant succeeded in extending the concept of defense to both higher and lower levels of maturity. As a consequence, the list of defenses has burgeoned; Valenstein (cited in Wallerstein, 1985) included 24 first-order mechanisms and 15 second-order complex behaviors. Wallerstein (1985) introduced a more general distinction between defenses as broad attitudes, such as sympathy, and defenses as more crystallized patterns of behavior, as exemplified by reaction formation.

Conceptual Revisions and Modifications

As these developments occurred, the concept of defense underwent a number of shifts and transformations. These changes, for the most part subtle and gradual, deserve to be articulated. Originally, Freud conceived the concept of defense as the result of the struggle by the ego against unpleasant ideas or affects (cf. Brenner, 1981). Specifically, Freud limited the scope of defense to sexual drives and motives (cf. Madison, 1961). Contemporary observers take a more inclusive view. According to Vaillant (1977, p. 9), the ego takes recourse to defense "to resolve conflict among the four lodestones of our inner life: instincts, the real world, important people, and the internalized prohibitions provided by our conscience and culture." In more specific terms, the ego makes use of defense mechanisms in the following five situations (Vaillant, 1977):

1. To keep affects within bearable limits during sudden life crises (e.g., following death).
2. To restore emotional balance by postponing or channeling sudden increases in biological drives (e.g., at puberty).
3. To obtain a time-out to master changes in self-image (e.g., following major surgery or unexpected promotion).
4. To handle unresolvable conflicts with people, living or dead, whom one cannot bear to leave.
5. To survive major conflicts with conscience (e.g., killing in wartime, putting a parent in a nursing home).

Thus defenses come into play in a wide variety of situations, some of them far removed from the conflicts over sexual expression in which Freud originally discovered them. Allport's (1937) concept of functional autonomy comes to mind as a possible explanation for the spreading of defenses beyond their original foci of conflict and discomfort. Behaviorists would invoke the concept of generalization to account for the mushrooming of defenses across situations and time. In any case, defenses have acquired the status of broad traitlike tendencies that are characteristic of a person and are relatively independent of their context. In this manner, the description, study, and evaluation of defenses has become an important topic of both theoretical and applied study of personality. In this connection, it should be remembered that the concept of personality was introduced into scientific psychology late in Freud's life (Allport, 1937). It played no role in the development of psychoanalysis, and Freud would have been very much surprised to be classified as a personality theorist. Nonetheless, Freud's concept of defense has come to represent an important interface between the explanatory scheme of psychoanalysis and the concerns of contemporary personality theorists with individual differences and their origin in the person's biographical experience. It is commonly recognized that defenses tend toward consistency across time and situation and thus constitute personality traits. Another change that has occurred pertains to the indicators and manifestations of defense. In the case of repression, Freud equated it with amnesia for painful events. Other defenses would presumably be expressed through avenues that would be equally dramatic, conspicuous, and disabling. Modern formulations, such as Goldin's (1964), capitalize on much subtler manifestations. Instead of active and motivated forgetting for whole sequences of events, repression is redefined as absence of reflective awareness of feelings that would bring about a reduction of a person's self-esteem. Its effect then would be selective rather than massive. This transformation of the criteria for defense poses a challenge for theoreticians and researchers. How can a defense mechanism be operationally defined without doing violence to the subtlety of its clinical manifestations? Resolving this issue is pivotal in transforming defenses from explanatory concepts invoked post hoc to constructs that are capable of being used in formulating and testing predictions.

Parallel to the issue of subtlety, there is the equally important consideration of generality. As originally conceived, defenses were manifested at specific times and contexts. What are the criteria of defense now that these mechanisms have been expanded in scope and have acquired the status of traitlike tendencies? In long-term investigations (e.g., Vaillant, 1977), the stability and generality of defense mechanisms is emphasized, in contrast to the activation of a defense at a specific and unique point in life. A special problem in this connection is posed by the relationship between defense mechanisms and cognitive styles. Both these constructs are embedded within the personality structure. In Freud's original formulation, defenses are triggered by anxiety; they are germane to conflict resolution and restoration of psychic equilibrium. Their operation and function then are linked to threatening and affectively arousing experience. By contrast, cognitive styles are construed as generalized tendencies habitually invoked regardless of the emotional valence of stimuli. As defenses are extended beyond their original focus of origin, they shade off imperceptibly into cognitive styles. More cautiously, can an empirical relationship be established between defense mechanisms and cognitive styles (e.g., repression and leveling), both of which involve glossing over the incongruous aspects of experience? This question was first broached by Klein (1954) and was thoroughly investigated by Hentschel (1980), who pinpointed a complex set of relationships between these two kinds of variables. As yet, all questions have not been answered, but the provisional conclusion is that cognitive styles are neither automatic extensions of defense mechanisms nor are they unrelated to the several modes of defense.

Defenses as Predictable and Observable Variables: From the Clinic to the Laboratory

As described in the preceding sections of the chapter, defenses are the observable tip of the psychoanalytic iceberg. As such, they rest on a conceptual foundation that is several steps removed from the data of the clinic or the laboratory. "Defense is the core of the dynamic aspect of the psychoanalytic theory" (Drews & Brecht, 1975, p. 128).[1] As Vaillant (1977, p. 77) put it: "Perhaps the concept of the unconscious defense mechanism was Freud's most original contribution to man's understanding of man." Conceptually pivotal, yet empirically demonstrable, defense mechanisms were virtually destined to serve as the point of contact between the empirical enterprise of modern psychology and the conceptual structure of psychoanalysis. Yet before establishing this point of contact, formidable obstacles had to be overcome. Freud's theory is explanatory and metaphorical. It is designed to elucidate the impact of the past upon the present. Experimentation is necessarily oriented toward the future and concerned primarily with the prediction of behavior. Once this fundamental task has been accomplished, its products can be applied to the explanation of the past and its effect on the present. Moreover, the raw material of Freud's theoretical formulations was based on the end results of prolonged and intensive intrapsychic processes. Experimentation of necessity is limited in duration, and the imperative of avoiding harm severely restricts the impact of experimental manipulations. More specifically, defense originates as a result of virtually intolerable conflict. How can it be reproduced in the laboratory, except in the form of "pallid facsimiles" (Kubie, 1952, p. 708) of the phenomena observed in the clinic? Finally, the manifestations of defense were first observed in the inextricable context of their antecedents and consequences. By contrast, the laboratory reproductions of defense were imbued with a peculiarly static quality. The objective of these studies was simply to prove that repression—or other defense mechanisms—exist. And this objective was often pursued by having normal volunteers perform tasks of limited duration and minimal personal relevance (cf. MacKinnon & Dukes, 1962). No wonder that Freud remained skeptical! His response to one of the earliest studies of repression is well known and is often quoted: "I cannot put much value on these confirmations because the wealth of reliable observations on which these assertions rest make them independent of experimental verification. Still, it (experimental verification) can do no harm." (MacKinnon & Dukes, 1962, p. 703) Thus, the early studies failed to satisfy either the experimenters or the psychoanalysts. If anything worthwhile emerged from these early attempts, it was in the form of offshoots and by-products. Differential recall of pleasant and unpleasant events, for example, is a legitimate and important problem in its own right, even though its relevance to the operation of repression is tenuous (cf. MacKinnon & Dukes, 1962).

Progress in the experimental study of defense was reached gradually, and at this time a great many obstacles have been overcome. Advances

---

[1] Translated from German by the author.

in experimental methodology and instrumentation, more flexible and complex research design, and just plain human inventiveness and creativity have helped narrow, even if they have not yet closed, the gap between experimental data and clinical phenomena. In the remaining space, some of the landmarks of this progression will be briefly indicated. The experimental investigation of defenses has moved from the general to the specific and interactive aspects of this research problem. No longer is the study of a defense mechanism an issue per se. Rather, animated by theoretical and applied considerations, the experimenters explore the operation of defense in a specific population and context, on the basis of explicit expectations and predictions. The question of whether defenses exist has been discarded in favor of more specific inquiry about how defenses operate and what consequences they bring about for their users. To this end, measures of defense had to be developed for standardized use in basic and applied research. Since a conceptual affinity exists between projective techniques and psychodynamic theories, it is not surprising that projective indicators of defense mechanisms were introduced. Schafer's (1954) analysis of the operation of various defenses in the Rorschach test stands as a landmark in this respect. What is puzzling is that the various proposals for deriving measures of defense mechanisms have not gained wider currency or more general acceptance and that they have not been more prominently used in research. The truth is that no projective technique nor any scoring scheme within it has acquired a predominant status as an operational measure of defense. Assessment of defenses by personality questionnaires has had more conceptual obstacles to overcome. Useful measures, such as those by Gleser and Ihilevitch (1969), have nonetheless been developed. By this time their status in the armamentarium of defense indicators is secure and they are widely used. Limitations of these paper-and-pencil measures for the tapping of characteristics that are essentially unconscious in their origins are readily apparent and not easily overcome. It would seem that the self-report avenue of measuring defenses is destined to remain an indispensable, but partial, avenue of assessing defense mechanisms.

Projective techniques and personality questionnaires share the feature of capturing the characteristics of persons at a frozen moment. Defense mechanisms, however, unfold in time. Sandler and Joffe (1969) pointed to the parallels between perceptual microgenesis and the sequences of conflict, anxiety, and defense observed in psychoanalysis. This parallel is basic to the percept-genetic approach, which was developed to investigate "events over time" (Smith, 1957, p. 306). Its contribution to research on defense mechanisms is twofold. First, its originators (Kragh & Smith, 1970) have designed methods that permit the observation of the emergence of defenses. Second, they have proposed operational definitions of most of the prominent defense mechanisms and have accumulated massive data on their manifestations. Percept-genetic contributions are amply represented in this volume. There is therefore no need to review them, especially since relatively recent presentations are available (cf. Smith & Westerlundh, 1980). It should, however, be pointed out that the prototypical percept-genetic instrument is the Defense Mechanism Test (Kragh, 1985), which construes the major Freudian defense mechanisms as distorted prerecognition responses to threatening stimuli. Thus the perceptual-genetic approach blends two traditions of investigation, the process-oriented and the psychodynamic, to reproduce macrotemporal developments in micro time. Along similar lines, Ehlers, as represented in this volume, and others have made great strides toward the systematic and objective investigation of the analysands' productions in the actual psychoanalytic hour. This approach permits the objective study of the phenomena that Freud, of necessity, was able to observe impression-istically. Thus the origins of psychoanalysis merge with the modern methods of investigating the same phenomena, and nine decades of interplay of theory, clinical observation, and experimentation have brought about a powerful spurt toward integration.

Unanswered Questions: Future Research Objectives

What remains to be done? Let me compress the multitude of unfinished tasks under a limited number of headings.

First, the transition of defense from an explanatory to a predictive concept is as yet incomplete. Two objectives can be envisaged. On the basis of antecedent variables, it should be possible to predict the emerg-ence of a specific defense mechanism under conditions of threat, conflict, and stress. Conversely, the appearance of a defense mechanism should be associated with predictable consequences in behavior. The identification of such links should place the application of defenses in a functional sequence, which could be articulated on the basis of theoretical formu-lations. Pinpointing these links would involve taking seriously the basic Freudian view of defense mechanisms as intermediate points between the challenges of and the responses to adaptation.

Second, the implementation of this proposal would entail laying bare and opening to empirical study the entire progression of threat, anxiety, defense, and its aftermath. As yet, in most of the studies extant the subjective experience of anxiety remains hidden from view. It is usually inferred from antecedent, presumably anxiety-arousing conditions, such as a peripheral threatening figure in the Defense Mechanism Test. The effectiveness of such stimuli is then inferred from the imposition of a defensive response, which follows the appearance of the stimulus designed to arouse anxiety. But how do we know whether anxiety has actually been experienced? What evidence do we have about the impact of such stimuli on the person's anxiety level? How is the reaction different upon the experience of a successful or unsuccessful defense? These questions could potentially be answered with the help of the available psychophysiological and psychological indicators of anxiety (cf. Johanson, Risberg, Silverskiöld, & Smith, 1986). To be sure, none of these measures is expected to stand in a one-to-one relationship to anxiety, as the term is understood clinically or invoked conceptually. Yet a pattern may be discerned from a complex relationship between a multiplicity of partially valid and relevant indicators and the manifestations of various defense mechanisms.

Third, research on defense mechanisms continues to be concentrated on psychopathology. At the same time, the adaptive function of defenses, recognized for several decades by both clinicians and theoreticians, has suffered at least partial neglect at the hands of experimenters. This imbalance is apparent in two ways. On the one hand, researchers have been more curious about the "traditional" defense mechanisms, readily linked to deficits and dysfunctions, than they are about the more "normal" defensive operations. Thus there is an extensive experimental literature about such defenses as repression, projection, or displacement and a paucity of experimental investigations on the more purely adaptive defenses like sublimation. Along the same lines, the level IV defenses, as identified and described by Vaillant (1977), have not been subjected to controlled investigation. The other aspect of this psychopathology bias is that "successful" defensive operations (i.e., those that result in the elimination of anxiety and other discomfort) are less often scrutinized than defenses that engender continuous or vicious cycles of aversive behavioral and effective consequences. A widely shared conclusion in theory and in the clinic is that defenses are indispensable and universal and that they "work" much of the time in reducing anxiety and facilitating coping. Is remains for these processes and their results to be scrutinized experimentally.

Related to the considerations above is the fourth unfinished task in the investigation of defenses. It refers to the concentration of the research effort on the "original" defenses named and described by Sigmund Freud and systematically presented in Anna Freud's classical monograph. By contrast, the newer patterns of defensive operations as described by contemporary psychoanalysts and other clinicians have as yet experienced much less investigation. Obstacles in correcting this imbalance include the absence of ready-made measures for the detection and identification of these less widely known defense mechanisms. Along similar lines, their conceptual status is not developed in sufficient detail, which poses obstacles in formulating theoretically meaningful predictions. Nonetheless, the panorama of defenses deserves to be investigated in all its variety and richness.

As the chapters in this volume demonstrate, the work of research and experimentation on defense mechanisms has moved a long way from its modest and, in retrospect, naive beginnings. Yet the clinical and theoretical understanding of defensive operations has also grown in sophistication and complexity. Interaction between systematic controlled study, naturalistic observation, and theoretical formulation involves continuous correction of imbalances and reciprocal catching up. Of necessity, throughout the findings may no longer exclusively confirm, invalidate, or illustrate clinical observations or theoretical concepts. The time has come for the results of experiments to have impact on theory and clinical practice.

References

Allport, G.W. (1937) *Personality: A psychological interpretation.* New York: Holt.

Brenner, C. (1981) Defense and defense mechanisms. *Psychoanalytic Quarterly*, *51*, 501–525.

Drews, S. & Brecht, K. (1975) *Psychoanalytische Ich-Psychologie.* Frankfurt/Main: Suhrkamp.

Fenichel, O. (1945) *The psychoanalytic theory of defense.* New York: Norton.

Freud, A. (1946) *The ego and the mechanisms of defense.* Madison, CT: International Universities Press. (Original work published 1936).

Freud, S. (1964) The neuro-psychoses of defense. In *The standard edition of the complete psychological works of Sigmund Freud: Vol. 3* (pp. 45–61). London: Hogarth Press. (Original work published 1894).

Freud, S. (1964) Further remarks on the neuro-psychoses of defence. In *The standard edition of the complete psychological works of Sigmund Freud: Vol. 3.* London: Hogarth Press. (Original work published 1896).

Freud, S. (1924) Further remarks on defence neuro-psychosis. In S. Freud *Collected papers: Vol. I* (pp. 155–182). London: Hogarth Press. (Original work published 1896).

Freud, S. (1948) The psychopathology of everyday life. New York: Macmillan. (Original work published 1901).

Freud, S. (1925) Repression. In S. Freud *Collected papers: Vol. IV* (pp. 84–97). London: Hogarth Press. (Original work published 1915).

Freud, S. (1963) Inhibitions, symptoms, and anxiety. In *The standard edition of the complete psychological works of Sigmund Freud: Vol. 20.* London: Hogarth Press. (Original work published 1926).

Gleser, G.C. & Ihilevich, D. (1969) An objective instrument for measuring defense mechanisms. *Journal of Consulting and Clinical Psychology*, *33*, 51–60.

Goldin, P.C. (1964) Experimental investigation of selective memory and the concept of repression and defense: A theoretical synthesis. *Journal of Abnormal and Social Psychology*, *69*, 365–380.

Hentschel, U. (1980) Kognitive Kontrollprinzipien und neurosenformen. [Cognitive control principles and varieties of neurosis]. In U. Hentschel & G.J.W. Smith (Eds.), *Experimentelle Persönlichkeitspsychologie: Die Wahrnehmung als Zugang zu diagnostischen Problemen* (pp. 227–321). Wiesbaden: Akademische Verlagsgesellschaft.

Johanson, A.M., Risberg, J., Silverskiöld, & Smith, G.J.W. (1986) Regional changes in cerebral blood flow during increased anxiety in patients with anxiety neurosis. In U. Hentschel, G. Smith, & J. Draguns (Eds.), *The roots of perception*. Amsterdam: Elsevier.

Jones, E. (1911) The psychopathology of everyday life. *American Journal of Psychology, 22*, 477–527.

Klein, G.S. (1954) Need and regulation. In M.R. Jones (Ed.), *Nebraska symposium on motivation*. Lincoln: University of Nebraska Press.

Kragh, U. (1985) *Defense Mechanism Test—DMT manual*. Stockholm: Persona.

Kragh, U. & Smith, G. (1970) *Percept-genetic analysis*, Lund: Gleerup.

Kubie, L.S. (1952) Problems and techniques of psychoanalytic validation and progress. In E. Pumpian-Mindlin (Ed.), *Psychoanalysis as science* (pp. 46–124). Stanford, CA: Stanford University Press.

MacKinnon, D.W. & Dukes, W.F. (1962) In L. Postman (Ed.), *Psychology in the making. Histories of selected research problems* (pp. 662–744). New York: Knopf.

Madison, P. (1961) *Freud's concept of repression and defense: Its theoretical and observational language*. Minneapolis: University of Minnesota Press.

Matte Blanco, I. (1955) *Estudios de psicología dinámica*. [Studies in the field of dynamic psychology]. Santiago: Ediciones de la Universidad de Chile.

Sandler, J. & Joffe, W.G. (1969) Toward a basic psychoanalytic model. *International Journal of Psychoanalysis, 50*, 79–90.

Schafer, R. (1954) *Psychoanalytic interpretation in Rorschach testing*. New York: Grune & Stratton.

Sjöbäck, H. (1973) *The psychoanalytic theory of defensive processes*. Lund: Gleerup.

Smith, G.J.W. (1957) Visual perception: An event over time. *Psychological Review, 64*, 306–313.

Smith, G.J.W. & Westerlundh, B. (1980) Perceptgenesis: A process perspective on perception-personality. *Review of Personality and Social Psychology, 1*, 94–124.

Vaillant, G. (1977) *Adaptation to life*. Boston: Little, Brown.

Wallerstein, R.S. (1985) Defenses, defense mechanisms, and the structure of the mind. In H.P. Blum (Ed.), *Defense and resistance. Historical perspectives and current concepts* (pp. 201–225). International Universities Press.

3
What Is a Mechanism of Defense?

HANS SJÖBÄCK

We are all agreed on this point: the theory of defense is a cornerstone of psychodynamic thinking. The analytical literature on various aspects of this theory is vast. Yet, there are few surveys of the theory as a whole (cf. Sjöbäck, 1973), and we find conspicuous confusion and salient dissent in the discussion of even its basic assumptions. Here are three instances of confusion and/or dissent.

1. Should the mechanisms of defense be described as "always pathogenic" (Freud's view, cf. Freud, 1937/1971, pp. 236–244), or perhaps labeled "pathologic" (cf. Sperling, 1958), or ought we to describe them as sometimes pathogenic, sometimes pathologic, and sometimes "normal" or adaptive, depending on the circumstances? (Cf. A. Freud, 1970, pp. 177–178; Hartmann, 1958; Loewenstein, 1967.) The discussion of this question reveals a confusion as regards both the immediate and the long-term consequences of countercathectic defensive processes, a confusion that contrasts with the fairly clear conceptions of their causal chains, and also with the assumptions of the characteristics of the basic defensive processes.

2. There is also confusion and disagreement as regards the definition of the various mechanisms of defense, their specific characteristics, their delimitation from each other, etc. The proper definition of denial has troubled many analysts (cf. Dorpat, 1985; Jacobson, 1957; Moore & Rubinfine, 1969; Sjöbäck, 1973, pp 209–238). Today the definitions of splitting and projective identification seem to share the same fate (splitting: see Blum, 1983; Dorpat, 1979; Lustman, 1977; Pruyser, 1975, etc.; projective identification, see: Grotstein, 1981; Ogden, 1979; Sandler, 1988).

3. A third bone of contention, finally, is quite simply the question of the ontological status of the mechanisms of defense and the defensive processes. What type of entity is a defensive process? What kind of reality ought we to assign to it? (The unclarity reigning here is of course but one facet of the basic uncertainty about the nature of psychoanalytic

theory, its concepts, and assumptions, from the point of view of the theory of science, and epistemology in general.)

One deplorable aspect of the analytical discussion of the nature of defense is actually a lack of clarity on a most basic point: a lack of delimitation between, on the one hand, the observed behaviors and reported experiences we wish to explain, and, on the other hand, the concepts and assumptions we use to transform the "explananda" (those behaviors, those experiences) we felt were insufficiently or inadequately explained by extant theories, into the empirical referents of the theory of defense. The basic rules of science teach us to proceed in this way: in the bewildering multitude of unexplained and unclassified phenomena, we single out some that we—in spite, sometimes, of their superficial disparity— explain in terms of identical or similar causal chains, postulated common process characteristics, and identical consequences. In this way we single out and delimit a class of phenomena from the mass of phenomena, and delimit and explain this class in terms of "common fate." Doing this, we obey the principle of explanatory parsimony: we use as few concepts and assumptions as possible to construe the causal chain, and its variations. Regarding these variations, we attempt to create definitions of as few basic types as possible, in the interest of clarity, and, above all, of facility of survey.

If we do not observe this basic precept, of distinguishing between explanatory terms and their explananda, the result is a perturbing confusion because one important aim of explanatory endeavors (i.e., theory making) gets lost, namely: that of subsuming a great and (as to varying observable characteristics) bewildering number of phenomena under a few classifying definitions. In the analytical discussion of these matters, the terminology unfortunately invites this confusion, since the term "defense" is often used to refer both to explananda (empirical referents) and to explanatory constructs. The result will be that we get lost in an unmanageable, endless list of "defenses" (because practically all types of experience and behavior may, according to the basic assumptions of the theory of defense, have defensive aspects, certain conditions prevailing). A notorious illustration of this confusion is the list of "defenses" offered by Bibring, Dwyer, Huntington, and Valenstein (1961). Some theorists have attempted to counteract this muddled thinking by insisting (a) on the basic distinction between empirical referent and explanatory entity, and (b) on the nature of the entity referred to by the explanatory term: it is a discretionary explanatory construct, and nothing else. Gill (1963, p. 96) is a pioneer here, it seems: "To say that defense itself is unconscious cannot mean that the defense *mechanism* is unconscious, since a defense mechanism is a theoretical abstraction of a way of working of the mind which of course cannot become conscious." (Gill's italics) (Cf. Sjöbäck, 1973, pp. 29–33.)

A theorist who insistently has stressed these important points is Wallerstein (1967, 1983, 1985). The core of his position seems to be as follows:

1. We must strictly observe the distinction between explananda, the empirical referents, on the one hand, and the propositions of the theory of defense, creating our explanatory constructs, on the other.

2. Explanatory constructs are not to be placed, ontologically, on a par with mental contents and events; rather, they are assumed to be discretionary patterns of contents ("structures," "defense mechanisms") or events ("processes," "defensive processes") created by the theorist to order and explain phenomena ("mental contents and events"). Thus, defense mechanisms and defensive processes are neither "conscious" nor "unconscious"; their ontological status as constructs, discretionary creations of the theorist, of course precludes the application of these terms to them.

This point of view is commendable and unobjectionable from the standpoint of the theory of science. It implies that the theorist creates hypothetical constructs as, above all, discretionary patterns of events, (a) to create primary regular sequences of events, "basic linear causal chains," (b) to construe patterns of complex interactions of mental contents and their ensuing transformations during and in the wake of the postulated interaction, the "mental process" as such, (c) to classify the events under scrutiny (the empirical referents) and separate them from other classes of events explainable by means of other hypothetical constructs, and (d) to create constructs describing subclasses of the basic process, thereby classifying the total class of empirical referents in subgroups (the empirical referents of the different mechanisms or processes). This position also has the advantage, not to say the unconditional precondition of good theory making, of directing, incessantly, the attention of the theorist to his aim, his sole task: of explaining observable, puzzling phenomena in as parsimonious a way as possible, and directing him away from the temptation to forget this in favor of theory making, as it were, for its own sake. These assumptions and observations are self-evident to every psychologist who has acquired a rudimentary understanding of the conditions of theory making, and the dangers of not taking them into account—dangers that become patent when we attempt to use theories whose construction has implied a neglect of these requisites. Yet, Wallerstein's views have, strangely enough, not gone uncontested in the recent analytical discussion.

The main aim of Gillett's article "Defense mechanisms versus defense contents" seems to be to question Wallerstein's view of the ontological status of defense mechanisms (defensive processes) and to propose another position which he deems better (Gillett, 1987). However, Gillett devotes a fair portion of his work to a discussion of the basic characteristics of the defensive processes—their main causes, their functional characteristics, and their consequences. I shall scrutinize neither these deliberations nor Gillett's terminology but concentrate on his main target: the ontological status of defense mechanisms and defensive processes. Gillett offers a somewhat confused discussion of the question of the nature of abstractions used in theoretical discourse in general. Then he proceeds to acknowledge the fundamental distinction between what he calls "defensive contents" (the empirical referents) and the "defense mechanisms" (the explanatory entities). As to the basic characteristics of these entities, he says that they cannot be regarded to be just hypothetical constructs—they must be assumed to exist in some way. I guess that Gillett means they exist in the sense that the theorist's task is to observe or/and describe them in some way or other, not construe them. The main point of reasoning seems to be this: the observable behavior (reported experience) we label "defensive" must have causes. These causes must then be defense mechanisms.

It is clear that theoretical terms and concepts, if they exist at all, clearly exist in a form different from the working of the mind they refer to. However, it is hard for me to see how Wallerstein's definition of a defense mechanism is compatible with the usual way the term is used in the psychoanalytic literature. The activity of the defense mechanisms is triggered by signal anxiety and has effects on observable behavior. How is this possible if defense mechanisms don't exist? How is this possible if they are concepts or terms in a theoretical statement? It seems to me more plausible to regard defense mechanisms as part of the "working of the mind" rather than *denoting* a way of functioning of the mind. (Gillett, 1987, p 266; Gillett's Italics) At other places in his article Gillett discusses the concept of causal chain, and the possible nature of causal chains, and it is obvious that the basic problem, as he sees it, is to construe (or to "find") the causal chain behind "defensive contents." "What I wish to stress is that there is no justification for claiming dogmatically that defense mechanisms do not exist, and on a commonsense level it is hard to see how they can have behavioral effects if they don't exist." (Gillett, 1987, p. 267).

Now, first, as to Gillett's answer to the question of the links of the causal chain, that defense mechanisms ought to be regarded as some sort of "workings of the human mind," this conception unfortunately will involve him in innumerable difficulties. He evades them by not defining what he means by a "working of the human mind," but it appears that he thinks there are some "functions" or "processes" that exist as sorts of mental entities in their own right and in some way or other interact with "mental contents." Wallerstein has pointed out some of the difficulties this kind of conception will lead to (Wallerstein, 1985, pp. 208–211). I shall not discuss the further difficulties encountered by all conceptions of this kind, the most well known being that of "form" or "structure" as a type of empty entity filled by "contents," but instead first concentrate on the question by which Gillett starts, about the nature of the causal chain behind experience and behavior said to be "defensive." Gillett repeats again and again, as if perplexed: What does cause them?

First we must do away with a confusion rampant in this context. Let us define a mental content (conscious) as some experienced mental entity, which is described as static, a snapshot from the stream of conscious experience. Then a mental event (conscious) is a portion of the stream of conscious experience (stream of contents) that goes on uninterruptedly during our waking hours. The basic characteristic of a mental event is a change in the qualities of a mental content or some mental contents. Conscious mental contents and conscious mental events are the target of most psychological research, but, as we know, Freud said that these contents and events often appear to be (a) inexplicable, and (b) fragmented, disconnected, and to understand the confusing stream of conscious mental contents, we must postulate that many aspects of conscious mental events are caused by preconscious or unconscious contents or events. The ontological status of preconscious and unconscious mental contents and events is identical with that of conscious mental contents and events, but their epistemological status is different: they are postulated, but we postulate that they "exist" in the same way as conscious mental contents and events exist. (There are theorists, both inside and outside psychoanalysis, who would object here, saying that unconscious mental contents and events cannot be said to exist in the same way as conscious ones, but let us leave this objection so far.)

Before we proceed, another question must be touched on: the question of the two temporal categories, of "contents" versus "events." It is evident that psychologists in general, and also psychoanalysts, work with two classes of concepts, namely: content; structure/event; process. The first level, that of "contents and events," causes us no trouble, but the second level does. Defense mechanisms are mostly described as something in abeyance, a potentiality, a structured readiness to respond in a specific way. This readiness is released when some specific conditions arise. Then a defensive process takes place. Defense mechanisms are, from this point of view, sometimes also described as "structures of the mind" (I need not repeat here, e.g., Rapaport's (1960) discussion of the concept of structure), and again we encounter obscurities. Structure as a term is used, to denote, among other things, (a) a phenomenal pattern of contents (i.e., what we also call a gestalt), (b) a pattern of mental contents (conscious and/or unconscious, etc.) that is not an experiential entity, and (c) specifically, a motivational or functional entity that is activated under specific conditions; its specific quality, as structure, besides its organization, is resistance to change. These various definitions of structure have played roles in the discussion of "defense mechanisms" and confuse our issue, the issue of causality. A simple solution has two steps: (a) to regard the concept of defense mechanism as a dispositional concept, which entails that a defense mechanism in no type of theory can be regarded as a cause of anything but the defensive process whose potentiality it is, and (b) to avoid using the term "defense mechanism" except when we must have recourse to the dispositional concept, and on the whole, to avoid the "static" concepts. Thus, in the following, I shall use only "mental event" and "process"; this is quite enough for the pursuance of the discussion.

Now we return to Gillett and his Gretchenfrage about the causes of mental events. Insofar as we wish to point to the antecedent links of the causal chains of conscious mental events and the sometimes ensuing behavior, they of course consist of other mental events, and nothing else. The basic object of study is a stream of mental events, and nothing else. This stream has, according to analytical assumptions, conscious, preconscious, and unconscious sectors, and we study the latter two only indirectly. Here Gillett of course immediately ripostes: but this to me simplistic assumption of the nature of the causal chain does not explain why some mental events are assumed to be defensive! Quite so, but the point is of course that on this stream of mental events (portions of which we may observe, portions of which we postulate) we superimpose patterns of causal connections, above all patterns of more or less complex interactions of mental contents—during which these contents are transformed in various ways. It is like having a stream of dots on a paper, and superimposing on this stream another, translucent paper, with a proposal for a pattern of the dots. (This simple analogy cannot include the concept of interaction and transformation, unfortunately; it only illustrates a simple static concept of "pattern.") Such a pattern may make a more or less "good fit," but after all it is only an invention of the maker of the pattern. This conceptualization, which of course is nothing but a transcription in another (in my opinion, more manageable) temporal mode of the conceptions of Gill and Wallerstein, invites some further clarifying comments.

1. This conception implies that a great portion of the "sequences of regularity and interdependency" with which we operate in theoretical deliberations are created by theorists rather than "existing as phenomena." Gillett here takes the opposite position. It seems to me reasonable that from all possible theories of the mind, some prove more useful in explaining and predicting the observable phenomena because they reflect sequences of regularities existing in the workings of the mind (Gillett, 1987, p. 267). Here, Gillett touches on some very difficult points of epistemology. How much order is inherent in the nature of things, and how much is a construct of the human theorist? More than two hundred years ago, David Hume attacked the position that we "experience" simple causal chains (those that refer to or are caused by, simple experiences of "before" and "after" in the world of material events) because they are "given" as "realities." Since the days of Hume, these problems have haunted philosophers and theorists of science; I shall not presume to pursue them;

I only point out that Gillett's position seems to lead to a naive epistemological realism of the kind few philosophers (apart from convinced Marxists) would care to defend. In any event, even though we may provisionally postulate that simple causal chains (of the "before–after" type) in the world of things are real characteristics of the events of this world, the concept of complex causal interaction of mental contents (which are a trifle more elusive than billiard balls) is not thereby much clarified.

2. Gillett (1987, p. 267) attempts to bolster his assumption of the ontological status of the defensive process by referring to an analogy with nuclear and elementary particle physics: "Many physicists believe in the existence of atoms, electrons, and even quarks, which are all theoretical entities of physics, with the same logical status as defense mechanisms in psychoanalytic theory. Perhaps defense mechanisms and other theoretical entities of psychology refer to physical processes of the brain." Now, first, the term "physicists" is vague, but if it is used to refer to researchers within the field of elementary particle physics, Gillett's statement is lamentably uninformed. But here we have first to compare primarily the status of "atoms, electrons, and even quarks" and that of the constructs of analysts. That is, it is necessary, before we try to construe analogies, to analyze what kinds of entity the physicists in question operate with. First, we have assumptions of different kinds of "protomatter," such as electrons, protons, and neutrons. Then we have assumptions about their characteristics, of which mass and charge are basic (and then further, "charm," etc.). Then we have, based on the assumptions about the characteristics of particles, the hypotheses of interactions and their results. It is palpably clear that if we attempt to attain any reasonable analogy between psychology and elementary particle physics here, the assumptions of "protomatter" (something in some way analogous to "things" in the perceptible world), are analogous to assumptions of unconscious mental contents, and to nothing else. The assumptions of the characteristics of elementary particles may be said to correspond to characteristics of mental contents, either in terms of protoexperience, such as "emotional charge," or in terms of a construct much more abstract, fetched from physics in a way, namely in terms of "cathexis," etc. As for the concept of defensive process, its only reasonable analogy is to "interaction of elementary particles, and their ensuing transformations."

3. With this question clarified, we might ask again, do many physicists really believe in the existence of elementary particles, as Gillett states? The term "physicist" delimits the class only in a vague way, but if we take it to refer to researchers within the field of elementary particle physics, Gillett is uninformed, to say the least. To be sure, in everyday talk, elementary particles are discussed as if really "existing" protomatter, but the researchers are of course well aware that even the particles, and the basic characteristics through which they are defined, are nothing but constructs. But, though constructs, are they thought to refer to some kind

of reality? Here is one answer, and I think it represents a position that for many reasons is unavoidable. In a recently published biography of Lord Rutherford, the author describes the physicist's attempts to build a model of the nucleus of the atom (consisting of positive and negative electrons). After describing Rutherford's endeavors, and his difficulties, the author concludes:

"But Rutherford was always honest and rarely, if ever, fudged an issue. He admitted here, for instance, that there was no evidence that negative electrons existed in any nucleus, but presumably they must be there for they were shot out as beta-rays in radioactive transformations which were certainly nuclear events. Here Rutherford shows that he was caught in a well-known philosophical trap: *it is not logically necessary that what comes out of something must have been inside it before it came out.* This fallacy was to lead Rutherford into a number of blind alleys in the years ahead, until the mathematics of quantum mechanics got him, and science in general, out of the impasse; and it remains true today that although electrons, as beta-rays, and helium nuclei, as alpha-rays emerge from the nucleus, we still have no evidence of their *independent existence as such within the nucleus.*" (Wilson, 1983, p. 389. *Italics added.*)

These statements, which represent the views of sophisticated physicists of the "existence" of elementary particles, should warn us not to seek facile but deceiving analogies between psychology and physics. Let me add: if physicists one day were to be able, by means of refined "prostheses of the sense organs" to "look into" the interior of the atom (instead of being reduced to observing what comes out of the atoms when subjected to violent influence from without, as they are in today's experimental particle physics), something that appears impossible, for different reasons, but if it, although impossible, were to happen: this would not strengthen Gillett's position, for simultaneously the analogy would break down, there being no possibility of psychologists finding prostheses of the sensorium enabling them to "look deeper into the mind." Thus, sensible physicists know well that their models of what happens in the atoms are "models," discretionary constructs, to explain what is observable under certain conditions, namely scatters of elementary particles apparently expelled from the interior of the atoms and of which "pictures" can be caught. Physicists I have discussed the matter with stress that there is incessant competition among differing models, the criterion of a good model being the combination of "good fit" and parsimony.

4. The foregoing quotation from Gillett ends with the suggestion that the theoretical entities of psychology refer to "physical processes in the brain." The comments on these cogitations of Gillett's need not be long: it is blatantly evident that Gillett confounds postulated ontological characteristics on the one hand, and levels of explanation, on the other (cf. Holt, 1975, esp. pp. 176 et seq., for an elementary exposition of this question).

5. Finally, what about the practical consequences of the two views discussed here, that of Gillett versus that of Gill, Wallerstein, and Sjöbäck? Gillett remarks, quite correctly (1987, p. 261): "It has been shown historically in science that theoretical understanding can have very practical implications which are only apparent at a later time."

What are the very practical implications of the two positions competing here? Gill's position leads to a clear conception of the task of the theorist: it consists of construing a discretionary system of propositions designed to explain as parsimoniously and as free of contradictions as possible as large a portion of the explananda as possible. Gillett's position leads to a much more equivocal description of the theorist's task, as is quite clear from the history of psychoanalytic thinking. This theorist is of course also aware of the task of explaining some preliminarily delimited class of puzzling phenomena, but he evidently thinks that his task is also to spy into the dark, hidden reality of "the workings of the mind" (which comprises not only concrete mental contents and events, but also the "realities" of their interaction), and his attention is then split, vacillating between two directions, that of the empirical referents to be explained and the "hidden reality" to be discovered. As is well known, this stance—which, unfortunately, is not rare among analysts, though seldom articulated with that frankness Gillett evinces—has led to dire results, that is, to a proliferation of concepts and assumptions that compete not on the basis of their explanatory range, their elegance, and parsimony, but on the basis of their alleged "truthfulness" as "descriptions" of a "hidden reality." Often enough, the empirical referents are almost neglected, or treated in a casual way, in discussions of assumptions of defense, because the author's interest is focused on the "exploration" of the "hidden reality." The quandary is of course that nobody is able to define this criterion of "truthfulness," since it is impossible to "demonstrate" (and no more possible to "prove") here, that is, to point to the "realities" as such or to point to empirical referents that logically and materially necessitate the existence of something not observable—or at least make the inference fairly compelling.

The muddle that we land in here is well illustrated by the contents of a recently published book, *Denial and Defense in the Therapeutic Situation* (Dorpat, 1985). This work contains many astute observations and assumptions that appear to be highly useful as components of an encompassing theory of defense, but unfortunately the usefulness of the endeavor is marred by the position Dorpat takes on "the nature of defense" (and the nature of mental processes in general), which in essence corresponds to Gillett's: he assumes that the defensive processes are "realities," which he "describes." Within this framework Dorpat puts forward three basic propositions: (a) there is (exists) one basic defensive process; (b) this basic defensive process can be described in detail, at a microlevel of mental processes, as a process of "cognitive arrest"; and (c) this basic defensive process is denial. The reification to which Dorpat adheres prevents him from considering the following questions.

1. Would it in some instances, taking into account the characteristics of some groups of explananda, be useful to postulate other basic defensive processes, or variants of the alleged basic process? This means, in other words: Does Dorpat's model of a defensive process "fit all instances" (of explananda), or does it not? In my opinion, his model cannot explain important aspects of some groups of explananda, for example, those connected with changes in reality feeling (cf. Freud, 1936/1971; Sarlin, 1962) and altered states of consciousness (cf. Dickes, 1965; Rohsco, 1967, etc.). From this point of view, Dorpat's picture of "the reality of the basic defensive process" appears to be a Procrustean bed for the explananda.

2. Throughout the history of psychoanalysis, from its inception in Freud's first analytical works until now, we find assumptions of a basic defensive process which, as is well known, Freud (and practically all analysts after him) called "repression." Dorpat now proposes that this basic process be called "denial." Why does he wish us to adopt this revision of analytical terminology, whose proposal alone causes confusion (not to speak of what would happen if it were adopted)? With regard to the basic differentiation of repression and denial (which ought to form the basis for a decision as to what to call a presumed "basic defensive process"), Dorpat first states (1985, p. 94): "Writings on primal repression do not give clinical referents, and they do not state what is and what is not primal repression." Now, this is a somewhat astonishing statement at least from one point of view, that which refers to the connection of primal repression and fixation (no primal repression without fixation), but we proceed: Dorpat offers us a chapter on "primal repression and denial," and here he concludes (1985, pp. 104–105):

"I proposed that the clinical referents of these theories of the primordial defense are the same as the clinical referents of denial. The primitive defense that analysts have called primal repression is, in my opinion, the basic defense of denial. One argument for the equivalence of primal repression and denial is that they have the same consequences, namely: the primitive defense prevents the formation of verbal representations; the content of what is defended against is unrememberable, and when it is later repeated, it occurs in the form of enactive memory; and developmental defects are consequences of the defense.

New cases of primal repression are said to emerge in early childhood, in traumatic states, and in the psychoses and borderline conditions. Clinical evidence obtained from studies of young children, traumatic states, and the psychoses and borderline conditions indicates that denial, and not primal repression, is the basic defense on which developmentally later and higher-level defenses such as repression and reaction formation are developed."

Apart from the contradictions unveiled here, the main question is of course why—if there be a basic defensive process—this ought to be labeled denial. The term "denial" is connected with more confusion and embarrassing contradictions than any other term in psychoanalytic thought (cf. Sjöbäck, 1973, pp. 209–238). Why choose it to designate the basic defensive process? Dorpat refers incessantly to "clinical referents" and "clinical evidence" which (a) are nonexistent as regards primal repression, (b) are the same for primal repression and for denial, and (c) demonstrate that denial, not primal repression, is the basic defense. When we search his text for these "clinical referents," we find only clinical vignettes from which no certain conclusions as to the specified characteristics of inferred or postulated defensive processes can be drawn. At no place in this work do we find enumeration and discussion of the differentiating clinical referents. This cavalier treatment of the question of the observations and the explananda the proposed theory should explain is explainable in only one way: Dorpat believes that there is an intrapsychic reality that he is able to describe; from this point of view, the empirical referents can be treated in a summary way. Only a deep commitment to reification of the sort Gillett recommends can cause a theorist to adopt a stance and a mode of processing like this.

What will be the consequences of such contributions as this on the development of analytical theorizing, here within the field of the theory of defense? Either Dorpat has demonstrated that his assumptions of the nature of the basic defense are "true" or so highly probable (as descriptions of "reality") that his colleagues (and all other psychologists interested in psychoanalysis) immediately are convinced, upon reading his work, or Dorpat has, in spite of his many valuable ideas, only added to the general confusion extant within the field of the theory of defense (and here especially within that portion of it associated with the term "denial"), because he can "convince" only a small number of friends, and other analysts who in advance happen to entertain ideas like his own, that he has created a "correct theory." Dorpat cannot demonstrate that his construct "exists"; this circumstance is so palpably evident that it demonstrates convincingly the untenability of Gillett's position. Instead of dividing their attention between the empirical referents and the attempt at spying into the "hidden dark reality" of mental events (and even "workings of the mind"),—with the dire consequences that this stance engenders—analytical theorists ought to accept the much more reasonable position that assumptions about the workings of the mind are discretionary constructs and that such assumptions ought always to be developed in close contact with the explananda, and to be as elegant logically and as parsimonious as possible. At the same time, their range of application should encompass the whole field of explananda preliminarily delimited, and perhaps later extended in accordance with rules agreed upon.

This way of seeing theories and theory making may initially represent a threat to the self-esteem of analytical theorists who feel they are called upon and uniquely equipped to gaze down into the secret depths of the human mind—real depths. But in the long run the result of the rejection of reification will result in a much improved psychoanalytic theory. This rejection will also bring to an end the ridicule that reification in theoretical matters calls forth in psychologists of all convictions outside psychoanalysis, a ridicule and a disdain that in an unfortunate way contribute to the isolation of psychoanalysts and their theories within the scientific community.

References

Bibring, G.L., Dwyer, T.F., Huntington, D.S., & Valenstein, A.F. (1961) A study of the psychological processes in pregnancy and of the earliest mother–child relationship. Appendix B. Glossary of defenses. *Psychoanalytic Study of the Child*, *16*, 62–72.

Blum, H.P. (1983) Splitting of the ego and its relation to parental loss. *Journal of the American Psychoanalytic Association*, Suppl., *31*, 301–324.

Dickes, R. (1965) The defensive function of an altered state of consciousness. *Journal of the American Psychoanalytic Association*, *13*, 356–403.

Dorpat, T.L. (1979) Is splitting a defense? *International Review of Psychoanalysis*, *6*, 105–113.

Dorpat, T.L. (1985) *Denial and defense in the therapeutic situation*. New York: Jason Aronson.

Freud, A. (1970) The symptomatology of childhood: A preliminary attempt at classification. In *The writings of Anna Freud: Vol. 7* (pp. 157–188). Madison, CT: International Universities Press.

Freud, S. (1971) A disturbance of memory on the Acropolis. In *The standard edition of the complete psychological works of Sigmund Freud: Vol. 22* (pp. 239–250). London: Hogarth Press. (Original work published 1936).

Freud, S. (1971) Analysis, terminable and interminable. In *The standard edition of the complete psychological works of Sigmund Freud: Vol. 23* (pp. 216–253). London: Hogarth Press. (Original work published 1937).

Gill, M.M. (1963) Topography and systems in psychoanalytic theory. *Psychological Issues*, *3*, Monogr. 2.

Gillett, E. (1987) Defense mechanisms versus defense contents. *International Journal of Psychoanalysis*, *68*, 261–269.

Grotstein, J.S. (1981) *Splitting and projective identification*. New York: Jason Aronson.

Hartmann, H. (1958) *Ego psychology and the problem of adaptation*. New York: International Universities Press.

Holt, R.R. (1975) Drive or wish? A reconsideration of the psychoanalytic theory of motivation. In M.M. Gill and P.S. Holzman (Eds.), *Psychology vs. metapsychology. Psychoanalytic essays in honour of G.S. Klein. Psychological Issues*, *9*, Monogr. 36, pp. 158–197.

Jacobson, E. (1957) Denial and repression. *Journal of the American Psychoanalytic Association*, *5*, 61–92.

Loewenstein, R.M. (1967) Defensive organization and autonomous ego functions. *Journal of the American Psychoanalytic Association*, *15*, 795–809.

Lustman, J. (1977) On splitting. *Psychoanalytic Study of the Child*, *32*, 119–154.

Moore, B.E. & Rubinfine, D.L. (1969) The mechanism of denial. *Monograph Series of the Kris Study Group of the New York Psychoanalytic Institute*: *Vol. 3*, pp. 3–57.

Ogden, T.H. (1979) On projective identification. *International Journal of Psychoanalysis*, *60*, 357–373.

Pruyser, P.W. (1975) What splits in splitting? A scrutiny of the concept of splitting in psychoanalysis and psychiatry. *Bulletin of the Menninger Clinic*, *39*, 1–46.

Rapaport, D. (1960) The structure of psychoanalyze theory: A systematizing attempt. *Psychological Issues, Monogr. 6.*. International Universities Press.

Rohsco, M. (1967) Perception, denial, and derealization. *Journal of the American Psychoanalytic Association*, *15*, 243–260.

Sandler, J. (Ed.) (1988) *Projection, identification, projective identification*. London: Karnac Books.

Sarlin, C.N. (1962) Depersonalization and derealization. *Journal of the American Psychoanalytic Association*, *10*, 784–804.

Sjöbäck, H. (1973) *The psychoanalytic theory of defensive processes*. New York: Wiley.

Sperling, S.J. (1958) On denial and the essential nature of defense. *International Journal of Psychoanalysis*, *39*, 25–38.

Wallerstein, R.S. (1967) Development and metapsychology of the defensive organization of the ego. Panel report. *Journal of the American Psychoanalytic Association*, *15*, 130–149.

Wallerstein, R.S. (1983) Self psychology and "classical" psychoanalytic psychology: The nature of their relationship. *Psychoanalysis and Contemporary Thought*, *6*, 553–595.

Wallerstein, R.S. (1985) Defenses, defense mechanisms, and the structure of the mind. In H.P. Blum (Ed.), *Defense and resistance. Historical perspectives and current concepts* (pp. 201–225). Madison, CT: International Universities Press.

Wilson, D. (1983) *Rutherford: Simple genius*. London: Hodder and Stoughton.

4
Percept-Genesis and the Study of Defensive Processes

BERT WESTERLUNDH

Microgenesis, Percept-Genesis, and the Theory of Perception

"Percept-genesis" is a term introduced by Kragh and Smith (e.g., 1970) and refers to the microdevelopment of percepts. The percept-genetic theory of perception is microgenetic. A general definition of microgenesis given by Hanlon and Brown (1989) reads: "Microgenesis refers to the structural development of a cognition (idea, percept, act) through qualitatively different stages. The temporal period of this development extends from the inception of the cognition to its final representation in consciousness or actualization (expression) in behavior."

Evidently, percept-genesis is a process theory of perception, which does not see the conscious percept as an immediate reflection of a given reality. Such theories were rare in psychology until the early 1960s. Thus, the "New Look" psychology of the 1940s and 1950s was very much oriented toward the study of nonveridical perception. But nonveridicality was explained as a secondary revision of an originally true copy of reality. This type of reflection theory was more or less supplanted in the 1960s by information processing models of perception, still very much with us. Typical such models (discussed by Marcel, 1983) can be said to be processual in the sense that they are sequential (proceeding in stages) and hierarchical (the stages become in some sense successively "higher" and more advanced). The process is generally thought to start with simple sensory information analysis and to end with perceptual meaning, the conscious end product.

This type of constructivist approach is radically different from that of microgenesis. Like most information processing models, microgenesis considers percept development to be a basically bottom-up, linear, sequential, and hierarchical process, and it states that all conscious percepts have such a prehistory. But the process is conceived of in quite a different way, where "primacy of meaning" and "biological development" are key concepts.

38

Thus the perceptual process is thought to follow the basic regulatory principle of biological development, the orthogenetic principle (Werner & Kaplan, 1956): "Wherever development occurs, it proceeds from a state of relative lack of differentiation to a state of increasing differentiation, articulation and hierarchic integration." Furthermore, meaning is considered to be the subjective aspect of organismic adaptation, existing from the inception of a perceptual process. The most important characteristic of such a process is that it is a sequence of transformations of meaning. For microgenesis, the early stages of perception are characterized by lack of self- and object differentiation, lack of sensory modality differentiation, and diffuse meaning spreading over a global semiotic field. In the continuation of the process, subjective components reflecting important aspects of life experience are successively eliminated, until at last, at a stimulus proximal, conscious stage, the intersubjective meaning of the stimulus predominates.

At this point, it is possible to articulate the relationship of microgenesis to information processing models. Early such models (e.g., Haber, 1969) were conceived of in terms of hierarchical serial processing, leading up to perceptual meaning. Data from the fields of subliminal perception and automatization cast doubt on this type of conceptualization, and more recent models, such as that of Marcel (1983) tend to be different. They stress parallel processing and play down the idea of hierarchical organization. In contrast, if we were to express the microgenetic model in information processing terms, we would have to use both the concept of hierarchy and that of extensive parallel processing. However, the biological and evolutionary orientation of microgenesis separates it from alternative conceptualizations.

Schools and Research Paradigms of Microgenesis

Psychological theories tend to be associated with specific methods and procedures of investigation. This is true also for microgenesis, where two such research paradigms have been fundamental. Both are illustrated in a classical paper by Heinz Werner: in "Microgenesis and aphasia," Werner (1956) discusses the symptomatology of a specific type of aphasic patient who has difficulty in word finding. When presented with some object, the patient is unable to find the word denoting the object. However, he often answers with a word from the semantic sphere to which the object belongs—for instance, "smoke" for "cigar." Werner thinks that this type of report reflects a universal early and primitive processing stage, which becomes manifest in such patients as a result of the neurological injury. He reasoned that such reports could be obtained from normals if conscious access to intersubjective stimulus meaning were made impossible by information reduction. Thus he studied the reports of normal subjects to verbal stimuli presented tachistoscopically a number of times at successively prolonged presentation times. At short such times, some subjects indeed gave reports that were nonveridical but belonged to the semantic sphere of the stimulus.

In this way, microgenetically oriented researchers in psychiatry and neuropsychology have observed the symptoms of neurologically injured patients. In their frame of reference, such symptoms are considered to be real stages in the microgenetic sequence, but on a primitive level not ordinarily reaching consciousness and motility. Clinical observation is thus one major research paradigm of microgenesis, often oriented toward the study of thought processes (and actions). Microgenetically oriented general psychologists and psychologists interested in personality and psychopathology have instead concentrated their interest on perceptual processing, and they have used information reduction techniques, especially iterated tachistoscopic stimulus presentations at successively prolonged exposure times.

With this, the major orientations of microgenetic research have been mentioned. The German Aktualgenese school, initiated by Friedrich Sander (Sander & Volkelt, 1962) and represented today by for example, Werner Fröhlich (1978) has a cognitive and general psychological orientation. The percept-genetic school of Lund, headed by Ulf Kragh and Gudmund Smith (Kragh & Smith, 1970; Smith & Danielsson, 1982), is oriented toward personality and psychopathology. Psychiatrical and neurological researchers with a microgenetic frame of reference include Paul Schilder (1951, 1953). Jason Brown (1988) is a leading researcher in this tradition today.

The Perceptual Process

For percept-genesis, the stimulus initiating a perceptual process initially gives rise to a global cognitive/affective configuration within the mind. Through the process, this is successively differentiated and delimited, and the more subjective components are excluded in favor of the intersubjective meaning of the stimulus. This implies that perceptual microgeneses initiated by different stimuli are originally rather alike but become successively more specific and stimulus proximal. The earlier parts of the process reflect subjective "personality" functioning, the later show a greater influence of the stimulus. This ordering is accompanied by a diminution of affect.

By studying a number of percept-geneses, it is possible to isolate hierarchical stages. In percept-genesis, it has been usual to speak of early, middle, and late levels of the process. From a theoretical point of view, the early level is characterized by extreme condensation of personal meaning and the use of primary process mechanisms. Its organization is influenced by drive functioning, and affect is not neutralized. The perceptual meaning configuration can take on a hallucinatory character. The middle level shows partly reduced affect. The differentiation between self and objects is greater, but not complete—objects are not completely objectified. The degree of condensation of meaning is lower. At this level, memory images with direct reference to significant life happenings are seen more often than in other parts of the process. The late level is more tied to the properties of the stimulus. Here, detailed analysis of fine form is possible. The differentiation of self and objects is complete. Affect is reduced, and the interpersonal meaning of the stimulus predominates.

Parallelisms

Microgenesis is conceived of as analogous to other processes of biological development and evolution. It has often been compared to two other such processes, namely phylogenesis and ontogenesis. As stated by Brown (1988), the physiological counterparts of the perceptual process are excitations starting at the upper brain stem and proceeding over limbic, temporal, and parietal areas to end in the visual cortex. This implies that there is a strict parallelism between the percept-genetic sequence and the phylogenetic acquisition of neural structure.

As regards the micro-ontogenetic parallelism, opinions are divided. The percept-genetic sequence shows a formal similarity over the levels to dream functioning, the functioning of small children and that of adults. Brown (1988) notices this but goes on to deny that it means that contents on different levels of the sequence belong to specific periods of life. He holds that position of a content in the sequence gives no information about its place in ontogenesis. In contrast, Kragh (Kragh & Smith, 1970, pp. 134–178) considers the percept-genetic sequence as the successive unfolding of personal history.

The question is somewhat complicated. It is clear that the occurrence of reports in percept-geneses referring to important life experiences is not too uncommon. But on a priori considerations, the initial probability of Kragh's hypothesis seems low. However, a recent attempt at a small but reasonably strict test of this hypothesis came out in favor of it (Westerlundh & Terjestam, 1990). But even if it were to receive further empirical support, it is clear that this must be limited to "episodic" memories and signs of psychic structure formation, while "procedural" skills (to revive Tulving's 1972 distinction) become automatized and can be found at very early process levels. Thus, subliminally presented words can activate a "sphere of meaning," as shown already by Werner (1956).

Determinants of the Percept

There is a successive determination whereby earlier contents are transformed into later in the perceptual process. From a descriptive point of view, the process is characterized by cumulation, elimination, or emergence—respectively, the continued existence, loss, or new appearance of elements of the percept.

In percept-genesis, "stimulus" and "sensations" are regarded as hypothetical determinants that influence but do not create the contents of the perceptual process. Generally, microgenetic theory is congruent with a critical epistemology, such as that presented by neo-Kantian and symbolic construction philosophers like Paul Natorp, Ernst Cassirer, and Susanne Langer.

Processes of a motivational order, such as drives and strong situational needs, can influence the attribution of meaning and thus reduce subjective variability in a percept-genesis. Generally, a percept-genesis always interacts with other microgenetic processes of the individual that have just taken place or are taking place at the same time. Motivational factors press toward microgenesis, that is, toward psychic representation. Such microgeneses will interact with perceptual adaptation. In the same way, spontaneous or induced sets will influence percept-geneses.

Individual regulations of access to consciousness, cognitive styles, put their mark on the process and influence the final conscious product. When such cognitive strategies are used to avoid unpleasure, they are called defense mechanisms. This is a final determinant of the perceptual process systematically distinguished in percept-genesis. The percept-genetic approach to the study of defenses will be treated more fully later.

The Technique of Information Reduction

Only the end stage of a percept-genesis, the stimulus-proximal, intersubjectively equivalent, "correct" configuration and meaning, ordinarily reaches consciousness. Of course, this is a necessity for efficient adaptation. The quasi-instantaneous, objectified character of percepts explains the long rule of the theory of perception as an immediate reflection of reality.

To study the ordinarily preconscious stages preceding the conscious percept, percept-genesis makes use of the technique of information reduction. The same stimulus is presented repeatedly at successively longer exposure times by means of a tachistoscope. Each time, the subject reports what has been seen, verbally and perhaps with a simple drawing. The shortest time used may be of the order of 10 milliseconds (ms). Such trials are continued until the subject is able to give a report of stimulus contents at an intersubjective level. The longest times used in a percept-genetic serial are about 2500 ms.

This way of protracting and fractioning the act of perception is in some ways not as unlike an ordinary perceptual act as might be imagined. Perception takes place in the "phenomenal now," a period of roughly a second. With stimuli depicting ordinary and unarousing objects, the sum total of tachistoscopic presentation times needed for correct recognition does not exceed this value.

Furthermore, the construction of a final, correct meaning and configuration from a number of discrete fixations, which is a feature of the fractioning technique, actually reflects the working of ordinary perception. As has been known for some decades, retinal stabilization of a stimulus input, which would in commonsense terms allow for a really "good look," actually leads to the breakdown of the percept (Pritchard, Heron, & Hebb, 1960). The phenomenal end product of a series of tachistoscopic presentations is in no way different from that of ordinary perception.

However, the instruction to verbalize experience sets up a microgenetic context, and the successive verbalizations of experience create a fading series of microgeneses, which will serve as a background for later experiences. The thrust of this background will be in the direction of cumulation (i.e., reports of the same experience). This is one factor reducing the variability of percept-geneses. Instructions stressing the reporting of new features and change are very important here.

Many of the factors mentioned as determinants of the percept actually reduce the subjective variability of perceptual reports. A compulsive cognitive style, to report objects and their characteristics (perhaps with increasing clarity) while excluding all reference to action and emotional valence, is not uncommon. Here, what can become conscious is limited to the last, stimulus proximal stage. Percept-geneses, series of reports to successively prolonged exposures of the same stimulus, vary from such constricted protocols to protocols showing an extreme richness of subjective material, with most falling in between.

The percept-genetic group is perhaps best known for research in two areas. One of these is the study of individual consistencies in cognitive processing. The process of adaptation to a new, unknown situation shows a pattern that is characteristic for the individual. Studies of such regularities can use the tachistoscopic fractioning technique presented above, but also repeated encounters with other, new, situations, which are not within the scope of adaptation to an average expectable environment. These have included the serial presentation of the Stroop Color-Word Test (Smith, Nyman, & Hentschel, 1986) and the serial afterimage technique (e.g., Smith & Danielsson, 1982). The other area in which well-known contributions have been made by the Lund group is the study of psychological defenses in perception.

The Theory of Defense

In contrast to a number of present-day endeavors in the field, percept-genesis takes its starting point in the classical psychoanalytic formulations of the theory of defense. As is well known, Freud used the concept quite early, but it came into prominence with his second theory of anxiety (1926/1971) and Anna Freud's monograph on the mechanisms of defense (1936/1961).

Defenses are part of potentially pathogenic intrapsychic conflicts. In Freud's formulation, a forbidden impulse—a temptation—strives toward consciousness and motility. On its way through the psychic apparatus, it activates an associated representation of a danger situation. This releases an anxiety signal, which is the proximal cause of the activation of defense mechanisms. Anxiety signals can also be released by threats associated to the danger situation—for example, fantasies activated by castration threats (A. Freud, 1936/1961). The aim of the defenses is to avoid conscious unpleasure. This is done by keeping the anxiety signal and the impulse from reaching consciousness. Sometimes this strategy must be supplemented by others, which allow for some veiled and transformed conscious representation of the contents of the impulse. This theoretical account led to a list of defenses, with repression as the basic one, accompanied by others (isolation, undoing, etc.).

Modifications of the Classical Theory

Three modifications and emendations of the classical view are of importance here. The first concerns the nature of pathogenic, neurosis-producing conflict. That such conflicts involved drive fixation and regression (due to frustration) was part of the classical view. However, the defenses were not thought to be part of this regressive pattern. Actually, in the clinical situation almost anything can serve as a defense against almost anything else, and the only basis for classification of a behavior as defensive is functional (see Wallerstein, 1985). But a study of the major defenses of the classical neuroses led Sandler and Joffe (1965) to the conclusion that these defenses were indeed general cognitive strategies that were used defensively but were on a developmental level corresponding to the forbidden impulses. This made these authors enunciate a principle of correlative drive and defense fixations in neurosis. This is of importance here, since the type and level of a defensive report in a percept-genesis will give information about the experience of danger and the type of impulse involved in the conflict.

Second, the classical theory concerned the mental representatives of a drive and their vicissitudes. From a microgenetic point of view, the fantasy images evoked by the drive are incomplete percept-geneses, in principle not different from parts of the genesis of full-blown percepts. This way of looking at the influence on mental functioning of drive stimuli and outer stimuli has become common among psychoanalysts, especially those who find the topographical model fruitful (see Sandler & Joffe, 1969; Westerlundh & Smith, 1983). On this view, in principle all defenses that are used against the representatives of impulses can be used against psychic representations of outer stimuli. This is of obvious importance for percept-genesis, which relies on the tachistoscopic presentation of special types of stimuli. There are far-reaching correspondences between the topographical ("Jacksonian") model, with its distinctions between unconscious, preconscious, and conscious functioning, and microgenetic theory. Brown (1988) states that the former puts more stress on inhibition, the later more on transformation of meaning. However, the study of defense through perception has demonstrated the importance of inhibition within a microgenetic framework.

Finally, intrapsychic conflict was classically described in the rather abstract terms of the structural theory—id impulses, ego defenses, and so on. With the increasing importance of object relation conceptualizations, the nature of the mental contents that are drawn into conflict has received more attention. Sandler and Rosenblatt (1962) stressed the importance of dyadic images involving the interaction of self and significant others in their concept of the representational world. Such representations play an important part in regulating behavior, constitute the content of drive representations and danger situations, and are the targets of defense. Kernberg (1976) used the same ideas in his concept of introjection. For him, introjection is the reproduction and fixation of an interaction with the environment, involving images of the object and the self in interaction with it, together with affective valence. These conceptualizations inform us about how stimuli intended to evoke the typical defensive processes of a subject must be constructed. They ought to be dyadic, with one person intended as a self and another as an object representation. They should represent temptations or threats referring to the danger situations presented in the theory of anxiety.

Percept-Genesis and the Study of Defensive Processes

The presentation of dyadic, interpersonal stimuli in the tachistoscopic information reduction research paradigm was introduced by Kragh. Already these early studies gave rise to conceptualizations in terms of defenses in the perceptual process (Kragh, 1955, 1959, 1960). Later, within the framework of a project for selecting aviation cadets by means of the percept-genetic technique, Kragh (1961) aimed at creating stimuli with a maximal relationship to the psychoanalytic theory of anxiety and defense. He devised two stimuli, structurally different but with the same content, for these young males. Both represented a scene with a neutral-looking, centrally placed young male (the self representation), and a peripheral, ugly and threatening older male person (the object representation). His idea was that stimuli of this type should activate signal anxiety, referring both to castration anxiety and to superego anxiety. Reports to them ought to reveal the defense mechanisms used by the subjects.

The Defense Mechanism Test

Kragh's early work was the starting point for one of the two reasonably standardized percept-genetic tests for the assessment of defenses, the Defense Mechanism Test (DMT: Kragh, 1985). This test is described in Chapter 7.

The Meta-Contrast Technique

Smith's Meta-Contrast Technique (MCT: Smith, Johnson, & Almgren, 1989) started as a way of studying how a stimulus is successively reported within the framework of an already stabilized perception. A coding system related to nosological entities and developmental levels was developed, and the instrument has been widely used in the clinical field. This test is also described in Chapter 7.

Validity of the Percept-Genetic Approach

The study of defensive processes has become increasingly popular in empirical psychology. Today, there are many such approaches. But it is reasonable to say that what is studied by most of them differs more or less radically from the original psychoanalytic formulations. This is probably most accentuated in the case of questionnaire approaches. What they study may be quite interesting from different points of view, but their relationship to the psychoanalytic theory of defense is tenuous. Naturally, this point is of importance practically. Quite conceivably, it would be possible to, for example, increase the power of the DMT as an instrument of selection by introducing scoring categories unrelated to conceptualizations of defense. The work of Cooper and Kline (1989) on an objectively scored version points in this direction. However, the question of the predictive and concurrent validity of the techniques concerns a body of research big enough to make separate treatment necessary.

What interests us in the present context is instead the relationship of the operationalizations to the theory of defense. The microgenetic and psychoanalytic formulations, and the basic methods of percept-genesis, have been presented above. It is of course suggested that the fit is better in this case than for the majority of other approaches.

Certain aspects of the question of validity have been taken up by Cooper and Kline. In their evaluation of the Defense Mechanism Test, Cooper and Kline (1986) discuss the face validity of the percept-genetic scoring of defense. While most such categories do indeed look as they ought to according to the theory, there is a notable exception, namely repression. In psychoanalysis, repression refers to the exclusion of contents from conscious representation. In percept-genesis, repression is scored when one or both of the persons in the stimulus are seen as rigid or lifeless.

It could be argued that the empirical referents of psychoanalysis and percept-genesis are not the same, and that rigidity and lifelessness could be indications of repression on a perceptual level. To bolster such an argument, it would be necessary to show that the percept-genetic scores appear when the determining conditions are such that one would expect repression. Now, repression is a mechanism linked to the phallic stage of drive organization. It is primarily directed against infantile sexual impulses and is the typical defense of hysterical neurosis (Fenichel, 1946).

What is known about the percept-genetic sign is the following: it is abundantly reported by patients suffering from hysterical neurosis (Kragh, 1985; Smith, Johnson, & Almgren, 1989). Children's reports of the sign increase dramatically at puberty (Carlsson & Smith, 1987; Westerlundh & Johnson, 1989). In experiments using percept-geneses as dependent variables, more subjects report the sign at experimental operations intended as sexual threats and temptations than in other conditions (e.g., Westerlundh & Sjöbäck, 1986). Whatever it is, the sign certainly works as repression is supposed to work. Cooper and Kline's discussion of face validity is important because it points out that percept-genesis studies a perceptual level of functioning and that the principles of representation on this level must be studied in their own right if valid conclusions are to be drawn.

The repression example above is of course an instance of construct validation, where data from different areas concatenate to give support to specific interpretations. This is the way that must be followed and has been followed in clinical, developmental, and experimental research oriented toward the study of the validity of percept-genetic scoring categories. To state that a certain report is defensive is to infer the activity of a defense mechanism for the purpose of avoiding unpleasure. Such an interpretation is always probabilistic, but the more we learn about the conditions that produce such reports, the better our interpretations will be. Much work has been done in this area; much remains. A reasoned judgment at present would be that a big part of percept-genetic interpretations stands up to such scrutiny. There are other areas of doubtful validity, where more research must be performed before a final verdict can be made.

References

Brown, J.W. (1988) *The life of the mind: Selected papers.* Hillsdale, NJ: Erlbaum.

Carlsson, I. & Smith, G.J.W. (1987) Gender differences in defense mechanisms compared with creativity in a group of youngsters. *Psychological Research Bulletin, Lund University, 27,* 1.

Cooper, C. & Kline, P. (1986) An evaluation of the Defense Mechanism Test. *British Journal of Psychology, 77,* 19–31.

Cooper, C. & Kline, P. (1989) A new objectively scored version of the Defense Mechanism Test. *Scandinavian Journal of Psychology, 30,* 228–238.

Fenichel, O. (1946) *The psychoanalytic theory of neurosis.* London: Routledge and Kegan Paul.

Freud, A. (1961) *The ego and the mechanisms of defense.* London: Hogarth Press. (Originally work published in 1936)

Freud, S. (1971) Inhibitions, symptoms and anxiety. In James Strachey (Ed. and Transl.), *The standard edition of the complete psychological works of Sigmund Freud: Vol. 20* (pp. 75–175). London: Hogarth Press. (Original work published 1926)

Fröhlich, W.D. (1978) Stress, anxiety, and the control of attention. In C.D. Spielberger & I.G. Sarason (Eds.), *Stress and anxiety: Vol. 5.* Washington, DC: Hemisphere.

Haber, R.N. (Ed.) (1969) *Information-processing approaches to visual perception.* New York: Holt, Rinehart and Winston.

Hanlon, R.E. & Brown, J.W. (1989) Microgenesis. Historical review and current studies. In Λ. Ardila & P. Ostrosky-Solis (Eds.), *Brain organization of language and cognitive processes* (pp. 3–15). New York: Plenum.

Kernberg, O. (1976) *Object relations theory and clinical psychoanalysis.* New York: Jason Aronson.

Kragh, U. (1955) *The actual-genetic model of perception-personality.* Lund: Gleerup.

Kragh, U. (1959) Types of pre-cognitive defensive organization in a tachistoscopic experiment. *Journal of Projective Techniques, 23,* 315–322.

Kragh, U. (1960) Pathogenesis in dipsomania: An illustration of the actual-genetic model of perception-personality. *Acta Psychiatrica Neurologica Scandinavica, 35,* 207–222, 261–288, 480–497.

Kragh, U. (1961) *DMT-Variabler som prediktorer för flygförarlämplighet* [DMT—Variables as predictors of pilot ability]. MPI rapport, 5.

Kragh, U. (1985) *Defense Mechanism Test. DMT manual.* Stockholm: Persona.

Kragh, U. & Smith, G.J.W. (1970) *Percept-genetic analysis.* Lund: Gleerup.

Marcel, A.J. (1983) Conscious and unconscious perception. *Cognitive Psychology, 15,* 197–300.

Pritchard, R.M., Heron, W., & Hebb, D.O. (1960) Visual perception approached by the method of stabilized images. *Canadian Journal of Psychology, 14,* 67–77.

Sander, F. & Volkelt, H. (1962) *Ganzheitspsychologie.* Munich: Beck.

Sandler, J. & Joffe, W. (1965) Notes on obsessional manifestations in children. *Psychoanalytic Study of the Child, 20,* 425–438.

Sandler, J. & Joffe, W. (1969) Towards a basic psychoanalytic model. *International Journal of Psychoanalysis, 50,* 79–91.

Sandler, J. & Rosenblatt, B. (1962) The concept of the representational world. *Psychoanalytic Study of the Child, 17,* 128–145.

Schilder, P. (1951) On the development of thoughts. In D. Rapaport (Ed.), *Organization and pathology of thought,* (pp. 497–518). New York: Columbia University Press.

Schilder, P. (1953) *Medical psychology.* Madison, CT: International Universities Press.

Smith, G.J.W. & Danielsson, A. (1982) Anxiety and defensive strategies in childhood and early adolescence. *Psychological Issues,* Monogr. 52. (Madison, CT: International Universities Press.

Smith, G.J.W., Johnson, G., & Almgren, P. (1989) *MCT—The Meta-Contrast Technique. Manual.* Stockholm: Psykologiförlaget.

Smith, G.J.W., Nyman, G.E., & Hentschel, U. (1986) *CWT-serialt färgordtest.* [*CWT- Serial Color-Word Test*]. Stockholm: Psykologiförlaget.

Tulving, E. (1972) Episodic and semantic memory. In E. Tulving & W. Donaldson (Eds.), *Organization of memory* (pp. 378–403). New York: Academic Press.

Wallerstein, R.S. (1985) Defenses, defense mechanisms, and the structure of the mind. In H.P. Blum (Ed.), *Defense and resistance: Historical perspectives and current concepts* (pp. 201–225). Madison, CT: International Universities Press.

Werner, H. (1956) Microgenesis and aphasia. *Journal of Abnormal and Social Psychology, 52,* 347–353.

Werner, H. & Kaplan, B. (1956) The developmental approach to cognition: Its relevance to the psychological interpretation of anthropological and ethnolinguistic data. *American Anthropologist, 58,* 866–880.

Westerlundh, B. & Johnson, C. (1989) DMT defenses and the experience of dreaming in children 12 to 13 years old. *Psychological Research Bulletin, Lund University, 29,* 6.

Westerlundh, B. & Sjöbäck, H. (1986) Activation of intrapsychic conflict and defense: The amauroscopic technique. In U. Hentschel, G.J.W. Smith, & J. Draguns (Eds.), *The roots of perception* (pp. 161–215). Amsterdam: North-Holland.

Westerlundh, B. & Smith, G.J.W. (1983) Perceptgenesis and the psychodynamics of perception. *Psychoanalysis and Contemporary Thought, 6,* 597–640.

Westerlundh, B. & Terjestam, Y. (1990) Memory activation and perceptual processing: On the idea of microgeny/ontogeny correspondence. *Psychological Research Bulletin, Lund University, 30,* 6.

Part II
Methodological Considerations

5
The Measurement of Defense Mechanisms by Self-Report Questionnaires

Uwe Hentschel, Wolfram Ehlers, and Rainer Peter

The Historical Roots of Defense Mechanisms: A Concept Formulated Without Any Intent of Its Quantification or Experimental Testing

In 1893 a new construct was introduced in psychology: repression. As far as psychology was concerned, the term "construct" still resided in the collective preconscious. Freud did not call it so but he described the phenomenon and how he thought this mechanism would work. "The basis for repression itself can only be a feeling of unpleasure, the incompatibility between the single idea that is to be repressed and the dominant mass of ideas constituting the ego. The repressed idea takes its revenge however by becoming pathogenic." (Freud, 1893, p. 116) In his report on the case of Miss Lucie R., Freud further postulated that it is primal repression that exerts some suction on all other ideas or affects later to be repressed: "When this process occurs for the first time there comes into being a nucleus and center of crystallization for the formation of a psychical group divorced from the ego—a group around which everything which would imply an acceptance of the incompatible idea subsequently collects." (1893, p. 123)

With the introduction of this new mechanism, the idea of defenses was born. In a paper about psychology for neurologists, Freud (1954) conceptualized also a hypothetical neuronal network for a generalized model of defense. In this first phase of the Freudian construction of the ego apparatus, the concept of repression and later the concept of defense in general for the modification of traumatic ideas (Freud, 1894, 1896) were described, with the potentially pathological mechanism of defense separating the unbearable idea from its affect. The same affect, however, which has not completely lost its strength, can become the unconscious source of energy in the formation of neurotic symptoms. Examples for early unbearable ideas are the incestuous impulses of the child directed at the parent of the opposite sex. The next steps in the sequence could be that the superego, evolving through the identification with parental authority, stimulates repression, with the possible result of an infantile amnesia of these impulses. This process is already part of repression proper, whereas primal repression was regarded by Freud as having an organic basis also (cf. the definitions and evaluation of the different defense mechanisms by Paul Kline in Chapter 1).

Besides the often pathogenic consequences, there are also examples of positive effects of defenses like the following almost monological discourse of a child (age 3.9) who dreamed of a ghost ready to swallow her: "There are no ghosts, no, really not" (denial of a subjectively believed fact). "When the ghost comes back my daddy will chase him away" (introjection). "Ghosts really like people, don't they?" (reaction formation). The defenses in this discourse obviously represent a nonpathologic cognitive effort to find reassuring support against the threatening dream images. This is a positive example of how the ego functions can counterbalance anxiety by means of defensive activity (Sandler, 1960) without regressive tendencies. In neurosis, instead, a regression of libido takes place simultaneously, leading to a reappearance of the repressed which, as a consequence, also can reactivate traumatic affects (Freud, 1911). All conflicts and defense mechanisms that can be reconstructed in clinical cases by means of psychoanalysis are elements of repression proper, and only this part of the defensive process can be a subject of clinical research.

The description and observation of defense mechanisms in psychoanalysis had from the beginning clear empirical perspectives. Defense was conceptualized as a behavior observation construct including the subjects' verbalizations but with no attempt at "measuring" them. Had there been an exchange of ideas between academic psychology and psychoanalysis, the chances for the concept of defense to be introduced to experimental psychology and psychological testing would not have been so poor. In academic psychology there was a keen interest in individual differences combined with an experimental approach introduced by Sir Francis Galton (1883). The first psychological laboratory was founded by Wilhelm Wundt in 1879, and the first testing laboratory and the term "mental test" were introduced by James McKeen Cattell in 1888, some years before Freud defined his basically empirical concept of defense. The history of psychology took another course, however, and the streams of these ideas did not merge until decades later. In their attempt to build the new psychology, Freud and his adherents stuck to their experience with neurotic patients. In this way the theory and application of psychoanalysis remained mainly in the clinical setting. The sprout of defense was developing in this atmosphere and gradually, with new layers, becoming part of a larger family. Contributions came from a range of different psychoanalytic theorists (cf. also other contributions in this book), which brought in interesting theoretical side issues regarding the breadth of definitions and dynamical roots of the term. The great disadvantage of giving too much space to interesting speculation, however, is evident in the often optional features of definitions and the looseness in terminology still characteristic of the field.

The far from optimal state of affairs is that we are confronted with different lists of defense mechanisms of various lengths ranging from 1 to 39 (Bibring, Dwyer, Huntington, & Valenstein, 1961), or 44 as postulated by Suppes and Warren (1975) (cf. also Chapters 7 and 11). There is of course no test available for the measurement of these defenses in this variety. Experimental psychologists were, often in a restricted way, focusing on the possible operationalizations of variables of all kinds, and their attempts to consider psychoanalytical concepts as well were not enthusiastically welcomed by psychoanalysis at first. There is the famous example of Rosenzweig's correspondence with Freud (cf. MacKinnon & Dukes, 1962), but also later there were many of new attempts to introduce the idea of empirical testing into the research on defenses. Eriksen (1950), for instance, designed an experimental analogy of repression that served as a model for a long series of experiments to test the psychoanalytic hypothesis of repression. Not only conservative psychoanalysts but also critical experimentally oriented psychologists like Klein (1970) have argued that experimentally induced anxiety is too trivial and artificial to form a relevant stimulus for repression in the psychoanalytic sense of the term. What seems necessary instead are designs that also make use of repressions that have already taken place as a result of the "natural" past experience of the subjects. The clash between psychodynamic concepts and traditional experimental methods could eventually be avoided with a more natural approach. It is in this light that we will also try to discuss the possibilities for the measurement of defense by means of self-report questionnaires.

The Full Scope of the Defensive Process and Different Methods for Its Registration

Freud arrived inductively at his concept of the unconscious through conclusions from observations of his patients. He used this concept as a common denominator for very different phenomena like forgetting of familiar names, slips of the tongue, dreams, and hysterical symptoms. The formation and use of this concept of the unconscious was a very important step in his theory building (Stagner, 1988), leading to a complex model of the mind. The general aim of the model was to describe behavior in terms of dispositions (e.g., fixation to a certain stage in the sexual development), situative aspects (e.g., fatigue), instigative causes (e.g., frustration), and the basic, essential causes (e.g., unconscious conflicts). It allowed also for the distinction of mental and material, reality-related causes in mental phenomena (e.g., the manifest contents of a dream) based on a recent perception as contrasted to its motivating force. Psychoanalysis thus clearly postulated a multiple causation for all observable behavior (Rapaport, 1960). With this perspective in mind, the criticism about a too simple, rigorous, and straightforward operationalization of predictor and criterion variables seems to be better understandable, and a necessary conclusion would be that to do justice to the complex theoretical model, a complex research design and/or complex model for the interpretation of empirical results is needed as well. The features that characterize most of the classical defense mechanisms are, of course, closely related to the psychoanalytic way of model building. Defense mechanisms are basically unconscious phenomena: they can be seen on the one hand as embedded in a situation-related process, which on the other hand also has clearly stable structural or dispositional components. Seen purely within the realm of psychoanalytic theory, the following points seem to make an experimental or quasi-experimental approach preferable: the fact that defense mechanisms are basically unconscious; their causal relatedness to epigenetic stages and psychic complexes; their process character and their actual relatedness to other psychic processes; and at least for the mechanisms at the lower end of a hierarchical conception (Vaillant, 1971), the fact that their observability is based on deviations from normal behavior, with the potential implication of image distorting consequences and an obstruction of adequate reactions.

At this point we want to stress how important the "milieu interne" is for an objective perception of the world and how eventual distortions of this objective perception can be conceptualized by referring to variables from the inner milieu. To do this, we will use the act of touching, which has been studied extensively by different gestaltkreis theorists (e.g., von Auersperg, 1947; von Weizsäcker, 1947) and to which von Auersperg (e.g., 1963a) has repeatedly referred. Perception and the represented reality join in what von Auersperg called "coincidental correspondence." With the first touching movement the actor usually has an idea of the whole (hypothesis-theory). The perceptual action develops in different phases involving preconscious processes (microgenesis); the whole sequence gets approved through its conscious labeling (retrograde determination). This process can be severely distorted when the temperature of the touching hand becomes lower. As gestalt psychology has shown, the material of the touched object (e.g., glass, porcelain, metal) is diagnosable through the heat conductivity of the object. When the temperature of the hand becomes lower, its discriminative ability diminishes. The conscious representation is the sensation of coldness with a loss of the neutral affect related to the object (von Auersperg, 1963b). Subject and object are clearly interrelated in this example. We have chosen the touching act because the hampering consequences are easier to demonstrate here, but in principle, the dependence of an objective perception on the milieu interne holds true for all sensory modalities.

According to percept-genetic theory, image distorting phenomena in the visual perception process can be regarded as representing defense mechanisms, mostly pathogenic, exerting some kind of filter function comparable to the cooler hand in the example of the touching act. Whereas percept-genetic theory is very process oriented (Draguns, 1984; Hentschel, 1984; Smith, 1984), the clinical observation is more directed to the pathogenic complex-related phenomenon. Vaillant's case of a hematologist is a remarkable example of how, for example, displacement and intellectualization can exert a filter effect on someone's behavior and experience: "His professional responsibilities were exclusively clinical but recently he had made a hobby of studying cell-cultures. In a recent interview he described with special interest and animation an interesting lymphocyte culture that he was growing from a biopsy from his mother. Only very late in the interview did he suddenly reveal that his mother had died from a stroke only three weeks previously. His description of her death was bland and without noticeable concern." (Vaillant, 1971, p. 113) In this vignette the effect of defense is very clear; the underlying process, however, is not explained. The process aspect of defenses will be discussed more extensively in the method chapter on percept-genetic techniques (Chapter 7).

None of the methods available for the registration of defenses can cover all the hitherto mentioned aspects. The different methods have specific advantages and weaknesses.

Basically there are four main empirical approaches for the registration of defense mechanisms:

1. The clinical method on the basis of behavior observation as introduced by Sigmund Freud and later elaborated by Anna Freud (1937). This method can still be a valuable and valid approach when applied properly with controls for reliability, as Vaillant (1974) has been able to show. In this volume the method is represented by the elaborate assessment technique of the Defense Mechanism Rating Scale (DMRS) by Christopher Perry (Chapter 8) and the Clinical Assessment of Defense Mechanisms (CADM) by Wolfram Ehlers (Chapter 17; cf. also Chapters 24 and 28).

2. Through the application of projective techniques by looking for special defense-related signs, which then can be combined to scales. (Falk Leichsenring covers this topic in Chapter 6 on the basis of inkblot techniques. Cramer (1991) has developed a special manual for registering defense by means of the TAT, and in Chapter 21 Phebe Cramer and Sydney Blatt give an example for a TAT application.)

3. By categorizing the answers and drawings of the subjects in percept-genetic techniques, which are represented in this volume by Chapters 9, 10, 14, 15, 20, 22, 26, and 27 and explained in more detail in the

methodological chapter by Smith and Hentschel (Chapter 7). A theoretical justification of the percept-genetic approach and its demarcation from other points of view is also given in Chapter 4. (There are other experimental approaches as well, some of them relying heavily on psychophysiological measures, like the augmenter–reducer typology as described in Chapter 13).

4. By the questionnaire approach, with which the present chapter is concerned, which probably can be seen as the most controversial of the four methods mentioned.

It might be added here that the content analysis of standardized verbal speech samples should be regarded as another independent approach for the registration of defenses. It has in a certain way links to the clinical and self-report approach, and we will describe it briefly in this chapter too.

The whole idea that it should be possible to represent the unconscious defensive process by means of questionnaires seems futile. In the vast majority of cases the actor without, for example, the help of a psychotherapist is not able to include the hypothetical transformations of unconscious or preconscious processes in his self-reflections. To elicit from subjects reliable statements like "I am often displacing" or "I am a repressor" therefore is inconceivable. That is one of the reasons for the opinion of many theorists that the registration of defense mechanisms through questionnaires is by definition impossible (cf. the critical remarks by Paul Kline in Chapter 1 and Bert Westerlundh in Chapter 4). Even if we might in principle agree with that assumption, this chapter's concern with the registration of defenses by questionnaires shows that we think that the method has some possibilities. In the proper sense of the meaning, it is true that questionnaires cannot be specifically complex-directed, nor can they register any aspects of the different stages that von Auersperg so vividly underlined in his theoretical descriptions of the microgenetic process. They are necessarily restricted either to cognitively represented behavior repertoires in respect to, for example, aggression, connected with defenses or other phenomena related to them, or pointing to the hypothesized relation between defenses and symptoms and/or personality traits. In both cases one is very likely to end up with a measurement of dispositions which at best can be regarded as a shadow of the dynamic concept of defenses. On the other hand, however, as already mentioned, defense mechanisms have beyond their situation-specific, process-oriented range of convenience, a more general structural aspect that can be of interest in its own right: isolation, for example, can also be seen as the habitual basic tendency to exclude one's affects. Freud (1936) pointed to the parallel of isolation and logical thinking. In regard to the measurement of dispositions of this kind, which also have implications for an objective reality perception, the application of questionnaires seems to us a viable approach.

To use once again the filter metaphor of defense mechanisms, it is conceivable that defense scores in self-report questionnaires represent rather linguistic filters, whereas the percept-genetic registration of defense mechanisms (cf. Chapter 7) could reflect the activation of perceptual filters. The perceptual mediation theory, as adopted by among others Bower (1970, p. 502), Shepard (1978), and Cooper (1975), takes as a point of departure the sensual input and its storage by a specific mode of perception. Bucci (1985) has elaborated on this idea to a model of dual coding for mental representations. Nonverbal and verbal information is stored in different specialized systems. Linguistic coding is evoked by verbal information, which is stored in abstract phonological or semantic units. Perceptual coding takes care of the information from the sensual channels. Feelings are also closely related to this system. Ehlers and his colleagues (Ehlers, Gitzinger, & Peter, 1988; Gitzinger, 1990) have developed a taxonomy of linguistic and perceptual coding of defense mechanisms. They postulated that mental representations of conflicts may take place within the linguistic coding system as well as within the perceptual system. Results of empirical studies showed that differences exist with respect to the subjects' preference for one of these coding systems in relation to defense as well. Different patterns of personality structure are involved in perceptual and linguistic coding of defense mechanisms.

Questionnaires and the Theory of Psychometric Measurement

The registration of intelligence is probably the most prominent field of applied measurement in psychology, but test construction theory is also very well represented by the attempt to register personality traits by means of questionnaires. The first one was Woodworth's Personal Data Sheet for screening American army recruits for maladjustment. This instrument was followed by a long string of questionnaires for very different purposes and closely related to the evolving theory of test construction based on statistical concepts. The central themes in this approach are reliability and validity, which themselves are subjected to quantitative assessment. The advantage is that you can give estimates independent from the conception of different observers as to how stable, consistent, exact, and similar a test score is to comparable scales and how useful it is in differentiating different groups (concurrent validity) and in predicting a certain behavior or performance (predictive validity). There are a number of additional criteria for the evaluation of tests, but we restrict ourselves to the basic terms to show the difference between a rather uncontrolled observational approach and a measurement approach for the registration of defense mechanisms and their applications. That it is possible to calculate an estimated error of your measurement (standard error of measurement) in the one approach in contrast to a subjective statement like "I think that this is true" can also underline our argument. Questionnaires are not completely unproblematic even within the realm of socially desirable behavior, due to some basic assumptions (cf. Wiggins, 1973) that are not always easy to check directly.

1. The assumption of the same or a similar meaning of the items for all subjects.
2. The assumption that people can describe themselves accurately.
3. The assumption that honest answers are given by the subjects on all test items.

Reliability and validity estimates however provide hints for indirect checking. As far as reliability is concerned, in spite of a great variation, a reasonable estimate of an average could be around .75 for questionnaire scales. It is impossible to give an estimation for an average figure for validity. There are too many ways of approaching the estimation of validity and, last but not least, there is the problem deciding to which criteria personality variables should be compared. It is a questionable assumption to view dispositions as the only determinants of actual behavior (Mischel, 1968). Situative aspects should also be taken into consideration (Magnusson & Endler, 1977), but traditional trait theorists have never claimed that a certain trait has the same impact under all conditions (Eysenck & Eysenck, 1980; Herrmann, 1980). Stagner (1977) has defined traits as generalized ways of perceiving a class of situations, which guide behavior in these situations. A dominant person can see, for example, a committee meeting as an opportunity to take over, whereas a submissive person may see it as a chance to let others make the decisions. A family discussion would not necessarily belong to the same class of situations. As, for example, Epstein (1977) and Wittmann and Schmidt (1983) have suggested, prediction can be improved by using averages of repeated measurements and paying more attention to the reliability of the criterion, covering a broader spectrum of situations also for behavior in the sense of multiple act criteria (Fishbein & Ajzen, 1974). It is self-evident that the criteria should be of some relevance with regard to the personality variables used as predictors (Monson, Hesley, & Chernick, 1982).

Summing up the debate on dispositions versus the impact of situations and the prediction of behavior, it seems as if almost all researchers have realized that dispositions alone are not enough. How to adequately include situative aspects is a problem of its own. Some strategies have already been mentioned, another well-known approach is the functionalistic one in the tradition of Brunswik (1955), which is also favored by many researchers in percept-genesis (cf. Hentschel & Schneider, 1986; Hentschel & Smith, 1980). Before dispositions can be combined with situative aspects, they themselves must be conceptualized, and an important tradition within the psychometric approach is to base this combination on the results of factor analysis. It was Cattell's (1945) aim to use a representative list of adjectives for personality description and then define the underlying dimensions of these words. Guilford and Guilford (1934) in a similar attempt have scrutinized all available items for extraversion/introversion in regard to their factor loadings. The continued search by way of multivariate methods for an "adequate taxonomy" of personality descriptive terms in their culturally shared meaning, comparable to the periodic table in chemistry, has led to a robust solution by the postulation of five basic factors (Digman, 1989; Goldberg, 1981) for which special tests are available (Costa & McCrae, 1989). They are replicable in other languages (Angleitner et al., 1990; De Raad, 1992) and also show some closer connections to the circumplex models worked out by the adherents of an interpersonal system in personality diagnosis (Wiggins, 1982; cf. also Chapter 18 by Conte & Plutchik). If it is true that the "big five" (neuroticism, extraversion, openness, agreeableness, and conscientiousness) cover a representative field of the culturally shared terms for personality description, an inevitable consequence is their hypothetical relationship to defense mechanisms as represented in self-report questionnaires, that is, the correlates of the actual process-oriented, complex-related psychodynamic constructs. We have no results for a direct test of this hypothesis, but we are able to provide an indirect argument, to which we will return later.

On the Theoretical Background for the Construction of Different Self-Report Questionnaires for Measuring Defense

The Projective Approach

The DMI

It is probably the projective approach within the test psychology movement that almost from the beginning had the closest contact with psychodynamic ideas. In this tradition, different defense mechanisms were operationalized in inkblot techniques (cf. Chapter 6), in the TAT (cf. Chapter 21), in the Color Pyramid Test (cf. Chapter 15), and in different drawing tests. In 1945 Rosenzweig introduced his Picture Frustration Test and subsequently discussed his scoring categories in terms of defense, but he refrained from defining the scales as such. Rosenzweig's way of presenting frustrating situations and asking the subjects for their subjective reactions is suitable for presentation in the form of a questionnaire. Gleser and Ihilevich (1969) were the first with this creative step and in the Defense Mechanism Inventory (DMI) confronted the subjects with little stories instead of pictures. They improved the technique even more by asking for answers on preformulated multiple-choice items, thus avoiding all further problems with interrater reliability. They adhered to the dynamic concept of defense with the basic idea that defense is activated only in the presence of a motivational conflict between, for example, the perception of an individual and his or her internalized values. Possible conflict solving in terms of defenses can take place in the form of a process in which the ego attacks, distorts, or becomes selectively unaware of certain aspects of the internal or external world. By grouping a number of defenses with a certain limitation in specificity, five clusters of defenses were conceptualized, being hypo- thetically evoked by conflicts centered around authority, independence, sex, competition, and specific situations. The final version of the DMI consists of 10 stories, each involving one of the above-mentioned frustrating conflicts. The subjects are confronted with preformulated reaction possibilities and are asked for their imagined reactions in such a situation, their actual behavior, impulsive fantasy, thoughts, and feelings.

The five clusters of defense to be discerned in the answers of the subjects, were called Turning Against Object (TAO), Projection (PRO), Principalization (PRN), Turning Against Self (TAS), and Reversal (REV). They can be summed up over the four levels or regarded separately on each level (e.g., TAO in impulsive fantasy). There is an impressive body of research with the DMI in the United States, and it is therefore not astonishing that it attracted the interest of researchers in other countries also. In Germany Hoffmann and Martius (1987) did research with the DMI with their own translation and in spite of interesting results criticized a number of points in the test construction: an overly differentiated set of instructions, problems with the scoring, an unequal distribution of emotional topics, and the classification of the defenses. Hentschel and Hickel (1977) did a pilot study with the DMI at roughly the same time, also with their own translation. The resulting test criteria and factor analyses were rather unsatisfactory, leading to the decision to develop a new test based on the same idea of presenting stories with a conflict and multiple-choice answers. Ehlers and Peter (1989), directing their attention to a theoretical foundation of test construction better than the DMI, have also presented a new German version of a defense questionnaire, the SEDCI (see below).

The Descendants of the DMI

The FKBS

In a pilot study with their own translation of the DMI, Hentschel and Hickel (1977) encountered the problem of subjects, above all those with a low level of education, who could not discern the four levels of reactions. The difference between thinking and fantasy in particular was often difficult for these subjects. As mentioned earlier, there were also problems with the resulting factor structure, which was neither congruent with the proposed clusters of defense nor representative of the majority of the items within the dimension to which they should hypothetically belong. It was assumed that the diversity of the items was too great and that the kind of scoring used, resembling a two-polar ipsative scaling, could have been a reason for this unsatisfactory factor solution. This resulted in a new instrument called Fragebogen zu Kon-fliktbewältigungsstrategien (FKBS [Questionnaire for conflict-solving strategies]: Hentschel, Kießling, & Wiemers, in press) with the following changes: most of the stories were rewritten, with the explicit aim of keeping the reported events close to daily experiences; only two levels of reactions were represented (viz., actual behavior and feeling), with a quantitative scoring asking for an estimation of certainty for each preformulated answer (sure, maybe, probably not, not at all). Whereas Gleser and Ihilevich (1969) tried to have a number of different defense mechanisms represented in all five clusters (e.g., REV: negation, denial, reaction formation, undoing, repression, reversal), for the FKBS all items were formulated as closely as possible according to the scale label. The main scales were kept congruent with those of the DMI (see Table 5.1). The reliability estimates for the five scales are given in Table 5.2. The FKBS is available in German, Dutch, English, Italian, and Georgian. Its validation has mainly been undertaken for the German and Dutch versions.

Attempts at Validation of the FKBS

The basic dimensions could be fairly well replicated by factor analysis (cf. Table 5.1) with a factor solution that explains 28.9% of the total variance. There is a clear separation of TAO, TAS, and PRO. PRN and REV, which also on the level of raw scores show a rather high intercorrelation (.71), collapse into one factor. Experts (psychologists and senior psychology students) had no difficulty in sorting the items correctly into the respective dimensions. The two levels (actual behavior and feeling) are highly correlated with each other. It was shown, however, in different experiments that feeling is the better predictor. Moreover, in some Dutch samples the discrepancy between the two levels was considerable. This was the reason for maintaining the option to have three scores (behavior, feeling, and an overall score), although the overall score seems to be sufficient for most purposes. This volume offers two chapters with empirical research on the FKBS (Chapters 16 and 25). Other evidence for its validity comes from clinical and experimental studies. Egle et al. (1989) have studied primary fibroneuralgia in comparison to a group with psychogenic pain and a control group. They started with Cremerius' characterization of primary fibroneuralgia patients as showing anal-retentional fixation with development of a "malicious humility": the

TABLE 5.1. The FKBS scales.

Theoretical concept			Identification by factor analysis[a]		
Scale		Content	No. of items from this scale	Have loadings	On factor[b]
TAO	Turning against object	Substitutive reactions of aggression against an external object	19 (95%)	5 > .30 5 > .45 7 > .60	1
TAS	Turning against self	Coping with the conflict is attempted by seeing oneself as the reason for the frustration, combined with guilt feelings	16 (80%)	7 > .30 4 > .45 5 > .60	2
REV	Reversal	Positive or neutral intentions are attributed to the person seen as the source of frustration	18 (90%)	7 > .30 10 > .45 1 > .60	3
PRN	Principalization/ intellectualization	Splitting off affects by intellectualization and rationalization	18 (90%)	7 > .30 9 > .45 2 > .60	3
PRO	Projection	Negative intentions or characteristics are attributed to the person seen as the source of frustration	13 (65%)	7 > .30 6 > .45	4

[a] Total variance explained 28.9%
[b] Explained common variance by factors: 1 (46%), 2 (27%), 3 (16%), 4 (11%).

submissive (depressive) behavior often shown by these patients is interpreted as implying a deep distrust of persons in their surroundings and as an outlet for their aggressive tensions. A hypochondriacal concentration on the body evoked by the pain serves as a substitute for real relationships with other people, from which they exclude themselves because of their lack of trust. The primary fibroneuralgia patients had much higher TAO, TAS, and PRO and lower REV and PRN scores than the control group. There were no significant differences between primary fibroneuralgia and

TABLE 5.2. Reliability estimates and discriminant values of the FKBS scales ($N = 273$).

	TAO	PRO	PRN	TAS	REV
Cronbach's alpha	.90	.79	.85	.85	.83
Mean r_{it} corrected	.53	.36	.44	.40	.41

psychogenic pain patients. In a study comparing insomniacs with controls (Herrmann-Maurer et al., 1992) the former showed less TAO and PRO. Differences between hypertensive patients and a control group are presented in Chapter 25.

Liedtke, Künsebeck, and Lempa (1990) used the FKBS to check the effects of an 8-week stationary psychotherapy with 54 psychosomatic and neurotic patients. They found significant evidence for a reduction of TAS and PRN and an increase of TAO. Their conclusion was that the form of psychotherapy applied had brought about a change in the preferred conflict-solving strategies of their patients in the desired direction and that the questionnaire to a great extent reflected the subjective experience with this therapy. A follow-up study one year later by the same authors (Liedtke, Künsebeck, & Lempa, 1991) with a sample comprising 50 of the original 54 patients showed that PRO and TAS were lower than directly after the therapy. PRN, REV, and TAO were at about the same level as at the time of intake, which means that TAO had gone down and PRN up, compared to the measurement at the end of the therapy. From the follow-up, the authors concluded that some important therapy effects, together with a reduction of symptoms, are still recognizable after one year. Other changes are regarded as less desirable: this concerns mainly the renewed increase of PRN.

The FKBS has also been applied in a number of experimental studies. On the basis of four FKBS scales (TAS, PRN, REV, and PRO), a neuroticism score, based on the difference in descriptions of self and ideal-self in a semantic differential (Hentschel & Klintman, 1974) and an achievement motivation score, derived from the Performance Motivation Test (Hermans, 1976) de Leeuwe, Hentschel, Tavenier, and Edelbroek (1992) classified a subsample of 30 subjects from a total sample of 83 computer operators into groups of non-stress-resistant (13) and stress-resistant (17). All subjects were confronted with a stressful two-channel task. Directly after this task, blood samples were taken to determine the subjects' levels of 3-methoxy-4-hydroxyphenylglycol (MHPG). The result supported the hypothesis of a significant difference in free MHPG between the stress-resistant and non-stress-resistant groups, with a higher MHPG level for the latter. Udenhout and Bekker (1990) used the FKBS for the prediction of learning in a coding and memory task. In the Coding Memory Test (de Zeeuw, 1980), the subject has to invent a system to order a series of letters and numbers in such a way that he or she knows the order by heart. Subjects are given 24 cards, each with a triple letter–number combination on it (e.g., ABA, Y2Z), which they have to order. Then the cards are turned around and the subjects are given a list with the same sign combinations in a random order; and are to choose the cards corresponding to the combination written on the list. Sixty subjects were given the task twice, and Udenhout and Bekker looked at the relation of learning (increase of correct responses from first to second trial) and defense. Subjects with high TAO scores (upper third of the distribution) compared to low TAO scores (lower third) showed more learning. Subjects with high REV scores (upper third) made more errors in general in the second trial and also more repetitive errors than subjects with low REV scores (lower third of the distribution).

The study on creativity performed by Hentschel and Schneider (1986) started with the assumptions that creativity is to a great extent unconscious and that susceptibility to subliminal stimulation should play a major role in the creative performance. Forty design students were given a number of supraliminal and subliminal slide presentations embedded in a series of control stimuli. The critical stimulus was a supraliminally shown neutral scene of two musicians, simultaneously presented with a subliminal slide with a changed meaning of the same scene—one musician performing an aggressive act on the other. Subjects had to describe what they had seen and fill in a semantic differential for the description of the atmosphere. Two scales were formed from the semantic differential "vicious aggression" and "dysphoria" to register possible deviations for the subliminal condition from the control condition. Creativity was estimated by means of the Creative Functioning Test (CFT) (Smith & Carlsson, 1990; Smith & Danielsson, 1980) using a tachistoscopically presented still life, first with increasing exposure times until recognition of the picture, and then again with decreasing exposure times. The main scores are the number of ideas that subjects produce during the ascending series and the ability to free themselves in the inverted percept-genesis from the objective meaning of the stimulus. Results showed that subjects with low TAO scores were less creative, irrespective of whether they were influenced by the subliminal stimulus. Subjects with high TAO scores were more creative (less adherence to the objective meaning of the stimulus in the inverted PG) only if they belonged to the subgroup that was not susceptible to the aggressive subliminal stimulus. Principalization exerted an influence on the "Richness of Ideas" (RI) variable in the ascending percept-genesis: subjects who either showed the combination of not being influenced by the subliminal stimulus in a dysphoric direction and low PRN scores or the combination of being subliminally influenced in this way and high PRN scores were more creative in terms of the RI score. A certain degree of aggression—maybe Vaillant's (1974) formulation of joyful expression of anger would fit here—without an oversensitive extraction of negative affective meaning seems to be positive for the creative performance. PRN can obviously counterbalance the oversensitive reaction to an aggressive subliminal stimulus in a dysphoric direction and in that combination still make a creative performance possible.

In a study on cognitive performance (Hentschel & Kießling, 1990) it was hypothesized that subjects with a different defense pattern would also show different correlates of psychophysiological measures during information processing. The 60 subjects taking part in that study were divided into groups with better and worse performance in a concept formation task (median splitting of the error score in the Symbol Maze Test [SMT], see Chapter 16). The subjects with the worst concept formation performance had higher TAS and PRN scores. In the Symbol Maze Test, decisions are required for choosing the right ways, leading to the center of the maze. For a right decision, indicated by the configuration of signs standing for the concept to be learned, no feedback is given. All errors are followed by a low tone. Since the exact times of the correct decisions were known for all subjects, the physiological reactions before and after the correct decisions could be compared, thus avoiding possible feedback-induced orientation reactions. Subjects with high TAS scores in comparison to subjects with low TAS scores (median split) showed lower skin conductance reactions after the correct decision than before and a tendency toward lower heart rate. Subjects with high PRN scores showed higher skin conductance reactions after making a correct decision in comparison to subjects with low PRN scores. In the concept formation experiment itself, no thinking aloud technique was used, but the results can be interpreted as if subjects with higher TAS scores had said to themselves "I can't manage this" and felt relief upon making no error at this point. Subjects with high PRN scores might have thought "This is too difficult" and might have been surprised that they succeeded with their choices. In the discussion of these results, the authors indicated a parallel to the field of psychosomatics, where clinicians often try to look for correlates of symptoms with defenses, whereas in this study defenses were the predictors and the psychophysiological reactions during information processing the dependent variables. A study on attention control that uses the FKBS scales in combination with the SMT error score as predictor variables is reported in Chapter 16.

The SEDCI

Theoretical Conception

The Self-Evaluation of Defense Concepts Inventory (SEDCI: in German, SBAK; Ehlers & Peter, 1989) is based on the psychoanalytic concept of reactivation of traumatic experiences. Freud (1926) distinguished between an individual traumatic situation and developmental risks, which can provoke traumatic situations. Both situations can result in defense provoked by states of helplessness, loss of love, castration anxiety, and the discrepancy between the pleasure principle and reality. The SEDCI operationalizes these theoretical postulates. In standardized conflict situations the stories are constructed to evoke originally traumatic situations and developmental risks by the reactivation of images. The resulting behavior alternatives, as expressed in the form of standardized items, can be interpreted as defense processes.

Test Construction

For the original construction of the SEDCI (Ehlers et al., 1988) 20 conflict situations with a total of 398 response alternatives were used. The item pool was reduced to 98 items after a first examination with 141 subjects, because many items were unclassifiable in separate dimensions by factor analysis. The new form of the inventory with 98 items was given to another sample of 560 patients recruited from the Therapeutic Clinic at Stuttgart-Sonnenberg. Again factor analysis and item analysis were performed. The present SEDCI version contains 17 stories with a total of 70 items scored on a five-point scale. For the 98-item version, a five- to six-factor solution seemed to be the most plausible, based on a Scree test. The psychoanalytic interpretation favored the five-factor solution. This solution explained 25.7% of the total variance. The scale construction was then further optimized using coefficients of consistency (Cronbach's alpha) and discriminant values (r_{it}). The means of these coefficients for the five scales are given in Table 5.3.

The Scales

Rationalization. This scale, which has good internal consistency, also explains the largest part of the total variance (cf. Table 5.3). It seems empirically and theoretically well founded. In this scale the defense mechanism of rationalization, which is defined as the justification of motivated behavior through reasonable explanations, is central. Other concepts included are the mechanisms of intellectualization, isolation and control of affect. The content of this scale thus consists of a defense pattern with a predominance of rationality directed against affective manifestations of behavior. A high score on this dimension means a marked superego-dominated attitude directed against affective impulses. The scale correlates with the following sociodemographic variables: age ($r = .14$) education ($r = -.24$), and sex ($r_{pbis} = -.10$). These correlations are very small but due to the size of the sample significant ($p = .001$).

Denial. This scale comprises answers in which the subject ignores or negates the conflictual context of motives. Defense mechanisms like

TABLE 5.3. The different SEDCI scales, their test criteria, and their variance explained by factor analysis.

	N (items)	Total variance	Cronbach's alpha	Difficulty value P_i	Index of discrimination r_{it}
Rationalization	15	11.22	.85	.41	.48
Denial	15	6.31	.77	.17	.37
Turning against object	15	3.26	.81	.53	.42
Regression	15	2.75	.73	.38	.34
Avoiding social contact	15	2.15	.77	.41	.43

reaction formation and displacement of aggression are also included. The reliability seems to be acceptable. The interpretation of the scale is more difficult because the test behavior of the subject shows not only denial in the proper sense of the term but also rejection of items, as can be inferred from the very high average index of item difficulty (cf. Table 5.3). This means that only a few subjects are willing to tackle the sexual connotation of the items in this scale. The correlation of this scale with sociodemographic variables are as follows: age ($r = .01$), education ($r = -.19$), and sex ($r_{pbis} = -.15$), from which the latter two are again small but significant ($p = .01$).

Turning Against Object. The dominating behavior pattern of this category is a spontaneous and direct expression of affect against a frustrating object without any reasonable justification or displacement of aggression on other objects. It represents to some degree the negative pole of rationalization and intellectualization. The reliability of this scale is good (cf. Table 5.3). The relation to the sociodemographic variables is similar to that of rationalization and denial.

Regression. Freud defined the defense mechanism of regression as the return to a fixation on a genetically earlier stage. In the SEDCI regression scale, only partial aspects of this classical definition are reflected. Primarily all receptive and passive resignative forms of coping with conflicts are covered here. Therefore relations to personality scales representing different aspects of depression can be expected, characterizing more passive and less action-oriented dispositions. There are no significant correlations with the sociodemographic variables. The internal consistency shows a moderate value (cf. Table 5.3).

Avoiding Social Contact. This scale is based on the defense against intimacy and heterosexual relations. Depending on the individual developmental fixation of impulses, the stories can stimulate aspects of impulse defense, phobic anxiety, and schizoid retreat. The correlation with the rationalization scale shows that this defense is based on the preference for rational behavior. The avoiding social contact scale is the most specific among all scales because women show significantly higher defense scores against the sexual connotations of the stories than men ($r_{pbis} = .25$; $p = .001$). The internal consistency of the scale is rather good (cf. Table 5.3).

Validation of the SEDCI Scales

Validation of the five scales was attempted by relating them to other questionnaires, clinical ratings of defense, differences between clinical groups, and therapy success. The results of these comparisons are given in Table 5.4. Of the two questionnaires given in Table 5.4, the Freiburger Persönlichkeitsinventar (FPI: Fahrenberg, Hampel, & Selg, 1984) is a conventional personality trait inventory. The PSACH (Psychoanalytic

TABLE 5.4. Validity estimates for the SEDCI.

	Correlations with personality questionnaires[a]			Comparisons between clinical groups[b]		Therapy outcome[c]			
SEDCI (N = 110)	FPI (N = 81)	PSACH (N = 77)	CADM (N = 105)	Healthy vs. neurotic subjects (N = 205 vs. N = 465)	Anorectic vs. bulimic subjects (N = 14 vs. N = 24)	Intake (I)	End of therapy (E)	Follow-up check 3 years' later (Fc)	Significant difference
Rationalization r = .36 avoiding social contact	r = −.34 aggressiveness	r = .34 control of feelings; r = −.33 anal impulsiveness	r = .34 denial; r = −.31 devaluation	p = 0.001	n.s.	M = 53.59 S = 15.48	M = 51.52 S = 15.48	M = 51.42 S = 13.12	
Denial				p = 0.001	n.s.	M = 17.51 S = 7.56	M = 17.14 S = 7.83	M = 17.73 S = 7.17	

70

				M = 33.28 S = 9.26	M = 33.01 S = 9.52	M = 35.08 S = 9.71	E-Fc and I-Fc
Turning against object		r = .42 need for prestige r = .39 sexual assertion r = .32 feeling of superiority			n.s.	n.s.	
Regression	r = −.23 composure r = .20 neuroticism	r = .22 basic distrust r = .24 fear of separation r = .22 control of feelings r = .22 need for prestige	r = .20 reaction formation	p = 0.05		n.s.	
Avoiding social contact	r = −.32 aggressiveness			n.s.	p = 0.05		

[a] Results from Ehlers and Peter (1989).
[b] Results from Ehlers and Peter (1989) and Peter (1993).
[c] Results from Schmidt (1991).

Character Typology: Meyer, Zenker, & Freitag, 1977) is a psycho-analytically inspired questionnaire also based on factor analysis for the final scale construction.

The rating scales of the Clinical Assessment of Defense Mechanisms (CADM) are described in more detail in Chapter 17. Like the DMSR (cf. Chapter 8), the CADM is a clinical rating system. The next two columns in Table 5.4 give results for the concurrent validity of the SEDCI for the comparison of neurotic patients versus control subjects and three types of eating disturbance. The last columns of Table 5.4 report results from therapy research with an earlier version of the SEDCI.

The SEDCI scales, with two exceptions, are independent of each other. Rationalization shows significant correlations with one FPI scale and two PSACH scales. The correlation with the clinical rating of denial could be taken as an indicator that rationalization also implies the tendency to deny affective motives. The negative correlation with devaluation could reflect the difference in maturity between the two defense mechanisms. Rationalization, however, shows a highly significant discrimination between healthy and neurotic subjects but no significant changes in the therapeutic process. The check for criterion validity for denial in relation to personality variables gave no significant correlations, and there were also no substantial correlations with the clinical ratings of defense mechanisms. The scale differentiates however between healthy and neurotic subjects. Turning against object shows correlations to three PSACH scales, indicating hysterical personality traits (viz., need for prestige, feeling of superiority, and sexual assertion). Furthermore, there is a significant tendency for a correlation with the aggressiveness scale of the FPI. It is assumed that this defense mechanism is more indicative of a healthy style of coping with conflicts so that it can be seen as a mature defense, although with no significant differences between healthy versus neurotic subjects.

Regarding psychotherapy outcome, Schmidt (1991) found a significant increase in turning against object for the comparisons of the follow-up check with the intake and the end of therapy. Regression shows a number of significant correlations with other variables at the 5% level of significance: fear of separation, control of feelings, and neuroticism and, in a negative direction, composure. There is a correlation for the clinical ratings with reaction formation. The correlations of the scale with the personality variables and the defense ratings demonstrate the validity of the regression scale because they indicate a general relation with variables reflecting an oral depressive character fixation (see Ehlers and Czogalik, 1984). In regard to concurrent validity, the difference between healthy and neurotic subjects is also significant at the 5% level. The results with respect to therapy outcome do not indicate any differences between the three points of time. Avoiding social contact shows a relation to a compulsive-depressive character disposition: self-pity, resignation, control of feelings, anal impulses, need for prestige, and aggressiveness. This pattern of variables is combined with signs of self-pity and resignation in the clinical ratings of defense mechanisms. The scale does not differentiate between healthy and neurotic subjects but between anorectic and bulimic patients. It was not used in the therapy outcome study.

The external validity can be evaluated as good for four of the scales (rationalization, turning against object, regression, and avoiding social contact). The denial scale needs further research. Rationalization, denial, and regression differentiate between neurotic patients and the control group. On the attempts to separate the two types of eating disorder, only the avoiding social contact scale showed a significant difference. As already mentioned, the therapy outcome study was done with an earlier version of the SEDCI, where in addition to the significances listed in Table 5.4, two other scales formerly used (reaction formation and turning against self) showed steadily decreasing values over time.

The Conventional Questionnaire Approach

Attempts at Constructing a One-Dimensional Scale

The Minnesota Multiphasic Personality Inventory (MMPI) can be regarded as a quarry for the construction of many new scales, so it is not surprising that it has also attracted the attention of psychologists interested in the concept of defense. We briefly describe below the most well known of these scales: Repression-Sensitization (RS), the construction problems of which are discussed in a separate chapter (cf. Chapter 12).

There are however other scales: for example, the manifest anxiety defensiveness scale by Milimet (1970), the admission and denial scales of Little and Fisher (1958), and the D-scale of Sarason, Ganzer, and Singer (1972). The interesting aspect for the measurement of defense is not so much that MMPI items are used here exclusively or partially but rather the application of straightforward self-description under the label of defense, as represented by the item "I sometimes feel that I'm about to go to pieces." The authors of the different questionnaires defend the use of their item forms with different arguments, but most of them see their scales as aimed at "derivates" or "correlates of defenses," not at defenses proper.

The research on perceptual defense by the Harvard studies (Bruner & Postman, 1947; Postman, Bruner, & McGuinness, 1948) had stimulated not only interest in finding out how this phenomenon could be explained but also the search for instruments for the prediction of a general behavior continuum, varying between extreme vigilance and an elevated threshold of reaction to threatening or emotional stimuli, corresponding to the defense mechanisms of intellectualization and repression, respectively. Projective techniques had been screened as well as behavior ratings, but the need for "an easily administered" method with good reliability and validity remained. This led to a number of attempts to construct new scales by means of MMPI items. Byrne's (1961) repression-sensitization scale aiming at such a general bipolar dimension of defensiveness was the first that had no overlap between items—in other versions, whole MMPI scales with overlapping items were subtracted from each other so that the same item could appear in the positive and negative ends. The first studies showed some convergent as well as discriminant validity. In 1964 Byrne presented the results of his extended research with the RS scale, at that time already in competition with 11 other scales of similar intention all derived from the MMPI. New issues arising from this line of research included the relations of the scale to defense ratings, selective forgetting, awareness of anxiety, and response to ambiguous stimuli, humor, and threat, as well as other measures of self-description, maladjustment, obstetric complications, child-rearing attitudes, and interpersonal behavior. It was Byrne's (1964) hope that psychological research including repression-sensitization would in the long run show more resemblance to physics than to psychoanalysis. Some time has passed since these programmatic statements, and Carl-Walter Kohlmann in Chapter 12 gives an overview of RS scale studies with special attention to the discrepancy between subjective and physiological stress reactions.

Multidimensional Approaches

Bond's Defense Style Questionnaire

Bond (1986a) started out with the construction of his defense style questionnaire with the similar idea that self-report methods for registering principally unconscious processes could be useful. He argued (Bond, 1986b) that under certain circumstances, defenses may become conscious and, more important, that even if someone is not aware of his or her defense, the behavior connected with it may be obvious to the people in the surroundings and eventually reflected back to the person. In this way, with statements such as "People tell me that I often take my anger out on someone other than the one at whom I am really angry," displacement could be registered even if a single act of displacement were unconscious. The specific assumption is that subjects can accurately comment on their characteristic style of dealing with conflicts: that is, give self-appraisals of the conscious derivates of defenses that are related to defenses (Bond, 1986a). Bond's questionnaire of defense style has 88 items and is constructed with the aim to measure 24 defenses. A factor analysis resulted in four factors, which Bond (1986b) interpreted against the background of a maturity dimension: 1, maladaptive action pattern (e.g., regression, acting out); 2, image distorting (omnipotence, splitting, primitive idealization); 3, self-sacrifying (reaction formation, pseudoaltruism); and 4, adaptive (suppression, sublimation, humor). This immaturity/maturity interpretation is supported by correlations in the respective direction with ego strength and ego development scales. A problem with this interpretation in terms of the construct validity of the scale is whether there is enough specific variance to interpret the four factors as qualitatively different phenomena and not just as four degrees of adaptation. Reister, Manz, Fellhauer, and Tress show that the German version of Bond's defensive style questionnaire with 88 items has a somewhat different structure, but they also present the results of a 35-item version (see Chapter 19).

The Life Style Index

Plutchik, Kellerman, and Conte (1979) have constructed their question-naire for the measurement of defense, the Life Style Index (LSI), on the basis of Plutchik's (1980) psychoevolutionary theory of emotions. According to that view, defenses are unconscious mechanisms to deal with conflicting emotions, which should be related to diagnostic categories also. The original 16 defenses in the LSI were later reduced in number of items and number of scales (8) so that they could be related to the 8 primary emotions of Plutchik's psychoevolutionary theory of emotions:

Trustful (denial)	Distrustful (projection)
Timid (repression)	Aggressive (displacement)
Discontrolled (regression)	Controlled (intellectualization)
Depressed (compensation)	Gregarious (reaction formation)

For the construction of the scale dimensions, ratings were made for different diagnoses in terms of defense, as well as for the appropriateness of the items. The maturity of the defenses and their direct and indirect similarity were also rated. A factor analysis was run to control the empirical overlap of the defenses. In Chapter 18 Conte and Plutchik present a more detailed report on the development of the LSI, as well as clinical studies on the prediction of readmission of schizophrenic patients, the outcome of long-term psychotherapy, the estimation of clinicians on which types of patient have a good prognosis in psychotherapy, and the risk of suicide and violence.

The Cognitive Orientation Questionnaire for
Defense Mechanisms and the Defense Mechanisms Questionnaire

In the theory of Cognitive Orientation (CO) by Kreitler and Kreitler (1976, 1982), defense mechanisms are conceptualized as cognitive strategies for the resolution of internal conflicts and are differentiated from the strategies for the resolution of purely cognitive inconsistencies and distress managing (coping) strategies. The internal conflicts are mainly localized to the stage of planning one's own action in response to a stimulus (What will I do?) and the beliefs connected with it. The defensive program resolves the conflict by producing a new behavioral intent: rationalization, denial, or projection. The questionnaire consists of four parts referring to norms (18 questions), general beliefs (11 questions), beliefs about self (12 questions), and goals (10 questions). It is a multiple-choice instrument with two or three response alternatives from which the subject is to check one. An example item is: "A person should try to guide his behavior according to logical rules which he can justify" (norms: rationalization). Kreitler and Kreitler also try to describe the role of the "cognitive programs" defined as defense mechanisms in the complete input–output chain of human information processing and behavior, that is, to localize the traces of defense in the meaning assignment process. In two of the studies reported in Chapter 11, the defense mechanisms questionnaire (Kreitler & Kreitler, 1972) was also used, in both cases comprising the dependent variable (i.e., as a criterion for the validation of the CO questionnaire of defense mechanisms). The defense mechanisms questionnaire consists of seven prototypical situations in which common moral standards are violated: for example, not returning the extra change given by mistake by a cashier at the grocery store. Each situation is followed by three items (rationalization, denial, projection) intended to represent possibilities of explaining to oneself or others this immoral behavior. The defense mechanism questionnaire clearly has elements of a projective test (see above) but is discussed here in the context of the general approach of Kreitler and Kreitler to measure defense mechanisms.

Content Analysis of (Standardized) Speech Samples

There is another approach for the registration of defenses that is not constrained by questions in the form of an inventory but allows the subjects to speak freely in interviews or in the context of a standardized task. Hilliard, Mauch, and Wittmann (1988) developed the Speech Characterization Coding System (SCCS), which can be used for the analysis of clinical interviews. The SCCS registers 11 speech variables which in empirical studies have shown a relation to defense mechanisms as measured by the FKBS. Since these results are based on small samples, further research is needed to ascertain the relation between the speech categories and defenses.

The system that allows for the inclusion of defenses in particular is the Gottschalk–Gleser method for measuring psychological states through the content analysis of verbal behavior (Gottschalk & Gleser, 1969). In the standard instruction, the subjects are asked to speak for 5 minutes about any interesting or dramatic personal life experience. The scales that have been constructed to categorize the recorded stories are described in greater detail in Chapter 23. A direct measure of defenses is applicable in those cases where the subject explicitly denies an affect or emotion ("I was not afraid.") or uses displacement by referring to others as being afraid. Furthermore, Gottschalk and Fronczek argue that some of the scales (hostility outward, hostility inward, and ambivalent hostility), which were actually not constructed for the measurement of defense, can under certain circumstances be regarded as defenses rather than as an expression of the respective emotion. Referring once again to the potential filter function of defenses, a result that relates scores on the hope scale to recovery of surgical patients (Gottschalk & Hooigaard-Martin, 1986) can also be seen within the context of defenses arranged on an immaturity–maturity dimension. Obviously the content analysis of speech is an independent approach and correlations with questionnaire scales on theoretical grounds (and supported by empirical results: Gottschalk & Gleser, 1969; van der Zee, 1992) cannot be expected to be very high.

Theoretical and Empirical Implications for Regarding Defense as a Complex Construct

Review of the correlations between the different variables in different techniques attempting to measure the same defenses gives a rather disappointing picture. Every psychologist knows of course that two variables with the same or a similar verbal label constructed on the basis of different operationalizations do not necessarily correlate with each other in a perfect manner; but by using the same verbal label, some sort of congruence is implicitly expected. We usually do not immediately realize that a characterization like "anxiety reactions" can be differentiated in physiological reactions of anxiety, anxiety in fantasy or dreams, and the subjective feeling of anxiety. Neither do we differentiate immediately the construct of repression as measured by a questionnaire and repression as measured, for example, by the DMT. To apply a complex model to the study of defenses could involve looking for the relationships of variables having a different label, relationships of variables with the same label at a higher level (second-order factors), and complex relationships of different sets of variables. The closest relationships can be expected of course between questionnaire scales. Unfortunately, there is to our knowledge no study in which the effort has been made to look systematically for the relationships between all or at least the most commonly used questionnaires.

Regarding some of the questionnaires included in this chapter, there is a study by Olff, Godaert, Brosschot, Weiss, and Ursin (1991) on the overall relationship between a Dutch five-story version of the DMI and a

Dutch translation of the LSI. In two samples (40 male undergraduate students and 110 male teachers), an overall score of the two inventories was used, representing some kind of "defensiveness," and the resulting correlations were $r = .52$ and $r = .55$. It is debatable whether an "overall score" of the kind used is the best way to test the relationship of the two inventories, but in any case the resulting 33% of common variance is not sufficient to permit us to speak of one and the same construct. Vickers and Hervig (1981) found a low convergent validity of the DMI to two other defense mechanisms questionnaires not discussed in this chapter, and Phebe Cramer (1988) in her overview of the DMI comes to the conclusion that REV is the only DMI scale that consistently shows the expected relationships with the criterion measures, most of them measures of other questionnaires including the results of the above-mentioned study by Vickers and Hervig.

The complex model argument includes the already mentioned possibility that defense should—at least in part—also be covered by the five scales regarded as representative for all culturally shared personality descriptions. According to a study by Borkenau and Ostendorf (1989), three of the big five factors (neuroticism, extraversion, and agreeableness) correspond to FPI scales. For the FKBS, in a study with 136 (77 females, 59 males) insomnia patients (Hermann-Maurer et al., 1992), significant correlations were found between extraversion (FPI: social orientation) and REV (.31), between neuroticism (FPI: irritability) and TAS (.22) and TAO (.33), and between agreeableness (FPI: aggressiveness) and TAO (.39); that is, the latter correlation due to the direction of the FPI scale is a negative one between agreeableness and TAO. The significant relationships of the SEDCI with the FPI scales are given in Table 5.4. The only relevant one indicates a positive relationship between agree-ableness and rationalization. On the whole, the overlap of the three of the big five with self-report defense scales seems to be weak to moderate (in one case), fullfilling the expectation that culturally shared personality dimensions cover some aspects of defense as measured by questionnaires, but defenses have obviously enough variance to give them the right to stand on their own.

Another interesting possibility in the comparison of self-report defense scales and personality questionnaires is the approach of Heilbrun and Schwartz (1979), who advocate taking defensive styles as moderator variables for the validity of personality scales. They could show that the validity of certain personality scales is partly determined by a certain defensive style. There is not much empirically based information available on the relation of questionnaire scales for the measurement of defense to projective techniques. A comparison of the DMI with the Blacky defense preference inquiry gave significant results for two of the DMI scales (cf. Massong, Dickson, Ritzler, & Layne, 1982). Since the direct relationship between projective inkblot test scores and questionnaire scales is not usually very high (cf. e.g., Walsh & Betz, 1990), even in multivariate comparisons (Rimoldi, Insua, & Erdmann, 1978), one cannot expect exceptional results for defense scales either. A better way to relate them might be to use the same target groups (e.g., carefully diagnosed neurotic patients) and then compare the contribution of the different techniques to the differentiation of the groups, a technique Hentschel and Balint (1974) have applied and summarized in the form of a "structurogram." The reader may refer to the SEDCI section concerning the empirical relationship of self-report defense scales with ratings of defense mechanisms.

Since in most contributions to this volume, defenses are registered by either percept-genetic methods or by questionnaires, the relationship of the variables across the two approaches seems to have special relevance. The correlations are very low on the level of single variables. In a sample of 92 normal subjects, there were no significant correlations between the FKBS scales and the DMT variables. Running an analysis with canonical correlations between the DMT and the FKBS gave no significant results either. With an earlier version of the SEDCI, 4 of 50 correlations with the DMT became significant in a sample of 70 neurotic or psychosomatic patients (Gitzinger, 1988), a result hardly better than what would be expected by chance.

The Implications of the Complex Model Interpretation of Defense for Further Research

As mentioned earlier, we think that the generally low correlations between single variables across different methods are a problem. A complex model interpretation offers a hypothetical conceptual solution. There is however no guarantee that it will suit common psychological thinking. Verbal labels of variables sometimes seem to be "imprinted" in our minds, and systems that try to avoid these labels usually pay a price for it. One might speculate, for example, whether the popular system of Cattell (1965) would not have become more popular if the author had not used his abstract index terms. Cattell's system with its oblique rotations, second-order factors, and complex equations for predicting actual behavior does show, however, that complex systems have a chance of acceptance if they are good. In reference to our topic it seems nevertheless easier to "think" in terms of simple variables than to try to remember by heart beta weights of multiple regressions and coefficients of the structure matrices of canonical factors. Since factor analyses over different methods might result primarily in method factors, factor analysis probably is not the optimal tool, but it can be used (e.g., in a confirmatory way) to check special hypotheses, and other multivariate methods can be used for screening the complex relations.

Further knowledge of an appropriate psychometric model for the relationship between different methods for the registration of defenses is in itself a very desirable goal. Unfortunately until now little support has been provided for a statistical relation of higher order between, for example, self-reported and percept-genetic defenses. There is, however, the possibility that the different approaches, in trying to understand how the other researcher's variables are constructed, will learn from each other in "interdisciplinary" research. The collaboration between neuroscience and the behavioral and computer sciences can be seen as a very sophisticated example. Neither behaviorism nor rule-based machine intelligence is able to explain brain functions, but neuroscientists should use both behavioral information in the concrete situation of the actor and knowledge of computer technology to analyze and reduce the immense amount of data. Applied to the topic of defense, this analogy could mean that, for example, psychoanalysts could learn from differential psychology and statistics how to better organize their observational data and, whenever deemed appropriate, to use it for the formation of hypotheses instead of retrospective explanations only, trying to avoid at the same time the danger of reductionism. The operationalization of the variables in experimental research—necessarily more formalized and reductionistic—should on the other hand also be based on clinical observations. The context of experience and unconscious motivation, very important aspects in psychodynamically oriented theorizing, should codetermine the empirical relevance and individual significance of the concepts used for variable construction.

A first step in the direction of replacing speculative discussions by "objective information" would be a sound and robust statistical model for a systematic mapping of the interactions among the different operationalizations, which till now often have unknown similarities. This could also enhance mutual learning and in the long run help the promising concept of defense to earn the place it deserves in academic psychology as well.

References

Angleitner, A., Ostendorf, F., & John, O.P. (1990) Towards a taxonomy of personality descriptors in German: A psycholexical study. *European Journal of Personality*, 4, 89–118.

Auersperg, A. von (1947) *Das Schema des getasteten Gegenstandes* [The schema of the touched object]. *Festschrift O. Pötzl* (pp. 82–97). Innsbruck: Wagner.

Auersperg, A. von (1963a) Großhirnpathologische Syndrome als Zeitigungsstörung der Aktualgenese [Brain pathological syndromes as disturbances in the timing during microgenesis]. In G. Schaltenbrand (Ed.), *Zeit in nervenärztlicher Sicht* [Time from a psychiatric perspective] (pp. 19–31). Stuttgart: Enke.

Auersperg, A. von (1963b) *Schmerz und Schmerzhaftigkeit* [Pain and painfulness]. Berlin: Springer.

Bibring, G.L., Dwyer, T.F., Huntington, D.S., & Valenstein, A.F. (1961) A study of the psychological processes in pregnancy and of the earliest mother–child relationship. *Psychoanalytic Study of the Child*, *16*, 62–72.

Bond, M. (1986a) Bond's defense style questionnaire (1984 version) In G.E. Vaillant (Ed.), *Empirical studies of ego mechanisms of defense* (pp. 146–152). Washington, DC: American Psychiatric Press.

Bond, M. (1986b) An empirical study of defense styles. In G.E. Vaillant (Ed.), *Empirical studies of ego mechanisms of defense* (pp. 2–29). Washington, DC: American Psychiatric Press.

Borkenau, P. & Ostendorff, F. (1989) Descriptive consistency and social desirability in self- and peer reports. *European Journal of Personality*, *3*, 31–45.

Bower, G.H. (1970) Analysis of a mnemonic device. *American Scientist*, *58*, 496–510.

Bruner, J.S. & Postman, L. (1947) Emotional selectivity in perception and reaction. *Journal of Personality*, *16*, 69–77.

Brunswik, E. (1955) Representative design and probabilistic theory in a functional psychology. *Psychological Review*, *62*, 193–217.

Bucci, W. (1985) Dual coding: A cognitive model for psychoanalytical research. *Journal of the American Psychoanalytical Association*, *33*, 571–607.

Byrne, D. (1961) The repression–sensitization scale: Rationality, reliability, and validity. *Journal of Personality*, *29*, 334–349.

Byrne, D. (1964) Repression–sensitization as a dimension of personality. In B.A. Maher (Ed.), *Progress in experimental personality research* (pp. 169–220). New York: Academic Press.

Cattell, R.B. (1945) The principal trait clusters for describing personality. *Psychological Bulletin*, *42*, 129–149.

Cattell, R.B. (1965) *The scientific analysis of personality*. Baltimore: Penguin.

Cooper, L.A. (1975) Mental rotation of random two-dimensional shapes. *Cognitive Psychology*, *7*, 20–43.

Costa, P.T., Jr. & McCrae, R.R. (1989) The NEO Personality Inventory (NEO-PI). In S.R. Briggs & J. Cheek (Eds.), *Personality measures*. Greenwich, CT: JAI Press.

Cramer, P. (1988) The defense mechanism inventory: A review of research and discussion of the scales. *Journal of Personality Assessment*, *52*, 152–164.

Cramer, P. (1991) *The development of defense mechanisms; Theory, research, and assessment*. New York: Springer.

Digman, J.M. (1989) Five robust trait dimensions: Development, stability, and utility. *Journal of Personality*, *57*, 195– 214.

Draguns, J.G. (1984) Microgenesis by any other name. In W.D. Fröhlich, G. Smith, J.G. Draguns, & U. Hentschel (Eds.), *Psychological processes in cognition and personality* (pp. 3–13). Washington, DC: Hemisphere.

Egle, E.T., Rudolf, M.-L., Hoffmann, S.O., König, K., Schöfer, M., Schwab, R. & Wilmowsky, H. von (1989) Persönlichkeitsmerkmale, Abwehrverhalten und Krankheitserleben bei Patienten mit primärer Fibromyalgie [Defenses and experience of illness with primary fibromyalgia patients]. *Zeitschrift für Rheumatologie*, *48*, 73–78.

Ehlers, W. & Czogalik, C. (1984) Dimensionen der klinischen Beurteilung von Abwehrmechanismen. [Dimensions of clinical ratings of defense mechanisms]. *Praxis der Psychotherapie und Psychosomatik*, *29*, 129–138.

Ehlers, W., Gitzinger, I., & Peter, R. (1988) *Experimental analysis of defense in a clinical setting.* Paper presented at the XXIV International Congress of Psychology, Sydney, Australia.

Ehlers, W. & Peter, R. (1989) *SBAK Testhandbuch* [SBAK Manual]. Ulm: PSZ-Verlag.

Epstein, S. (1977) Traits are alive and well. In D. Magnusson & N.S. Endler (Eds.), *Personality at the crossroads: Current issues in interactional psychology.* Hillsdale, NJ: Erlbaum.

Eriksen, C.W. (1950) *Perceptual defence as a function of unacceptable needs.* Unpublished doctoral dissertation. Stanford University, Stanford, CA.

Eysenck, M.W. & Eysenck, H.J. (1980) Mischel and the concept of personality. *British Journal of Psychology, 71,* 191– 204.

Fahrenberg, J., Hampel, R., & Selg, H. (1984) *Das Freiburger Persönlichkeitsinventar, Handbuch zum FPI-R [The Freiburg Personality Inventory,* Manual for the FPI-R]. Göttingen: Verlag für Psychologie.

Fishbein, M. & Ajzen, I. (1974) Attitude toward objects as predictors as single and multiple behavioral criteria. *Psychological Review, 81,* 59–74.

Freud, A. (1937) *The ego and the mechanisms of defense.* London: Hogarth Press.

Freud, S., with Breuer, J. (1893) On the psychical mechanisms of hysterical phenomena: Preliminary communication. In *The standard edition of the complete psychological works of Sigmund Freud: Vol. 2* (pp. 3–181). London: Hogarth Press.

Freud, S. (1894) The neuro-psychoses of defence. In *The standard edition of the complete psychological works of Sigmund Freud: Vol. 3* (pp. 45–61). London: Hogarth Press.

Freud, S. (1896) Further remarks on the neuro-psychoses of defence. In *The standard edition of the complete psychological works of Sigmund Freud: Vol. 3* (pp. 162–185). London: Hogarth Press.

Freud, S. (1911) Psychoanalytic notes on a autobiographical account of a case of paranoia (dementia paranoides). In *The standard edition of the complete psychological works of Sigmund Freud: Vol. 12* (pp. 9–79). London: Hogarth Press.

Freud, S. (1926) Inhibitions, symptoms and anxiety. In *The standard edition of the complete psychological works of Sigmund Freud: Vol. 20* (pp. 87–172). London: Hogarth Press.

Freud, S. (1936) *The problem of anxiety.* New York: Norton.

Freud, S. (1954) *The origins of psychoanalysis: Letters to Wilhelm Fließ, drafts and notes: 1887–1902,* M. Bonaparte, A. Freud, & E. Kris (Eds.). London: Imago.

Galton, F. (1883) *Inquiries into human faculty and its development.* London: Macmillan.

Gitzinger, I. (1988) *Operationalisierung von Abwehrmechanismen: Wahrnehmungsabwehr und Einstellungsmessung psychoanalytischer Abwehrkonzepte* [Operationalization of defense mechanisms: Perceptual defense and attitude measurement of psychoanalytical defense concepts]. University of Freiburg, unpublished thesis.

Gitzinger, I. (1990) Perceptual and linguistic coding of defense mechanisms in a clinical setting. *PPmP Diskjournal, 1.* no. 1, 197 [*Psychotherapie, Psychosomatik, Medizinische Psychologie, 40*].

Gleser, G.C. & Ihilevich, D. (1969) An objective instrument for measuring defense mechanisms. *Journal of Consulting and Clinical Psychology*, *33*, 51–60.

Goldberg, L.R. (1981) Language and individual differences: The search for universals in personality lexicons. In L. Wheeler (Ed.), *Review of Personality and Social Psychology: Vol. 2* (pp. 141–165). Beverly Hills, CA: Sage.

Gottschalk, L.A. & Gleser, G.C. (1969) *The measurement of psychological states through the content analysis of verbal behavior*. Berkeley, Los Angeles: University of California Press.

Gottschalk, L.A. & Hoigaard-Martin, J. (1986) The emotional impact of mastectomy. *Psychiatry Research*, *17*, 153–167.

Guilford, J.P. & Guilford, R.B. (1934) An analysis of the factors in a typical test of introversion–extraversion. *Journal of Abnormal and Social Psychology*, *28*, 377–399.

Heilbrun, A.B. & Schwartz, H.L. (1979) Defensive style and performance on objective personality measures. *Journal of Personality Assessment*, *43*, 517–525.

Hentschel, U. (1984) Microgenesis and process description. In W.D. Fröhlich, G. Smith, J.G. Draguns, & U. Hentschel (Eds.), *Psychological processes in cognition and personality* (pp. 59–70). Washington, DC: Hemisphere.

Hentschel, U. & Balint, A. (1974) Plausible diagnostic taxonomy in the field of neurosis. *Psychological Research Bulletin*, no. 2, monograph series.

Hentschel, U. & Hickel, U. (1977) *German translation of the Defense Mechanism Inventory—DMI*. University of Mainz, unpublished.

Hentschel, U. & Kießling, M. (1990) Are defense mechanisms valid predictors of performance on cognitive tasks? In G. van Heck, S. Hampson, J. Reykowski, & J. Zakrzewski (Eds.), *Personality psychology in Europe: Vol. 3* (pp. 203–219). Amsterdam: Swets & Zeitlinger.

Hentschel, U., Kießling, M., & Wiemers, M. (in press) *Fragebogen zu Konfliktbewältigungsstrategien—FKBS* [Conflict-solving strategies inventory—FKBS]. Weinheim: Beltz.

Hentschel, U. & Klintman, H. (1974) A 28-variable semantic differential. I. On the factorial identification of content. *Psychological Research Bulletin, Lund University*, *16*, no. 4.

Hentschel, U. & Schneider, U. (1986) Psychodynamic personality correlates of creativity. In U. Hentschel, G. Smith, & J.G. Draguns (Eds.), *The roots of perception* (pp. 249–271). Amsterdam: North-Holland.

Hentschel, U. & Smith, G. (1980) Theoretische Grundannahmen und Zielsetzung des Buches [Theoretical frame of reference and aims of the book]. In U. Hentschel & G. Smith (Eds.), *Experimentelle Persönlichkeitspsychologie. Die Wahrnehmung als Zugang zu diagnostischen Problemen* [Experimental personality psychology. The perceptual approach to diagnostic problems] (pp. 15–29). Wiesbaden: Akademische Verlagsgesellschaft.

Hermans, H.J.M. (1967) *Handleiding bij de Prestatie-Motivatie Test* [Manual for the Performance Motivation Test]. Amsterdam: Swets & Zeitlinger.

Herrmann, T. (1980) Die Eigenschaftskonzeption als Heterostereotyp [The trait concept as hetero-stereotype]. *Zeitschrift für Differentielle und Diagnostische Psychologie*, *1*, 7–16.

Hermann-Maurer, E.K., Drews, U., Imhof-Eichenberger, E., Knab, H., Schneider-Helmert, D., Hentschel, U., & Schoenenberger, G.A. (1992) *Schlafstörungen: Konfliktbewältigungsstrategien von Insomniepatienten* [Conflict-solving strategies of insomniacs]. *Zeitschrift für Klinische Psychologie, Psychopathologie und Psychotherapie, 40*, 34–46.

Hilliard, R., Mauch-Puhalak, I., & Wittman, L. (1988) *The Speech Characterization Coding System (SCCS): A new tool for psychotherapy research*. Paper presented at the 19th annual SPR meeting, Santa Fé, NM.

Hoffmann, S.O. & Martius, B. (1987) Zur testdiagnostischen Erfassung des Abwehrstrukturen von Patienten mit Angstneurosen, paranoiden Syndromen und karzinomatösen Erkrankungen [On testing the defense structure of anxiety neurotic, paranoid, and cancer patients]. *Psychotherapie, Psychosomatik, Psychosomatische Medizin, 37*, 97–104.

Klein, G.S. (1970) *Perception, motives, and personality*. New York: Knopf.

Kreitler, H. & Kreitler, S. (1972) The cognitive determinants of defensive behaviour. *British Journal of Social and Clinical Psychology, 11*, 359–372.

Kreitler, H. & Kreitler, S. (1976) *Cognitive orientation and behavior*. New York: Springer.

Kreitler, H. & Kreitler, S. (1982) The theory of cognitive orientation: Widening the scope of behavior prediction. In B. Maher & W.B. Maher (Eds.), *Progress in Experimental Personality Research: Vol. 11* (pp. 101–169). New York: Academic Press.

Leeuwe, J. de, Hentschel, U., Tavenier, R., & Edelbroek, P. (1992) Prediction of endocrine stress reactions by means of personality variables. *Psychological Reports, 70*, 791–802.

Liedtke, R., Künsebeck, H.-W., & Lempa, W. (1990) Änderung der Konfliktbewältigung während stationärer Psychotherapie. Eine psychometrische Untersuchung zum Abwehrverhalten [Changes in coping with conflicts during inpatient psychotherapy]. *Zeitschrift für Psychosomatische Medizin und Psychoanalyse, 36*, 79–88.

Liedtke, R., Künsebeck, H.-W., & Lempa, W. (1991) Abwehrverhalten und Symptomatik ein Jahr nach stationärer psychosomatischer Therapie [Defense and symptoms one year after in-patient psychotherapy]. *Zeitschrift für Psychosomatische Medizin und Psychoanalyse, 2*(37), 185–193.

Little, K.B. & Fisher, J. (1958) Two new experimental scales of the MMPI. *Journal of Consulting Psychology, 22*, 305– 306.

MacKinnon, D.W. & Dukes, W.F. (1962) Repression. In L. Postman (Ed.), *Psychology in the making* (pp. 662–744). New York: Knopf.

Magnusson, D. & Endler, N.S. (1977) *Personality at the crossroads: Current issues in interactional psychology*. Hillsdale, NJ: Erlbaum.

Massong, S.R., Dickson, A.I., Ritzler, B.A., & Layne, C.C. (1982) A correlation comparison of defense mechanism measures: The Defense Mechanism Inventory and the Blacky Defense Preference Inventory. *Journal of Personality Assessment, 46*, 477–480.

Meyer, A.-E., Zenker, R., & Freitag, D.E. (1977) *Psychoanalytische Charakter-Typologie in faktoranalytischen und itemanalytischen Überprüfungen* [Psychoanalytic character typology empirically controlled by factor analysis and item analysis]. University of Hamburg, unpublished.

Milimet, C.R. (1970) Manifest anxiety-defensiveness scale: First factor of the MMPI revisited. *Psychological Reports, 27*, 603–616.

Mischel, W. (1968) *Personality assessment*. New York: Wiley.

Monson, T.C., Hesley, J.W., & Chernick, L. (1982) Specifying when personality traits can and cannot predict behavior: An alternative to abandoning the attempt to predict single-act criteria. *Journal of Personality and Social Psychology*, *43*, 385–399.

Olff, M., Godaert, G., Brosschot, J.F., Weiss, K.E., & Ursin, H. (1991) The defense mechanism test and questionnaire methods for measurement of psychological defenses. In M. Olff, G. Godaert, & H. Ursin (Eds.), *Quantification of human defense mechanisms* (pp. 302–317). Berlin: Springer.

Peter, R. (1993) *Selbst- und Objekt-repräsentanzen von Eßstörungspatientinnen* [Self- and object-representations of female patients with eating disorders]. University of Ulm, Germany.

Plutchik, R. (1980) *Emotion: A psychoevolutionary synthesis*. New York: Harper & Row.

Plutchik, R., Kellerman, H., & Conte, H.R. (1979) The structural theory of ego defenses and emotions. In C.E. Izard (Ed.), *Emotions in personality and psychopathology* (pp. 229–257). New York: Plenum.

Postman, L., Bruner, J.S., & McGinnies, E. (1948) Personal values as selective factors in perception. *Journal of Abnormal Social Psychology*, *43*, 142–154.

Raad, B. de (1992) *The cross word-class replicability of the Big Five personality dimensions in the Dutch language*. Paper presented at the Fifth Congress of the European Association for Personality Psychology, Rome, June 1990.

Rapaport, D. (1960) The structure of psychoanalytic theory. *Psychological Issues: Monogr. 6*. Madison, CT: International Universities Press.

Rimoldi, H.J.A., Insua, A.M., & Erdmann, J.B. (1975) Personality dimensions as assessed by projective and verbal instruments. *Journal of Clinical Psychology*, *31*, 524–539.

Rosenzweig, S. 1945/1946. The picture-association method and its application in a study of reactions to frustration. *Journal of Personality*, *14*, 3–23.

Sandler, J. (1960) The background of safety. *International Journal of Psychoanalysis*, *41*, 352–356.

Sarason, I.G., Ganzer V.J., & Singer, M. (1972) Effects of modeled self-disclosure on the verbal behavior of persons differing in defensiveness. *Journal of Consulting and Clinical Psychology*, *39*, 483–490.

Schmidt, J. (1991) *Evaluation einer psychosomatischen Klinik*. [Evaluation of a psychosomatic clinic]. Frankfurt: Verlag für Akademische Schriften.

Shepard, R.N. (1978) The mental image. *American Psychologist*, *33*, 125–137.

Smith, G.J.W. (1984) Stabilization and automatization of perceptual activity over time. In W.D. Fröhlich, G.J.W. Smith, J.G. Draguns, & U. Hentschel (Eds.), *Psychological process in cognition and personality* (pp. 135–142). Washington, DC: Hemisphere.

Smith, G.J.W. & Carlsson, I. (1990) The creative process: A functional model based on empirical studies from early childhood to middle age. *Psychological Issues, Monogr. 57*. Madison, CT: International Universities Press.

Smith, G.J.W. & Danielsson, A. (1980) Von offen gezeigten Fluchttendenzen zu symbolischen und wahrnehmungsmäßigen Strategien [From open flight to symbolic and perceptual tactics: A study of defenses in preschool children]. In U. Hentschel & G.J.W. Smith (Eds.), *Experimentelle Persönlichkeitspsychologie* [Experimental personality psychology] (pp. 64–93). Wiesbaden: Akademische Verlagsgesellschaft.

Stagner, R. (1977) On the reality and relevance of traits. *Journal of General Psychology*, *96*, 185–207.

Stagner, R. (1988) *A history of psychological theories*. New York: Macmillan.

Suppes, P. & Warren, H. (1975) On the generation and classification of defense mechanisms. *International Journal of Psychoanalysis*, *56*, 405–414.

Udenhout, M. & Bekker, F.J. (1990) *Defense mechanisms—A barrier in the learning process*. Leiden University, unpublished.

Vaillant, G.E. (1971) Theoretical hierarchy of adaptive ego mechanisms. *Archives of General Psychiatry*, *24*, 107–118.

Vaillant, G.E. (1974) *Adaptation to life*. Boston: Little, Brown.

Vickers, R.R. & Hervig, L.K. (1981) Comparison of three psychological defense mechanism questionnaires. *Journal of Personality Assessment*, *45*, 630–638.

Walsh, W.B. & Betz, N.E. (1990) *Tests and assessment* (2nd ed.). Englewood Cliffs, NJ: Prentice Hall.

Weizsäcker, V. von (1947) *Der Gestaltkreis* [Gestalt region theory] (3rd ed.). Stuttgart: Thieme.

Wiggins, J.S. (1973) *Personality and prediction: Principles of personality assessment*. Reading, MA: Addison-Wesley.

Wiggins, J.S. (1982) Circumplex models of interpersonal behavior in clinical psychology. In P.C. Kendall & J.N. Butcher (Eds.), *Handbook of research methods in clinical psychology* (pp. 183–221). New York: Wiley.

Wittman, W.W. & Schmidt, J. (1983) *Die Vorhersagbarkeit des Verhaltens aus Trait-Inventaren. Theoretische Grundlagen und empirische Ergebnisse mit dem Freiburger Persönlichkeitsinventar (FPI)* [The predictability of behavior from trait inventories. Theoretical basis and empirical results with the Freiburg Personality Inventory (FPI)]. Research report no. 10. Department of Psychology, University of Freiburg.

Zee, M. v.d. (1992) *De invloed van defensie mechanismen en affectief-emotionele houdingen op psycho-fysiologische stress indikatoren* [On the effects of defense mechanisms and affective-emotive attitudes on psycho-physiological stress indicators]. Leiden University, unpublished thesis.

Zeeuw, J. de (1980) *Coderingsmemoriseringstest—CMT* [Coding Memory Test—CMT]. Unpublished, Leiden University.

6
The Assessment of Primitive Defense Mechanisms by Projective Techniques

FALK LEICHSENRING

Defense mechanisms are regarded as means by which the ego protects itself against such unpleasurable experiences as anxiety, depression, guilt, and shame (e.g., Fenichel, 1945; A. Freud, 1936/1959; S. Freud, 1972b). A symptom is seen as the result of the failure of a defense against instinctual drive derivatives (Freud, 1972b). Various constellations of defense mechanisms are regarded as more or less specific to the different types of neurosis (A. Freud, 1936/1959; S. Freud, 1972b). However, defense mechanisms are not regarded as pathogenic per se, but only when used in exaggeration (Freud, 1972a, 1972c) or in a rigid or overgeneralized way (Loewenstein, 1967). The adaptive functions of defense mechanisms were stressed by Anna Freud (1936/1959), Hartmann (1939), and others. According to A. Freud, each person chooses a limited number of defense mechanisms to protect oneself against unpleasurable experiences. The constellation of defense mechanisms habitually used contributes to what is called a person's "character" (A. Freud, 1936/1959; Hoffmann, 1984; Reich, 1933). According to Millon (1984, p. 460), a systematic assessment of defense mechanisms "is central to a comprehensive personality assessment."

A. Freud (1936/1959) described 10 defense mechanisms (repression, regression, reaction formation, isolation, undoing, projection, introjection, turning against the self, reversal, and sublimation); however, a growing number of mechanisms are listed by later authors (e.g., Bibring, Dwyer, Huntington, & Valenstein, 1961; Laughlin, 1970). In addition to intrapsychic defense mechanisms, interpersonal ones have been described (Heigl-Evers, 1972; Richter, 1967; Willi, 1975). The glossary of the recent revision of the *Diagnostic and Statistical Manual of Mental Disorders* (DSM-III-R: American Psychiatric Association, 1987) includes 18 defense mechanisms. Various authors have tried to systematize the growing number of defense mechanisms (e.g., Plutchik, Kellermann, & Conte, 1979; Vaillant, 1971, 1976).

Kernberg (1977, 1984) differentiates two levels of defensive organization: neurotic, versus borderline or psychotic. The former is characterized by an advanced defensive constellation centering around repression and other advanced defensive operations (e.g., reaction formation, isolation, and undoing). In contrast, borderline or psychotic defensive organization is characterized by a constellation of primitive defensive operations centering around the mechanism of splitting. Subsidiary mechanisms are projective identification, primitive denial, devaluation, idealization, and fantasies of omnipotence. By Kernberg's definition splitting means the active keeping apart of the libidinally determined and the aggressively determined self- and object representations. This mechanism serves to protect the ego core built around positive introjection. Thus, Kernberg emphasizes the defensive function of splitting, whereas other authors regard splitting not as an active defense but as a passive fragmentation (e.g., Benedetti, 1977). For a discussion of splitting, see also Lichtenberg and Slap (1973). According to Arlow and Brenner (1964), a regression of particular ego functions in the service of defense against anxiety may lead to psychotic symptoms.

The Empirical Assessment of Defense Mechanisms

It is difficult to assess defense mechanisms empirically: these processes are conceptualized as unconscious. Furthermore, the presence of a defense mechanism has to be judged from the absence or the distortion of a certain drive derivative or affect (Beutel, 1988). Self-report instruments, rating scales, content analytic methods, and projective techniques are usually used for the assessment of defense mechanisms, each method being associated with specific methodological problems (Beutel, 1988). This chapter describes and discusses the assessment of defense mechanisms by projective techniques. The focus is on the so-called primitive defense mechanisms and their assessment by the Rorschach test and the Holtzman Inkblot Technique (HIT: Holtzman, Thorpe, Swartz, & Herron, 1961). The assessment of defense mechanisms by means of the Thematic Ap-perception Test (TAT) is described by Bellak (1975), Cramer (1987; Cramer & Blatt, 1990), and Rauchfleisch (1989). Projective techniques are assumed to assess "deeper" (i.e., less conscious) levels of psychological functioning. Thus these methods seem to be especially appropriate for the assessment of defense mechanisms. For this purpose, it is necessary to specify test indicators that can be scored reliably and are valid with regard to the respective defense mechanisms.

As demonstrated below, sufficient interrater reliability could not be demonstrated for all defense mechanisms examined and their respective Rorschach scores. A variable purportedly indicative of a specific defense mechanism may often be interpreted with regard to another hypothetical construct. Thus validation becomes difficult. This aspect is discussed later on. In my view, this ambiguity stems from the impossibility of gaining "pure" indicators of defense mechanisms: these indicators are complex products of different psychological functions.

The Assessment of Low Level Defense Mechanisms by Means of the Rorschach and the Holtzman Inkblot Technique

Rorschach scoring systems for defense mechanisms were developed by Schafer (1954), Gardner, Holtzman, Klein, Linton, and Spence (1959), Baxter, Becker, and Hooks (1963), and Bellak, Hurvich, and Gediman (1973). In recent years some authors have tried to assess defense mechanisms considered to be characteristic of borderline patients by means of the Rorschach (H. Lerner, Albert, & Walsh, 1987; H.D. Lerner, Sugarman, & Gaughran, 1981; R. Lerner & H. Lerner, 1987). Lerner and collaborators developed a content-based Rorschach scoring system focusing on the human responses: splitting is scored, for example, if two human figures are described and the affective content of the description of one figure is clearly opposite to the other (H.D. Lerner et al., 1981, p. 710): "Two figures, a man and a woman. He's mean and chanting at her. Being rather angelic, she's standing there and taking it." Devaluation is scored on a five-point scale. Low level devaluation (scale value 5) is scored if the dimension of humanness is lost: for example, figures are seen as robots, puppets, or as humans with animal features. Denial is scored on a three-point scale. Low level denial (scale value 3) is scored if something is added that is not there or an aspect is not taken into account that can be seen clearly. Incompatible descriptions are included here, too (H.D. Lerner et al., 1981, p. 711): "A person but instead of a mouth there is a bird's beak." Idealization is scored on a five-point scale. Low level idealization (scale value 5) is scored if the dimension of humanness is lost, but an enhancement of identity is implied: for example, if statues of famous figures, giants, and superheroes are described (H.D. Lerner et al., 1981, p. 710): "A bust of Queen Victoria." Projective identification is scored if confabulatory responses involving human figures are given in which the form level is weak or arbitrary (H.D. Lerner et al., 1981, p. 711): "A huge man coming to get me. I can see his huge teeth. He's staring straight at me. His hands are up as if he will strike me."

Details of the scoring rules were described by R. Lerner and H. Lerner (1980) and H.D. Lerner et al. (1981). According to their findings, sufficient interrater agreement can be obtained in scoring those indicators (also Gacano, 1990). With regard to validity Lerner and Lerner (1980) found significantly more Rorschach indicators of splitting, projective identification, low level devaluation, and low level denial in borderline patients than in neurotics. However, no differences could be detected concerning indicators of idealization. Indicators of splitting and projective identification were found in the borderline group only. However, in another study, H. Lerner et al. (1987) could demonstrate no differences between neurotics and borderline outpatients with the exception of indicators of projective identification. Borderline inpatients, however, had significantly more indicators of splitting, projective identification, and omnipotence than neurotics. This result is in contrast to the assumption and empirical findings that the borderline personality disorder is a long-term condition (Carr, 1987; Koenigsberg, 1982). The differences found between in- and outpatients may result from decompensation leading to hospitalization and may or may not be connected with differences in defense mechanisms. Unfortunately, the criteria used to classify neurotics and borderline outpatients were not specified by H. Lerner et al. (1987), a fact already criticized by Carr (1987).

H.D. Lerner, Sugarman, and Gaughran (1981) demonstrated that a mixed group of patients with schizotypal and borderline personality disorder (DSM-III: American Psychiatric Association, 1983) showed significantly more Rorschach indicators of splitting and projective identification and a significantly higher weighted sum for devaluation, idealization, and denial than a group of schizophrenic patients. However, combining borderline and schizotypal patients is questionable, because these disorders are considered to be quite different by authors of different theoretical orientations (Akiskal et al., 1985; Carr, 1987; Kernberg, 1984; McGlashan, 1983; Stone, 1980). Indicators of projective identification were found only in the borderline group (see also H. Lerner et al., 1987). As a weighted sum is used for devaluation, idealization, and denial, it is not clear from the data presented by H.D. Lerner et al. (1981) whether the indicators of the "primitive" forms of these defense mechanisms differentiate significantly between the groups. The results obtained by comparing borderline and schizophrenic patients are in contrast to Kernberg's (1977, 1984) conclusion that borderline patients and psychotics differ in reality testing but not in primitive defense mechanisms. However, in psychotics those mechanisms serve a different purpose: They help to prevent the further disintegration of self–object boundaries (Kernberg, 1977, 1984). Furthermore, the failure to find projective identification in schizophrenics is in contrast to the conclusions of authors familiar with that topic (Kernberg, 1977, 1984; Ogden, 1982; Rosenfeld, 1954). As Carr (1987) points out, the unexpected differences between borderline and schizophrenic patients may result from the fact that according to the data of H.D. Lerner et al. (1981), schizophrenics give less human and quasi-human responses. It is on these variables that the Lerner scoring system is based.

P.M. Lerner (1990, p. 35) spoke of "the general hypothesis that borderline patients exhibit a defensive structure significantly different from that of schizophrenics and neurotics." The kinds of source from which he draws that conclusion are not clear to me. I suppose that Lerner uses only his data based on human responses, but he does not specify the defense structure he assumes schizophrenics to have. The results of the studies reported question the validity of the Lerner scoring system of primitive defense mechanisms, at least in borderline outpatients and schizophrenics. Furthermore, the data published by Lerner and collaborators are not sufficient to decide whether the differences found can be used for differential diagnosis of individual patients: significant differences on a group basis are necessary, but not sufficient for this purpose. This is true for some other studies using the Lerner system—for examples, that of Gacano (1990), which does not even include a control group. To decide whether differential diagnosis of individual patients is possible, additional research is necessary, classifying individual patients on the basis of indicators proposed by Lerner and collaborators. Referring to object relation theory, Carr (1987) argues in favor of scoring not only human and quasi-human responses for defense mechanisms, but all responses, human or nonhuman, and all behavioral evidence related to the testing situation.

In one of my own studies with borderline patients (Leichsenring, 1991a) I applied the Lerner scoring system to HIT responses of 30 borderline and 30 neurotic inpatients. The patients had been classified on the basis of Diagnostic Interview for Borderlines (DIB: Kolb & Gunderson, 1980). However, the scoring of defensive operations was not restricted to human or quasi-human responses. Splitting was scored, for example, if the response "paradise, butterflies, and birds in the sky" was followed by the response "a hangman, cutting off the head of man sentenced to death." Concerning the assessment of projective identification by means of projective techniques I see a fundamental problem: recent definitions of projective identification by Kernberg (1977) and Ogden (1979, 1982) necessarily imply an interactional component by which the external object is influenced in a way that it feels, thinks, or behaves like the externalized parts of the self. Since inkblots cannot "react," the indicators proposed by Lerner and colleagues for projective identification can be assumed to indicate projection rather projective identification (Leichsenring, 1991a).

In the above-mentioned study, sufficient interrater agreement with a blind rater could be demonstrated both for the DIB and for the scoring of indicators of splitting, "projective identification," low level denial, and low level devaluation (Leichsenring, 1990, 1991a). According to the results, borderline patients showed significantly more indicators of these defense mechanisms than neurotics. However, no difference concerning indicators of low level idealization could be found, a result supporting Lerner and Lerner's (1980) findings. Furthermore, no differences could be found for all other levels of idealization, devaluation, and denial (Leichsenring, 1991a). Referring to the defense mechanisms that significantly discriminated between the two groups, it was possible to classify individual patients with quite good results for sensitivity and specificity: by a criterion of at least one indicator of splitting, 80% (24/30) of the borderline patients (sensitivity) and 70% (21/30) of the neurotics (specificity) were classified "correctly," that is, in agreement with the DIB diagnoses. By a criterion of at least one indicator of "projective identification," the corresponding percentages are 77 and 80%. The diagnostic classifications in regard to specificity are insufficient when low level devaluation and denial are used as predictors (Leichsenring, 1991a).

According to these data, the Lerner indicators of primitive defensive operations can be scored on the HIT with sufficient interrater agreement and will yield a high discriminative power. Nevertheless, the question remains whether these indicators measure primarily defense mechanisms; there is a considerable overlap between these indicators and several "classical" Rorschach and Holtzman variables. Indicators of both low level devaluation and of low level denial overlap with "fabulized combinations" and "contaminations," indicators of projective identification overlap with "confabulations," the form level, and the hostility and anxiety variable. For definitions of these variables see Rapaport, Gill, and Schafer (1950), Elizur (1949), Murstein, (1956), and Holtzman et al. (1961). In contrast, the Lerner indicators of splitting do not correspond to any other Rorschach variable. It is possible that the Lerner indicators of low level devaluation and low level denial do not measure these defense mechanisms, but fabulized combinations and contaminations (i.e., thought-related variables). It is also possible that indicators of projective identification do not measure this defense mechanism, but confabulations, form level, anxiety, and hostility. This problem is similar to the interpretation of fabulized combinations and contaminations as indicators of boundary disturbances (Blatt & Ritzler, 1974; H.D. Lerner, Sugarman, & Barbour, 1985).

In my own study the patients were administered not only the HIT, but also the Borderline Syndrome Index (BSI: Conte, Plutchik, Karasu, & Jarret, 1980; Leichsenring, 1992) and a self-report instrument that I had developed to assess borderline personality organization via the three structural criteria given by Kernberg (Borderline Personality Inventory, BPI: Leichsenring, 1991b). According to the data, the HIT indicators of "projective identification" and of low level denial showed significant correlations with the BSI score ($r = .37, .38$). This was not true for indicators of splitting and low level devaluation ($r = .13, -.02$). However, the BSI is not a measure of defense mechanisms. Furthermore, the differential diagnostic validity of the BSI seems to be questionable as far as classification of individual patients is concerned (Leichsenring, 1992). Reliability and discriminative validity of the Borderline Personality Inventory are promising (Leichsenring, 1991b). The HIT indicators of splitting, "projective identification," low level devaluation, and low level denial showed significant correlations with the low level defense score, but also with the two questionnaire scores representing the other structural criteria (Leichsenring, 1991b) (see Table 6.1). These data indicate that

TABLE 6.1. Correlations of HIT indicators for primitive defenses with the three subscales of the Borderline Personality Inventory.

HIT Indicators for Primitive Defenses	Borderline Personality Inventory Categories[a]		
	Low level defenses	Identity diffusion	Reality testing
Splitting	.29*	.47**	.46*
"Projective identification"/ projection	.52**	.55**	.56**
Low level devaluation	.42*	.38*	.47**
Low level denial	.50**	.54**	.59**

[a] * $p \pm .05$, ** $p \pm .01$
SOURCE: Leichsenring (1991c).

the HIT variables of low level defense mechanisms are not "pure" indicators of these mechanisms; rather, considerable aspects of reality testing and identity diffusion are involved. Further ego functions may be involved, as well (e.g., the function of primary vs. secondary process thinking) (Leichsenring, 1991c).

On the level of items, the HIT indicator of splitting correlates highest (.50) with the BPI items "Sometimes there is another person appearing in me, that does not belong to me" (identity diffusion subscale) and "I have heard voices talking about me, although nobody was there" (reality testing subscale). The HIT indicator of "projective identification" correlates significantly (.56, .52, .55) with the items "Sometimes I have murderous ideas," "Sometimes I feel that people or things change their shape, although they really do not," and "I have seen strange figures, although nobody was there." Both low level devaluation and low level denial correlate highest with the latter item (.65, .58).

Various relationships can be demonstrated between certain defense mechanisms and cognitive styles (Gardner et al., 1959; Klein & Schlesinger, 1949). Cognitive styles resemble character defenses in that they are ways of contacting reality (Bellak, et al., 1973; Klein & Schlesinger, 1949). According to Gardner et al. (1959, p. 128) cognitive styles may be "preconditions for the emergence of defensive structures." In another study (Leichsenring, Roth, & Meyer, 1992) Ertel's (1972) DOTA dictionary and Günther and Groeben's (1978) method of assessing the level of abstractness of speech were applied to the responses of borderline and neurotic patients on the HIT. By these content analytic methods, borderline patients could be discriminated from neurotics with quite good results for sensitivity and specificity (Leichsenring et al., 1992). For the present context it is interesting that the HIT indicators of splitting, "projective identification," low level devaluation and low level denial correlate significantly ($r = .42, .41, .26, .47$) with a variable of Ertel's (1972) DOTA dictionary, the so-called A terms (e.g., "always," "never,"

"total," "complete," "certain," "naturally," "only," "must," "must not"),
which is interpreted as indicating cognitive dynamics characterized by
a tendency to avoid cognitive ambiguity (Leichsenring et al., 1992).
According to these results, there seems to be a connection between low
level defense mechanisms assessed by the (modified) Lerner criteria and
avoidance of cognitive ambiguity. These results are in accord with the
above-mentioned general expectations and findings of Klein, Gardner,
and colleagues.

In another study (Leichsenring & Ardjomandi, 1992), the discriminative
power of Kernberg's (1967) "presumptive diagnostic elements" of a borderline disorder and of other psychiatric symptoms was examined empirically
in the foregoing sample of borderline and neurotic patients: according to
the data, by a criterion of at least three of Kernberg's "presumptive
diagnostic elements," 76% (19/25) of the borderline and 89% (17/19) of
the neurotic patients could be classified "correctly," that is, in agreement
with Gunderson's Diagnostic Interview for Borderlines. The HIT indicators
of splitting and low level devaluation correlate significantly with the
clinical diagnosis (presence or absence) of "impulse neurosis and addictions" ($r = .30, .33$), "suicidal attempts" ($r = .38, .32$), "mutilation of
self or damaging others" ($r = .32, .51$), and a "prepsychotic personality
structure" ($r = .32, .40$). Indicators of low level devaluation correlate
significantly with the clinical diagnosis of disturbances of manifest object
relations ($r = .33$). Indicators of low level denial correlate significantly
with "suicidal attempts" ($r = .40$) and a "prepsychotic personality structure" ($r = .48$). The indicators of "projective identification" correlate
significantly only with the latter criterion ($r = .53$). However, all correlations are significant, but only of moderate size. These results seem to
indicate that the Lerner indicators of defense mechanisms are meaningfully
associated with severe psychiatric symptoms. However, not all correlations
are conceptually clear: for example, the correlation between indicators
of low level denial and "suicidal attempts." On the other hand, some
variables that can be expected to be correlated are not (e.g., indicators of
splitting and "projective identification" with disturbances of manifest
object relations).

Summing up, the data presented are in favor of the validity of the
modified Lerner criteria with the exception of primitive idealization,
but further research is necessary to determine whether these indicators
measure primarily primitive defense mechanisms and whether these indicators are valid for primitive defense mechanisms in psychotics.

Cooper, Perry, and Arnow (1988) developed a Rorschach scoring system
for 15 defense mechanisms that they grouped into three categories:
neurotic (according to Fenichel, 1945; Schafer, 1954), borderline (according
to Kernberg, 1967), and psychotic (according to Semrad, Grinspoon, &
Feinberg, 1973). This system relies primarily on content, too, but is not
restricted to human responses. In its scoring criteria of neurotic defenses
it is strongly influenced by Schafer (1954), Holt (1960), and Weiner

(1966). In scoring borderline defenses, some criteria of Lerner and collaborates were utilized; others were developed by the authors. Referring to Semrad et al. (1973), "hypomanic" and "massive" denial are scored as "psychotic" defense mechanisms that involve major distortions in perception or extreme affective or associative elaborations of perceptions. Unfortunately, the criteria used for scoring neurotic, borderline, and psychotic defense mechanisms were not published by Cooper et al. (1988). However, in an earlier paper (Cooper & Arnow, 1986) scoring criteria of "borderline defenses" were presented, referring to response content and remarks about the examiner, the testing situation, and the self.

Cooper et al. (1988) reported interrater agreements between .45 (rationalization) and .80 (primitive idealization), with a median of .62. Interrater agreement for the three categories of neurotic, borderline, and psychotic defense mechanisms is .71, .81, and .72.

Only for one defense mechanism (primitive idealization) did interrater agreement exceed .80; six defense mechanisms were scored with an interrater agreement of at least .70 (isolation, Pollyanna-ish denial, devaluation, projection, massive denial). The interrater agreement for repression as the central neurotic defense mechanism was only .58; for reaction formation it was .57.

The validity of the Rorschach Defense Scales was tested by Cooper et al. (1988) in three samples of patients: borderline and antisocial personality disorder according to DSM-III, and bipolar Type II patients according to the Research Diagnostic Criteria. According to the results, indicators of splitting, devaluation, projection, and hypomanic denial correlate significantly with external criteria of borderline personality disorder, Perry 's (1982) Borderline Personality Disorder Scale (BPD), and the sum of the positive DSM-III criteria of the borderline personality disorder. These correlations, however, are only of moderate size (.24 to .40). The indicators of projective identification do not correlate significantly with these external criteria. Contrary to the expectations, hypomanic and massive denial do not correlate significantly with the bipolar criteria. The significant correlation of hypomanic denial with the borderline criteria makes the classification of this defense mechanism as "psychotic" questionable. Furthermore, none of the 15 defense mechanisms studied correlated significantly with the external criteria of antisocial personality disorder and bipolar Type II. Discriminant function analysis with the borderline defense indicators as predictors failed to discriminate the three diagnostic groups significantly. Cooper et al. (1988, p. 197) attribute this result to the presumed close relationship between these three disorders. However, at least for the bipolar disorder the conceptual relationship to the other disorders is not yet clear.

If the percentage of observed indicators of a defense mechanism relative to the total number of all defenses for each subject is used in correlation analyses, the Rorschach splitting indicator correlates significantly with BPD subscales for splitting of object ($r = .29$) and of self images ($r =$

.31). However, the authors' conclusion (p. 200) that "bipolar Type II diagnosis showed a strong association with defense mechanisms of intellectualization and isolation of affect" seems to me a little bold: The correlation between the bipolar diagnosis and the subjects' ranks on both intellectualization and isolation is insignificant. If the relative percentage of these defenses is used for calculation, this correlation is .23 for both, intellectualization and isolation. Probably by a mistake, .23 is indicated as significant for isolation and as insignificant for intellectualization.

Summing up the findings concerning the Cooper scoring system, the reliability for the scoring of special defense mechanisms is not sufficiently high. For some of the defense mechanisms this may be due to the low base rates as assumed by Cooper et al. (1988). According to the data presented by the authors, the validity of the indicators of projective identification as a borderline defense mechanism and of massive and hypomanic denial as psychotic defense mechanisms seems to be questionable. However, hypomanic denial seems to be associated with borderline pathology. To establish the validity of neurotic defense mechanisms, studies with neurotics are necessary. According to the results, it is not possible to assess primitive defense mechanisms by the Cooper criteria in antisocial personalities—given that antisocial personalities are considered to be a subgroup of borderline patients (Kernberg, 1975), a classification supported by the findings of Pope, Jonas, Hudson, Cohen, and Gunderson (1983).

Summing up, the findings presented here give some evidence that primitive defense mechanisms may be assessed by Rorschach or HIT scores. However, I agree with Carr (1987, p. 353) that ". . . convincing validation will have to come from evidence that shows that a Rorschach measure for a specific defense is correlated adequately with some clinical or behavioral evidence for that particular defense, rather than that a plethora of defenses differentiates large diagnostic groups that, on the basis on somebody's theory, presumably use these defenses." Thus, further research assessing defense mechanisms by independent measures and correlating the findings is necessary.

References

Akiskal, H.C., Chen, S.E., Davis, G.C., Puzantian, V.R., Kashgarian, M., & Bolinger, J.M. (1985). Borderline: An adjective in search of a noun. *Journal of Clinical Psychiatry*, *46*, 41–48.

American Psychiatric Association (1983). *Diagnostic and statistical manual of mental disorders* (3rd ed.). Washington, DC: Author.

American Psychiatric Association (1987). *Diagnostic and statistical manual of mental disorders* (3rd ed., rev.). Washington, DC: Author.

Arlow, J. & Brenner, C. (1964). *Psychoanalytic concepts and the structural theory*. Madison, CT: International Universities Press.

Baxter, J., Becker, J., & Hooks, W. (1963). Defensive style in the families of schizophrenics and controls. *Journal of Abnormal and Social Psychology*, *5*, 512–518.

Benedetti, G. (1977). Das Borderline-Syndrom. Ein kritischer Überblick zu neueren psychiatrischen und psychoanalytischen Auffassungen [The borderline syndrome. A critical review of recent psychiatric and psychoanalytic concepts]. *Nervenarzt*, *48*, 641–650.

Bellak, L. (1975). *The TAT, CTA and SAT in clinical use*. New York: Grune & Stratton.

Bellak, L., Hurvich, M., & Gediman, H.K. (1973). *Ego functions in schizophrenics, neurotics and normals*. New York: Wiley.

Beutel, M. (1988). Bewältigungsprozesse bei chronischen Krankheiten [Coping mechanisms and chronic disease]. In U. Koch (Ed.), *Psychologie in der Medizin*. Weinheim: Edition Medizin, VCH.

Bibring, G.L., Dwyer, T.M., Huntington, T.S., & Valenstein, A.F. (1961). A study of psychological processes in pregnancy and the earliest mother–child relationship. *Psychoanalytic Study of the Child*, *16*, 25–72.

Blatt, S.J. & Ritzler, B.A. (1974). Thought disorder and boundary disturbances in psychosis. *Journal of Consulting and Clinical Psychology*, *42*, 370–381.

Carr, A.C. (1987). Borderline defenses and Rorschach responses: A critique of Lerner, Albert and Walsh. *Journal of Personality Assessment*, *51*, 349–354.

Conte, H.R., Plutchik, R., Karasu, T.B., & Jerrett, I. (1980). A self-report borderline-scale. Discriminative validity and preliminary norms. *Journal of Nervous and Mental Disease*, *168*, 428–435.

Cooper, S.H. & Arnow, D. (1986). An object relations view of the borderline defenses: A Rorschach analysis. In M. Kissen (Ed.), *Assessing object relations phenomena*. Madison, CT: International Universities Press.

Cooper, S.H., Perry, J.C., & Arnow, D. (1988). An empirical approach to the study of defense mechanisms. I. Reliability and preliminary validity of the Rorschach defense scales. *Journal of Personality Assessment*, *52*, 187–203.

Cramer, P. (1987). The development of defense mechanisms. *Journal of Personality*, *55*, 597–614.

Cramer, P. & Blatt, S. (1990). Use of the TAT to measure change in defensive mechanisms following intensive psychotherapy. *Journal of Personality Assessment*, *54*, 236–251.

Elizur, A. (1949). Content analysis of the Rorschach with regard to anxiety and hostility. Rorschach Research Exchange, and *Journal of Projective Techniques*, *13*, 247–287.

Ertel, S. (1972). Erkenntnis und Dogmatismus [Cognition and dogmatism]. *Psychologische Rundschau*, *23*, 241–269.

Ertel, S. (1981). Prägnanztendenzen in Wahrnehmung und BewuBtsein [Tendencies of Prägnanz in perception and consciousness]. *Zeitschrift für Semiotik*, *3*, 107–141.

Fenichel, O. (1945). *The psychoanalytic theory of neurosis*. New York: Norton.

Freud, A. (1959). *Das Ich und die Abwehrmechanismen* [The ego and the mechanisms of defense]. Munich: Kindler. (Original work published 1936).

Freud, S. (1972a). *Studien über Hysterie* [Studies on hysteria]. Gesammeltz Werke, Vol. 1 (pp. 75–312).

Freud, S. (1972b). *Hemmung, Symptom und Angst* [Inhibitions, symptom and anxiety]. Gesammeltz Werke, Vol. 14 (pp. 111–205). Frankfurt: Fischer, 1972.

Freud, S. (1972c). *Die endliche und die unendliche Analyse* [Analysis terminable and interminable]. Gesammeltz Werke, Vol. 16 (pp. 57–99). Frankfurt: Fisher, 1972.

Gacano, C.B. (1990). An empirical study of object relations and defensive operations in antisocial personality disorder. *Journal of Personality Assessment, 54,* 589–600.

Gardner, R., Holzman, P.S., Klein, G.S., Linton, H., & Spence, D.P. (1959). Cognitive control. A study of individual consistencies in cognitive behavior. *Psychological Issues, 4.*

Günther, U. & Groeben, N. (1978). Abstrakheitssuffixverfahren. Vorschlag einer objektiven und ökonomischen Erfassung der Abstraktheit/Konkretheit von Texten [The suffix method of abstractness. Proposal of an objective and economical assessment of the abstractness/concreteness of texts]. *Zeitschrift für experimentelle und angewandte Psychologie, 25,* 5–74.

Hartmann, H. *Ego psychology and the problem of adaptation.* Madison, CT: International Universities Press, 1939. [Deutsch: *Ich-Psychologie.* Stuttgart: Klett, 1972.]

Heigl-Evers, A. (1972). *Konzepte der analytischen Gruppenpsychotherapie* [Concepts of the psychoanalytic group therapy]. Göttingen: Vandenhoeck & Ruprecht.

Hoffmann, S.O. (1984). *Charakter und Neurose* [Character and neurosis]. Frankfurt: Suhrkamp.

Holt, R. (1960). *Manual for scoring primary process on the Rorschach.* Unpublished manuscript.

Holtzman, W.H., Thorpe, J.S., Swartz, J.D., & Herron, E.W. (1961). *Inkblot perception and personality.* Austin: University of Texas Press.

Kernberg, O.F. (1967). Borderline personality organization. *Journal of the American Psychoanalytic Association, 15,* 641–685.

Kernberg, O.F. (1975). *Borderline conditions and pathological narcissism.* New York: Jason Aronson.

Kernberg, O.F. (1977). The structural diagnosis of borderline personality organization. In P. Hartocollis (Ed.), *Borderline personality disorders. The concept, the syndrome, the patient.* Madison, CT: International Universities Press.

Kernberg, O.F. (1984). *Severe personality disorders. Psychotherapeutic strategies.* New Haven, CT: Yale University Press.

Klein, G. & Schlesinger, H. (1949). Where is the perceiver in perceptual theory? *Journal of Personality, 18,* 32–47.

Koenigsberg, W.H. (1982). A comparison of hospitalized and non-hospitalized borderline patients. *American Journal of Psychiatry, 139,* 1292–1297.

Kolb, J.E. & Gunderson, J.G. (1980). Diagnosing borderline patients with a semistrucured interview. *Archives of General Psychiatry, 37,* 37–41.

Laughlin, H.P. (1970). *The ego and its defenses.* New York: Appleton-Century-Crofts.

Leichsenring, F. (1990). Discriminating borderline from neurotic patients. *Psychopathology, 23,* 21–26.

Leichsenring, F. (1991a). "Frühe" Abwehrmechanismen bei Borderline- und neurotischen Patienten ["Early" defense mechanisms in borderline and neurotic patients]. *Zeitschrift für klinische Psychologie, 20,* 75–91.

Leichsenring, F. (1991b). *Zur Entwicklung eines Fragebogens zur Borderline-Persönlichkeitsstörung* [The development of a questionnaire for borderline personality disorder]. Manuscript submitted for publication.

Leichsenring, F. (1991c). Primary process thinking, primitive defensive operations and object relationships in borderline and neurotic patients. *Psychopathology*, *24*, 39–44.

Leichsenring, F. (1992). Zur differential-diagnostischen Validität des Borderline-Syndrom-Indexes [On the differential diagnostic validity of the Borderline Syndrome-Index]. *Diagnostica*, *38*, 155–159.

Leichsenring, F. & Ardjomandi, M.E. (1992). "Gibt es borderline-verdächtige Symptome?" [Are there presumptive symptoms of a borderline disorder?]. Gruppenpsychotherapic und Gruppendynamik, *28*, 29–39.

Leichsenring, F., Roth, T., & Meyer, H.A. (1992). Kognitiver Stil bei Borderline-im Vergleich zu neurotischen Patienten: Ambiguitätsvermeidung und verminderte Abstrakheit [Cognitive style in borderline compared to neurotic patients: Avoidance of ambiguity and reduced abstractness]. *Diagnostica*, *38*, 52–65.

Lerner, H., Albert, C., & Walsh, M. (1987). The Rorschach assessment of borderline defenses: A concurrent validity study. *Journal of Personality Assessment*, *51*, 334–348.

Lerner, H.D., Sugarman, A., & Gaughran, J. (1981). Borderline and schizophrenic patients. A comparative study of defensive structure. *Journal of Nervous and Mental Disease*, *169*, 705–711.

Lerner, H.D., Sugarman, A., & Barbour, C.G. (1985). Patterns of ego boundary disturbance in neurotic, borderline and schizophrenic patients. *Psychoanalytic Psychology*, *2*, 47–66.

Lerner, P.M. (1990). Rorschach assessment of primitive defenses: A review. *Journal of Personality Assessment*, *54*, 30–46.

Lerner, R. & Lerner, H. (1980). Rorschach assessment of primitive defenses in borderline personality structure. In J. Kwawer, H. Lerner, P. Lerner, & A. Sugarman (Eds.), *Borderline phenomena and the Rorschach test*. Madison, CT: International Universities Press.

Lichtenberg, J. & Slap, J. (1973). Notes on the concept of splitting and the defense mechanism of splitting of representations. *Journal of the American Psychoanalytic Association*, *21*, 772–787.

Loewenstein, R. (1967). Defensive organization and autonomous ego functions. *Journal of the American Psychoanalytic Association*, *15*, 795–809.

Murstein, B.I. (1956). *Handbook of projective techniques*. New York: Basic Books.

McGlashan, T.H. (1983). The borderline syndrome: Is it a variant of schizophrenia or an affective disorder? *Archives of General Psychiatry*, *40*, 1319–1323.

Millon, T. (1984). On the renaissance of personality assessment and personality theory. *Journal of Personality Assessment*, *48*, 450–466.

Plutchik, R., Kellermann, H., & Conte, H.R. (1979). A structural theory of ego defenses and emotions. In C. Izard (Ed.), *Emotions in personality and psychopathology* (pp. 229–257). New York: Plenum.

Schafer, R. (1954). *Psychoanalytic interpretation in Rorschach testing. Theory and Application*. New York: Grune & Stratton.

Ogden, T.H. (1979). On projective identification. *International Journal of Psychoanalysis*, *60*, 357–373.

Ogden, T.H. (1982). *Projective identification and psychotherapeutic technique.* New York: Jason Aronson.

Rapaport, D., Gill, M., & Schafer, R. (1950). *Diagnostic psychological testing: Vols I & II.* Chicago: Year Book Publishers.

Perry, C. (1982). *The borderline personality disorder scale: Reliability and validity.* Manuscript submitted for publication.

Pope, H.G., Jonas, J.M., Hudson, J.I., Cohen, B.M., & Gunderson, J.G. (1983). The validity of DSM-III borderline personality disorder. *Archives of General Psychiatry, 40,* 23–30.

Rauchfleisch, U. (1989). *Der Thematische Apperzeptionstest (TAT). in Diagnostik und Therapie* [The Thematic Apperception Test (TAT). in diagnostics and therapy]. Stuttgart: Enke.

Reich, W. (1933). *Charakteranalyse. Technik und Grundlagen* [Character analysis]. Berlin: Selbstverlag.

Richter, H.E. (1967). *Eltern, Kind und Neurose* [Parents, child and neurosis]. Stuttgart: Klett.

Rosenfeld, H. (1954). Considerations regarding the psychoanalytic approach to acute and chronic schizophrenia. *International Journal of Psychoanalysis, 35,* 135–147.

Semrad, E., Grinspoon, L., & Feinberg, S. (1973). Development of an ego profile scale. *Archives of General Psychiatry, 28,* 70–77.

Stone, M.H. (1980). *The borderline syndromes.* New York: McGraw-Hill.

Vaillant, G.E. (1971). Theoretical hierarchy of adaptive ego mechanisms. *Archives of General Psychiatry, 24,* 107–118.

Vaillant, G.E. (1976). Natural history of male psychological health. The relation of choice of ego mechanism of defense to adult adjustment. *Archives of General Psychiatry, 33,* 535–545.

Weiner, I.B. (1966). *Psychodiagnosis in schizophrenia.* New York: Wiley.

Willi, J. (1975). *Die Zweierbeziehung* [The dyadic object relation]. Reinbek: Rowohlt.

7
Percept-Genetic Methodology

GUDMUND J.W. SMITH AND UWE HENTSCHEL

Sigmund Freud's original idea about the operation of defense (repression) is illustrated by Fig. 7.1. The percept-genetic tests described in this chapter are built on an analogous conception. Figure 7.2 shows that in these tests, a subliminal picture, eventually becoming supraliminal, is introduced as a threat to a hero figure, with whom the viewer is supposed to identify. How the viewer handles the subconscious anxiety generated by this situation, registered as bodily reactions, verbal reports, or drawings, forms the basis for the interpretation of these reactions as defensive.

Defenses are, of course, theoretical constructs: they cannot be seen or touched, either in clinical settings or in everyday life or experimental situations (cf. also the warnings by Hans Sjöbäck in Chapter 3 against reification of the construct). If you share your kitchen with a mouse you do not have to spot the animal itself, only such traces of it as black droppings or a gnawed flour bag, to be convinced of its existence. In the case of defense mechanisms you must be content with the traces only. But these can be obvious enough, ranging from perceptual distortions to avoidance reactions. Moreover, they have a nonrandom distribution over situations and patients, manifesting themselves as severe symptoms, operating in one way in histrionics, in another in compulsives, differing between young and old, or remaining only latent possibilities. Freud himself vacillated in his view of defenses as purely pathogenic, finally settling for the pathogenic perspective. To some of his followers, the ego psychologists, the adaptive possibilities of defensive strategies were as interesting as the pathogenic ones. The introduction of defensive hierarchies with Gedo and Goldberg (1973) and Vaillant (1971) implied that some defenses, the mature ones, seen from the perspective of an adult way of functioning had to be considered to be less pathogenic than the immature ones. One of the methods presented below, the Meta-Contrast Technique (MCT), has been particularly adapted to a developmental perspective, because both behavioral and perceptual manifestations can be registered, the former being more typical of young children and impulse ➡ conflict ➡ defense ➡ symptom

or :

impulse ➡ conflict ➡ defense ➡ character

FIGURE 7.1. The operation of defense in the psychoanalytic frame of reference.

considered to be prestages of the well-known adult mechanisms (Smith & Danielsson, 1982).

The MCT was introduced as a diagnostic tool in psychiatric settings but has lately also been applied in neuropsychology (cf. Hanlon, 1991). The Defense Mechanism Test (DMT) originally proved to be a useful instrument for the selection of stress-tolerant subjects but is now more and more adapted also to psychiatric problems. These applications should not be allowed to obscure the fact that defense manifestations are not only typical of the field of abnormal psychology but also appear in the protocols of so-called normals, perhaps in a more varied and flexible way than in psychiatric patients, cases of cerebral dysfunction, stress-intolerant people, etc. The scoring principles adopted for the DMT (Kragh, 1985) attest to this difference between adaptive and pathogenic uses of defenses. It thus seems obvious that defenses are employed not only to parry ominous anxiety signals but much more broadly to serve the maintenance of our general mental comfort. When using them we may feel better and less bothered by vague uneasiness, and we may be able more easily to concentrate on the task at hand, to be spared feelings of guilt for neglect of others, etc. It is instructive to learn that total absence of defenses in our experiments (Smith & Danielsson, 1982) was most typical of children and youngsters who were unable to control their anxiety and were generally viewed by their therapists as having very bleak prospects. Also among patients who had attempted suicide, those who showed no signs of defense were, retrospectively evaluated, most at risk for a new fatal attempt (Berglund & Smith, 1988). Perhaps defenses are also utilized for keeping at bay some of the subliminal influences constantly impinging on us, threatening to disturb our efficiency or equanimity. One aspect of defensive functioning that is often neglected is tolerance of anxiety. Signals of anxiety do not automatically trigger defensive reactions if the person can tolerate a certain level of discomfort. Studies in creativity (Smith & Carlsson, 1990) have shown that creative people are more tolerant of anxiety and less susceptible to subliminal influences of a negative, aggressive kind (Hentschel & Schneider, 1986), perhaps because they have the means to resolve conflicts in a productive way. Their defensive reactions

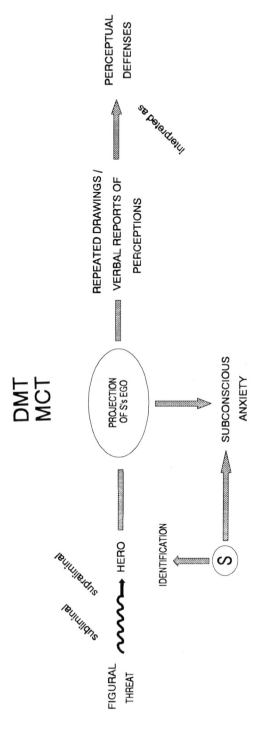

FIGURE 7.2. The operation of defense in percept-genetic tests.

tend toward the mature end of the continuum and seldom dominate their percept-geneses in a one-sided way.

One problem connected with the concept of defense is the tendency of defenses to multiply over the years—in the writings on defenses. If we think of defenses as acting on different manifestations of our mental life—affects, ideas, percepts, motilities—it is a complex construct. Holland (1973) suggested that all defensive strategies are steered by a few or just one general operation in a quasi-algebraic way and proposed displacement as this general operator. He differentiated between displacement of direction (in the sense of a change in the self–nonself "localization": e.g., projection–introjection), displacement in time (e.g., regression), displacement in number (e.g., repression, denial), and displacement in similarity (e.g., sublimation, reaction formation). The idea of displacement as a central operation seems in a certain way similar to the central concept of reality distortion in percept-genetic techniques (cf. Chapters 22, 27). A schematic, parsimonious concept like this should not be used to rule out all specificity but rather as a help to explain the phenomena in their acknowledged variety. Holland has explicitly stated it in this way, and in percept-genesis the value that is given to the specific kind of reality distortion is already obvious from the scoring instructions of, for example, the DMT or MCT. Suppes and Warren (1975) have made another attempt to provide a comprehensive classification of defense mechanisms. They use the basic idea that "transformations" are constituent for all defenses. They relate these transformations, however, not to physical or quasi-physical dimensions but to the "actor", the "action," and the "object" (cf. Fig. 7.3). Restricting their idea to the self as actor, and allowing also for the condition of no transformation, they can, on theoretical grounds, postulate a list of 29 different mechanisms of defense, which when identification as a basic principle is added, is extended to 44. An example for three transformations (on the actor, the action, and the object) would be, for example, the combination of projection plus reaction formation and turning against self which, in a verbalized form, could imply change from

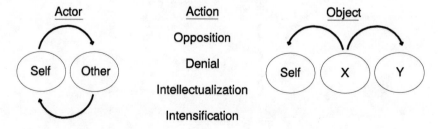

FIGURE 7.3. Defenses as transformations on the actor, the action, and the object. (After Suppes and Warren, 1975.)

the nonacceptable unconscious proposition of "I love him" to the consciously acceptable one "He hates me."

From verbalizations given as examples, the transformations postulated by Suppes and Warren (1975) seem to be very sensible because they reflect the consequences of the whole defensive process. In reality an additional inference is needed because the unconscious proposition is not so easily available to the observer. Percept-genetic methods can help to uncover the unconscious proposition on the basis of a comparison of the subjectively perceived (and reported) content with the objectively presented stimulus. There are two inherent restrictions to this general statement. Whereas for example the object in the system of Suppes and Warren can be anybody ranging from mother, brother, or friend, to someone on the street, the application of a specific percept-genetic technique as a standardized test requires one stimulus or a restricted set of standardized stimuli, thus also limiting the range of potentially conflictual object representations. Restricting the object relation to the "Oedipal situation" as, for example, in the DMT and its modified version, DMTm (Andersson & Bengtsson) can, however, be defended with the argument that this is a very important and "prototypical situation" potentially influencing all other relations. The second restriction concerns the role of the actor, which in real life is the acting person, whereas in percept-genetic techniques, the identification of the responding subject with the hero must be postulated as an intermediate process to explain the transformations as defense mechanisms. Although an indirect proof for the feasibility of this latter assumption can be taken from all studies with results supporting the concurrent or predictive validity of percept-genetic tests, it could and should, as Martin Johnson (1986) has argued, be submitted to critical tests. Adding to Holland's (1973) remarks on the paradoxical thinking in psychoanalysis, the "paradox" in percept-genetic techniques lies in the need for the subject first to have an idea of the objective stimulus before he or she can distort it, which however is an elementary process in all defense mechanisms. The effect or idea that is repressed or denied must necessarily have gained some representation before it is repressed or denied. The percept-genetic process in its beginnings thus necessarily comprises elements from subliminal perception, and the theoretical links between the two approaches have repeatedly been underlined (e.g., Dixon, Hentschel, & Smith, 1986; Hentschel, Smith, & Draguns, 1986).

The Defense Mechanism Test (DMT)

In 1955 Ulf Kragh started out to describe personality in its present functioning via perception in terms of perceptual construction and reconstruction processes. At the same time his intent was to overcome the restriction of a mere conscious conception of personality. After having experimented with different tachistoscopically presented TAT and TAT-like pictures, he published his DMT in 1969 (see also Kragh, 1960). From the beginning on, within the theoretical frame of references of perception–personality, the main aim of the DMT was the registration of defense mechanisms conceptualized in close relationship to the classical concept of defense (A. Freud, 1936/1946). Within the microgenetic tradition, the DMT can be characterized as a hologenetic procedure presenting repeatedly one and the same stimulus in a tachistoscopic device to the respondent starting with very short (subliminal) exposure times up to an exposure time of 2 seconds, at which a conscious representation is or at least should be possible.

The theoretical conception of perception–personality was worked out further by Kragh and Smith in 1970, and the first revision of the DMT was published in 1985 (Kragh, 1985). Thousands of subjects have been tested with the DMT, mainly with the purpose of selecting stress-resistant job applicants for jobs like jet pilot and frog man (Kragh, 1962). Ulf Kragh and others had also selected a number of case histories describing clinical cases (e.g., Kragh, 1970, 1980, 1984) and the DMT, although on a small scale, started to be used also for purposes of clinical diagnosis (Hentschel & Balint, 1974; Sharma, 1977). Today there are clinical research projects with the DMT going on in Sweden (Armelius & Sundbom, 1991), in the Netherlands (Godeart, Hagenaars, Olff, & Brosschot, 1991), in Italy (Rubino, Pezzarossa, & Grasso, 1991; cf. also Chapter 20), and in Germany (Gitzinger, 1988; cf. also Chapter 27; and Hentschel et al.; cf. Chapter 22). Hentschel and Kießling (1990) and Hentschel, Kießling, and Hosemann (1991), have also used the DMT for the prediction of the performance in cognitive tasks and attention control. Another important topic has become the relation of DMT categories to psychophysiological and endocrine variables, especially also in stress research (e.g., Ursin, Baade, & Levine, 1978; Endresen & Ursin, 1991). A bibliography edited by Sjöbäck and Bäckström (1990) lists more than 100 publications on the DMT, documenting the steadily increasing interest in the technique. We refer to the DMT manual (Kragh, 1985) for most of the technical details of the testing procedure. The test is given in a darkened room (2.8 lux); the subject is told that he or she will see some pictures (this is explained with a demonstration slide) and is instructed to tell everything that is seen (including impressions) and to make a simple drawing of the exposed stimulus. There are strict rules for follow-up questions in which all kinds of suggestion are to be avoided. Each subject is tested with two sex-specific test slides showing a male or female hero with an "instrument" and a threatening male or female figure peripheral to the hero. The answers of the subject reflecting the subjective meaning of the stimulus are regarded as "phases" and registered as P1 (the first description with a meaningful structure), T1 a threshold phase in which for the first time a threat from the peripheral person is seen, and the C-phase, when the stimulus structure in all details is correctly represented in the subjective interpretation. The whole perceptual process reconstructed from the drawings and verbal answers from the respondent is subject of the DMT scoring procedure. The deviations from the objective content of the pictures shown are interpreted in terms of 10 main categories of defense mechanisms:

1. Repression, signified by the report of an inanimate hero or peripheral person.
2. Isolation, inferred from signs of separation of the hero and the peripheral person.
3. Denial, given on the basis of reports that deny or diminish the threat.
4. Reaction-formation, scored on the basis of answers turning the threat into its opposite.
5. Identification with the aggressor, standing for reports of an aggressive hero.
6. Turning against the self, scored when the hero or the instrument is hurt or worthless.
7. Introjection of the opposite sex, inferred from reports of the hero with another sex.
8. Introjection of another object, given in cases of duplication or multiplication of the hero.
9. Projection, interpreted on the basis of specific changes in the process of the hero perception during the P-phases.
10. Regression, scored in cases of breakdown of an earlier intact pictorial structure.

Within these main signs there are various numbers of other sign variants. Isolation has, for example, 14 variants, reaction formation has 4, turning against the self 2. Examples of the scoring of the subjects' drawings are given in Fig. 7.4. There are different models for the psychometric treatment of the signs. Kragh (1969) has worked with ratings for the severity of maladaptation, and Neuman (1978) has proposed a phase-related weighing model. The manual of the revised DMT (Kragh, 1985) mentions the possibility of partitioning the whole process into three sections (early, middle, and late phases), which is empirically applied in Chapter 22. In clinical applications comparisons between diagnostic groups are often also made on the basis of sign variants (Rubino et al., 1991). A phenomenological approach, basically without the need to use the psychodynamic theoretical frame of reference was chosen by Cooper (1991), who has tried to "construct" the basic variables by means of G-analysis (Holley & Guilford, 1964).

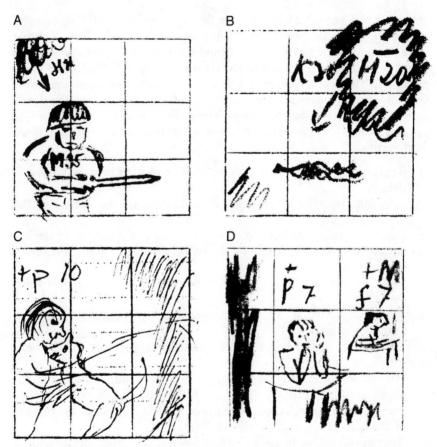

FIGURE 7.4. Examples for different DMT drawings and categorizations. (A) Identification with the aggressor: "A soldier with a gun. In winter dressing." (B) Turning against the self: "Maybe patient on the operation table during stomach operation. A male assistant and a female doctor?" (C) Repression and reaction formation: "A boy playing with a puppy." (D) Reaction formation: "A girl sitting at the other table, writing."

Reliability and Validity of the DMT

From the whole test procedure it is obvious that a simple retest within a short period of time is as inadequate as the calculation of a split-half coefficient. Reliability estimates thus can be made on interrater comparisons and retests using, for example, one test picture at the first instance and another for the retest. Interrater reliability has a range from .65 to .95, depending on the pretraining of the scorers. Stability over time for defensive signs estimated by parallel test results seems to be also very good ($r = .81$ after one year; cf. Kragh, 1985). Concerning validity, the

1985 manual lists 18 studies (16 with significant results) in which the group test version has been applied; this could be up-dated by more recent studies listed in the bibliography by Sjöbäck and Bäckström (1990) (cf. also the contributions in this volume using the DMT: Chapters 10, 15, 20, 22, 27). Concerning the selection of pilots especially, the incremental validity of the DMT is worth mentioning. The DMT has been used repeatedly in this context with highly preselected groups. Given very low correlations also to the other tests in the test battery used for selection, the resulting validity can be claimed almost exclusively for the DMT (cf. Kragh, 1985). The DMT results did not reach significance in a study with British Air Force pilots for the prediction of their success in flight training (Stoker, 1982).

Problems with the DMT

Olff (1991) has made an inquiry about the DMT procedures used by different researchers and has concluded that the procedures are far from standardized (differences in types of projector, illumination in the room and on the screen, distance to the screen, questions asked, etc.). Hans Sjöbäck (1991) has written a paper with the provocative title, "The Defence Mechanism Test: What pictures do you use?" also revealing an unexpected variety. Sjöbäck claims that many of these variants are un-authorized. The variance in the test material used and in the skill of the experimenters represents a serious problem for the accumulation of knowledge and impedes a conclusive judgment regarding the value of the test. However, for the selection of Scandinavian air force pilots, which provides the strongest support for the validity of the test, the test pro-cedure is quite well standardized. Critical evaluations of the test from other psychological laboratories often concern the difficulty of learning the scoring system, unwillingness to accept the psychoanalytical frame of reference and, if the standards of the selecting institution so require (see Stoll, 1990), the difficult if not impossible task of explaining the test results to the testees.

Modifications of the DMT

In the DMT the defensive process in the subject is stimulated according to the basic process as outlined in Fig. 7.2. The threat stems from a situation reminding one of the one-sided oedipal situation with the parental figure of the same sex as a punishing agent. In psychoanalysis the complete oedipal situation has been formulated with libidinal and aggressive impulses for both parents, thus also including the possibility of both parents as punishing agents. In line with this basic idea and the additional elaboration of a theoretical model based on Heinz Kohut's and Melanie Klein's psychoanalytical conceptions, combined with a developmental perspective,

Alf Andersson (Andersson & Bengtsson, 1986) has proposed a change of the test pictures confronting both males and females with a male and a female threat figure. Affect-defenses are described as a dialectical series represented in developmental order as reification, personification, and annihilation. These affect-defenses correspond to the following signs in the modified DMT version (DMTm): repression, introaggression, and isolation of affect. The three qualitatively different forms of handling the "evil" are directed by basic instrumental proficiencies. The main aim of Andersson (Andersson & Bengtsson, 1986) is to demonstrate that it is not enough to name various forms of defense; one must also deepen the analysis of motives underlying the defensive activity bound to a verbal symbolic medium and thus protracted in relation to the original triggering situation. Most of the studies using the DMTm have not been published in English, but this test, with its elaborated theoretical frame of reference, seems to be useful in the clinical context when studying states of identity crises, neurotic and narcissistic problems, and psychotic states, yet not alleging, to have introduced a new test. DMT-like pictures without the claim that a new test has been constructed have been used among others by Westerlundh (e.g., Westerlundh and Sjöbäck, 1986; cf. also Chapter 14; Kline & Cooper, 1977). Gitzinger (1991) has changed the basic testing device by showing, compared to the DMT, slightly changed stimuli on a computer monitor and providing an interactive computer program for the scoring procedure that then follows. Since Gitzinger's contribution to this volume is the first written report about the new technique, a final evaluation of its advantages or disadvantages seems premature, but she is able in Chapter 27 to present some results in support of the concurrent validity of the new version. Brand, Olff, Hulsman, and Slagman (1991) have also experimented with digitized pictures for measuring defense. But their perceptual defense test (PD-test) does not pretend to replace the DMT. It is obvious that the new technical possibilities will stimulate other attempts to present DMT or DMT-like pictures on a computer screen or a video monitor. It should be kept in mind however ·that generating new stimuli is one thing and the introduction of a new "test" is another. This is as every test author knows a very laborious task. The concept of defense in our view would profit more from a few well-standardized, reliable and valid test instruments than from a great number of experimental versions.

New Thematic Innovations Based on the DMT Device

The Mother–Child Picture Test (MCPT)

The MCPT utilizes the DMT presentation device. The stimulus is a picture of a woman feeding a child with a spoon. The child is sitting in a high chair. Both woman and child are seen in half profile. The feminine characteristics of the woman are quite obvious. Behind the woman, part of a half open window is showing. Preliminary studies by S. Balint indicated that when subjects viewed this picture in a tachistoscope they often described it in such a way as to reveal their own very personal and deep-seated conflicts around mother–child relations. In the first systematic validation studies, the test was administered to 100 mothers and their children aged 7–8 years (Smith et al., 1980, 1981, 1984). The scoring scheme partly referred to mothers and children together, partly to these groups separately. Only a selection of possible scoring categories is presented here.

Mother not reported even in the final phase (for children); the child in the picture reported to have disappeared from one phase to the next (for mothers and children).
The child is seen as a doll, an animal, an object, etc. (for mothers).
The child is seen as naughty, dirty, unkempt, etc. (for mothers).
Picture reported as frightening, mother as aggressive, etc. (for children).

The first two of these groups of signs, in particular, could be classed as defensive; the latter two as more open expressions of disgust for the child or fright of the mother. These signs, together with signs not accounted for here, were arranged into strong, medium, and marginal categories. There was a high correlation between mothers and children in half of the groups ($p < .001$) and, still, in the other half when it was cross-validated ($p < .01$). The scoring categories were also validated against results of the parallel mother–child study and in a later study (Ryde-Brandt, 1992).

The Meta-Contrast Technique (MCT)

The original purpose of the MCT was to study the development of a new percept within the context of an old percept, stabilized beforehand, when the meaning of the new percept was at variance with or implied a threat against the old percept. The introduction of antagonistic material made the MCT a test of coping mechanisms concerned with mediation of conflict. These mechanisms, it has turned out, are the core of what we call defenses. As thus indicated, the MCT implies repeated tachistoscopic presentations of pairs of stimuli, one of them exposed immediately before the other. The second stimulus (B) in a pair is intended to offer a constant perceptual frame of reference to which the viewer has been adapted in advance. Within this frame the development of the first stimulus (A) is going to be followed step by step. A is either incongruent with B or represents a threat to a person depicted in B. To begin with, A is exposed very rapidly and does not manifest itself as a perceptual structure in its own right, but sometimes as changes in the B-percept. With subsequently prolonged exposure times, however, A gradually penetrates B, often in "disguise," to begin with. The test session is concluded when A+B have been correctly reported or when the longest exposure time has been reached. It would be unnecessary to dwell on the technical details (given in Smith, Johnson, & Almgren, 1989). Let us just repeat the three basic phases of the test session:

1. Starting with .01 s (somewhat longer with the new TV device), B is presented at gradually prolonged exposure times until it has been correctly reported.
2. Thereafter, B is exposed at a standardized level alone five times in a control series.
3. A is then introduced before B at .01 s (again somewhat longer with the new device). The time of B is held constant and that of A prolonged every second time (according to a geometric scale with a constant of the square root of 2).

There are presently eight stimulus pictures divided up into two tests that have proved to be parallel. Each test includes two tasks or two pairs of pictures (A+B). Each of the four pairs is assigned a number from 1 to 4. Stimulus B2 is a thoroughly revised version of card 1 in the Thematic Apperception Test. The other pictures are either original drawings or photo montages. The two picture pairs in the first test are: A1 = a car, B1 = interior of a room, A2 = apelike human, B2 = boy (hero) and background window. The original tachistoscopic contrivance allowed the second stimulus in a pair to be exposed on a semitransparent projection screen directly after the first one. Exposure times ranged from 10 ms upward (cf. Fig. 7.5). A new contrivance exploits a computer program and a swift TV screen. Stimuli are projected in front of the subject, who describes what she has seen after each presentation. The experimenter not only records what the subject says but also how she behaves (shutting the eyes, yawning, looking obviously panic-stricken, becoming restless, etc.).

Scoring

The scoring refers to changes in reports of B and interpretations of A and, not least important, the subject's behavior. The sequential aspect is always in focus. What is scored late in a series is supposed to represent more manifest tendencies than what is reported early, the reason being that late phases are closer to the individual's habitual level of experiencing. There are two main groups of signs: signs of anxiety and signs of defense against anxiety and conflict. The former signs are ordered in a scale from open manifestations of panic to less severe forms of anxiety (internalized fear). The defensive signs range from primitive, behavioral forms to more advanced meaning transformations of A. They are grouped in the following categories: repressive strategies, isolation and negation strategies, projective strategies, depression, regressions, and self-referential sign variants.

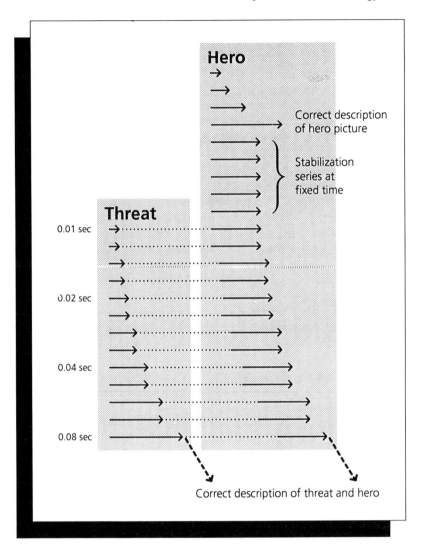

FIGURE 7.5. The general design of the Meta-Contrast Technique (MCT).

In some instances the differentiation between various defenses, on the one hand, and cognitive style, on the other, can be difficult to ascertain.

1. The group of anxiety signs (mainly in the threat series). Signs of anxiety are organized in a hierarchy ranging from open fear or primary anxiety; via grave signs like broken structures, leaking (inefficient) defenses, zero-phases (without meaningful content); to moderate or mild signs like black structures reported late or early in the test series.

2. The group of defensive signs. Defensive activity in the individual is, of course, connected with fear and anxiety and a gradually progressing internalization during childhood. Still, at an age of 4–5 years and particularly in cognitively less mature children, external defenses dominate: it is the child itself who shuts its eyes, etc., later the hero as seen by the child. Behavioral defenses may, however, be registered even in normal adults, who often resort to them when more mature strategies prove inefficient. Primitive defenses are particularly common in psychologically disturbed people.

a. The group of repressive strategies (mainly in the threat series). The grouping presupposes that the adult strategy of repression originates in direct denial at the behavioral level in children of preschool age. Even more advanced and transformed signs imply a symbolic denial of danger. The signs range from direct denial like eye-shutting behavior; overinternalized but primitive strategies like eye-shutting reports; middle level strategies, when the threat becomes lifeless or is masked; to more transformed threats, like reports of a house, a tree, or a bike at the place of the threat.

b. The group of isolation and negation strategies (mainly in the threat series). This group of strategies does not attain full strength until late latency. The different strategies have an important characteristic in common: the separation of the hero from the threatening emotion. The most primitive isolation occurs when the subject isolates literally (hands on the screen, etc.). Spatial distortion and negation represent the next level. Genuine signs of isolation imply that the threat is whitened or covered. Empty geneses, where nothing happens, also belong in this group of signs.

c. The group of projective strategies (in both series). These strategies occur early in the development. The projectively functioning individual does not let a disturbing A become established as a structure in its own right, but interprets it via the habituated B-perception (which is affected more or less, e.g., by becoming almost unrecognizable or by just appearing in a new perspective—sensitive change). The subliminal influence of A on B often can be noted during the first exposures after the control series.

d. The group of depressive strategies (mainly in the threat series). Inhibition is the central, anxiety-dampening defense strategy in this group. In its massive variants it often indicates a psychotic "inhibition depression." Among the most common signs are stereotypies (i.e., reports at least five times in a row of an unchanged noninterpretation or wrong interpretation of A). Other severe signs of depression include reports of the threat as old, ill, etc. until the end.

e. The group of regressive strategies (in both series). All regressive reactions involve retreats from a habitual level to a more immature level. When a mature defense like genuine isolation fails (because anxiety is breaking through), the subject may try a more primitive strategy like eye-shutting. The depth of the regression may be defined as the difference between the baseline level and the final level. There are regressions to infantile ways of experiencing, discontinuities of a nonprojective type like zero-phases, leaking defenses (where the subject may see a statue but still think that the statue is dangerous), and defensive regressions.

  f. The group of self-referential signs or variants (in the threat series) where, for instance, the threat may be represented by a duplicate of the hero.

Standardization Data

The most recent manual (Smith, Johnson, & Almgren, 1989) offers standardization data in detail. Let it just be said here that not only interrater but also test–retest correlations have been generally high, often close to the statistical ceiling. Validation data have been presented in more than 30 mutually independent studies, typical test criterion correlation coefficients ranging from .50 to .85. The first validation studies showed, for instance, that people with histrionic characters had more signs of what was called repression than other clinical groups, compulsive–obsessive subjects more signs of isolation–negation, psychotics more signs of regression, etc. The criterion groups were carefully selected. Later validations also refer to correlations with other tests, to change as a result of therapy, to differences between young children and older ones, etc. The MCT has also been applied in neuropsychological studies (e.g., in groups of demented people suffering from Alzheimer's or Pick's diseases, in brain tumor cases, and people suffering from exposure to organic solvents). The differentiating power of the test has proved to be surprisingly high (see Hanlon, 1991; Johanson et al., 1990; Lilja, Smith, & Salford, 1992).

New Thematic Innovations Based on the MCT Device

A Test of Flight Phobia

In her attempts to analyze the problem of flight phobia Gunilla van der Meer (Andersson, 1989) constructed special thematic pictures. "The B stimulus depicts the interior of a transportation vehicle, not necessarily a cabin, with four chairs, arranged in two rows of two chairs each, and with a person of indeterminate sex (hero), sitting in a front-row chair, next to a window. The window was drawn in relatively large size in order not to limit the possibilities of interpretation only to an airplane. Stimulus A depicts an airplane, seen from the outside, through the window." The stimuli were presented as in the ordinary MCT. All subjects in the criterion groups tested in the validation studies reported themselves to be severely afraid of flying. They were prepared to fly only if absolutely necessary and then with great discomfort, anxiety, and somatic symptoms before and during the flight. The following scoring dimensions were most effective in differentiating flight phobics and controls:

Grave anxiety, open fear, defined in accordance with the original MCT.

Primitive forms of repression, including avoidance behavior of the subject him- or herself or of the hero in the picture, and also reports of A reduced to only part of the aircraft.

Primitive forms of isolation. This category refers to magic behavior as described in the MCT, spatial distortions with changes of the distance between hero and threat, and denial of the threat.

Stereotypies. These are defined as in the original MCT.

Negative comments about the hero. Reports of hero as sad, lonely, bowed down, badly cut, curvy legs, etc.

Grave regression, as in the MCT.

Comforting strategies. All reports in which the subject seeks consolation or support: hero is strengthened, extra persons are seen in the cabin, the subject turns to the experimenter for support, the event does not take place in the air, not even in an aircraft.

There was generally more defensive activity in the flight phobia group than in the control group in the first study. By means of a general defense score, the investigator registered a highly significant difference ($p = .002$, Andersson, 1989).

The Body Self Test

The Body Self Test was developed as a means of differentiating various types of psychological reaction after induced abortion (Terjestam, 1989).

Picture B depicts a nude woman and picture A a uterus, to be projected on the lower part of the woman's body; 25 scoring dimensions were tried.

The validation study included 58 Scandinavian women, 20–38 years old, who had no children and visited an abortion clinic to have an early elective abortion. They were interviewed 1 to 7 days before abortion. Immediately after the abortion and during the following 8 weeks they answered a mood scale. Nine weeks after the abortion they took the Body Self Test and were again interviewed. The test to some degree measured fairly stable aspects of the body self. The following scoring categories significantly discriminated between subjects with abortion reactions codetermined by different types of conflicts, and subjects with more positive reactions.

The total structure in picture B disappears and the subject reports having seen nothing. This type of report was typical of women who had a negative abortion reaction as a result of a disturbed relation to men.

Picture A is seen as a rigid and lifeless object. In these women the negative reaction was due to generalized mental discomfort.

The woman in picture B is more than 45 years old. Here the negative reaction was codetermined by a conflict-laden sexual identity.

The woman in picture B is hurt. This type of answer seemed to reflect an experience of injury induced by the operation.

Among scoring categories with at least seemingly positive postabortion implications, the following deserve to be mentioned.

There are more than 15 exposures without any report of picture A.

The woman changes identity (is reported as "new").

The woman in picture B is reported as more than 45 years old, worn-out, and wrinkled.

The Body Self Test has been shown to be a means by which the actual abortion reactions can be studied and differentiated in terms of underlying psychodynamic conflicts. In addition, the test appears to reveal aspects of the self that are related to the abortion experience.

DMT and MCT: A Comparison

The two tests may appear to be similar because both employ tachistoscopic techniques and anxiety-arousing stimulus pictures. But the different presentation devices make them obviously dissimilar. And even though both tests were developed from percept-genetic assumptions, the DMT was more clearly influenced by the psychoanalytic theory of defenses and the MCT by an interest in coping strategies for the mediation of conflict. After its implementation, the DMT was validated as a test of stress tolerance in groups of fighter pilots and frog men. Systematic attempts at clinical validation are relatively recent (see Armelius and Sundbom, 1991; Sundbom, 1992; Hentschel et al., Chapter 22).

The MCT was originally tried as a diagnostic instrument. It appears to be less differentiating than the DMT in normals and is particularly efficient in spotting regression, projection, psychotic dissociation, depressive inhibition, and cerebral dysfunction. Even if the DMT explicitly refers to the psychoanalytic model of defense as initiated by signal anxiety, signs of anxiety are not scored. In the MCT, anxiety is one of the main scoring dimensions. Many signs with identical labels are scored differently in the two tests (e.g., zero-phases and depression). A zero-phase in the MCT (i.e., the disappearance of an established B-percept) is obviously a more serious sign than in the DMT. Neurotic signs in the DMT may concern the threat as well as the hero and the hero's attribute. This has been particularly exploited in the modified DMT and most notably concerns repression. In the MCT, repression only pertains to the threatening A. The DMT in its original form misses the behavioral aspect. In the MCT behavioral defenses represent the most primitive level in the hierarchically organized defensive categories. The hierarchical organization is empirically based on the results of extensive developmental studies, from the age of 4 years upward (Smith & Danielsson, 1982).

To Sum Up the Differences

In the DMT the hero is alone with the evil from the very beginning, the question being where the evil is localized (inside me or outside me) and how it is handled. The MCT, rather, represents an inventory of the possible defensive strategies of a subject who, via the picture material, is confronted with a contradiction or a threat insidiously creeping into his sheltered existence.

References

Andersson, A.L. & Bengtsson, M. (1986) Percept-genetic defenses against anxiety and a threatened sense of self as seen in terms of the spiral aftereffect technique. In U. Hentschel, G. Smith, & J.G. Draguns (Eds.), *The roots of perception* (pp. 217–246). Amsterdam: North-Holland.

Andersson, G. (1989) A psychodynamic approach to flight phobia: Evaluation of a new percept-genetic instrument. *Psychological Research Bulletin, Lund University*, *29*, no. 4–5.

Armelius, B. & Sundbom, E. (1991) Hard and soft models for the assessment of personality organization by DMT. In M. Olff, G. Godaert, & H. Ursin (Eds.), *Quantification of human defense mechanisms* (pp. 138–148). Berlin: Springer.

Berglund, M. & Smith, G. (1988) Post-diction of suicide in a group of depressive patients. *Acta Psychiatrica Scandinavica 77*, 504–510.

Brand, N., Olff, M., Hulsman, R., & Slagman, C. (1991) Perceptual defense: The use of digitized pictures. In M. Olff, G. Godaert, & H. Ursin (Eds.), *Quantification of human defense mechanisms* (pp. 293–301). Berlin: Springer.

Cooper, C. (1991) G-analysis of the DMT. In M. Olff, G. Godaert, & H. Ursin (Eds.), *Quantification of human defense mechanisms* (pp. 121–137). Berlin: Springer.

Dixon, N.F., Hentschel, U., & Smith, G.J.W. (1986) Subliminal perception and microgenesis in the context of personality research. In A. Angleitner, A. Furnham, & G. van Heck (Eds.), *Personality psychology in Europe: Vol. 2. Current trends and controversies* (pp. 239–255). Lisse, The Netherlands: Swets & Zeitlinger.

Endresen, I.M. & Ursin, H. (1991) The relationship between psychological defence, cortisol, immunoglobulins, and complements. In M. Olff, G. Godaert, & H. Ursin (Eds.), *Quantification of human defense mechanisms* (pp. 262–272). Berlin: Springer.

Freud, A. (1946) *The ego and the mechanism of defense.* Madison, CT: International Universities Press. (Original work published 1936).

Gedo, J.E. & Goldberg, A. (1973) *Models of the mind. A psychoanalytic theory.* Chicago: University of Chicago Press.

Gitzinger, I. (1988) *Operationalisierung von Abwehrmechanismen: Wahrneh-mungsabwehr und Einstellungsmessung psychoanalytischer Abwehrkonzepte* [Operationalization of defense mechanisms: Perceptual defense and attitude measurement of psychoanalytical defense concepts]. University of Freiburg, unpublished thesis.

Gitzinger, I. (1991) *DCT (Defense mechanisms computer test).* Unpublished manuscript, Center for Psychotherapy Research, Stuttgart.

Godaert, G., Hagenaars, J., Olff, M., & Brosschot, J.F. (1991) Defensiveness and cardiovascular reactions. In M. Olff, G. Godaert, & H. Ursin (Eds.), *Quantification of human defense mechanisms* (pp. 273–281). Berlin: Springer.

Hanlon, R.E. (Ed.) (1991) *Cognitive microgenesis: A neuropsychological perspective.* New York: Springer.

Hentschel, U. & Balint, A. (1974) Plausible diagnostic taxonomy in the field of neurosis. *Psychological Research Bulletin, Lund University, no. 2.* Monograph Series.

Hentschel, U. & Kießling, M. (1990) Are defense mechanisms valid predictors of performance on cognitive tasks? In G. van Heck, S. Hampson, J. Reykowski, & J. Zakrzewski (Eds.), *Personality Psychology in Europe: Vol. 3. Foundations, models and inquiries* (pp. 203–219). Amsterdam: Swets & Zeitlinger.

Hentschel, U., Kießling, M., & Hosemann, A. (1991) Anxiety, defense and attention control. In R.E. Hanlon (Ed.), *Cognitive microgenesis: A neuropsychological perspective* (pp. 262–285). New York: Springer.

Hentschel, U. & Schneider, U. (1986) Psychodynamic personality correlates of creativity. In U. Hentschel, G. Smith, & J.G. Draguns (Eds.), *The roots of perception* (pp. 249–271). Amsterdam: North-Holland.

Hentschel, U., Smith, G., & Draguns, J.G. (1986) Subliminal perception, microgenesis, and personality. In U. Hentschel, G. Smith, & J.G. Draguns (Eds.), *The roots of perception* (pp. 3–38). Amsterdam: North-Holland.

Holland, N.N. (1973) Defence, displacement and the ego's algebra. *International Journal of Psychoanalysis, 54,* 247–257.

Holley, J.W. & Guilford, J.P. (1964) A note on the G-index of agreement. *Education and Psychological Measurement, 24,* 749–753.

Johanson, A., Gustafson, L., Smith, G.J.W., Risberg, J., Hagberg, B., & Nilsson, B. (1990) Adaptation in different types of dementia and in normal elderly subjects. *Dementia, 1,* 95–101.

Johnson, M. (1986) Percept-genesis and the "scientific method". In U. Hentschel, G. Smith, & J.G. Draguns (Eds.), *The roots of perception* (pp. 403–417). Amsterdam: North-Holland.

Kernberg, O.F. (1977) The structural diagnosis of borderline personality organization. In P. Hartocollis (Ed.), *Borderline personality disorders* (pp. 87–121). Madison, CT: International Universities Press.

Kline, P. & Cooper, C. (1977) A percept-genetic study of some defense mechanisms in the test PN. *Scandinavian Journal of Psychology, 18,* 148–152.

Kragh, U. (1955) *The actual-genetic model of perception-personality.* Lund: Gleerup.

Kragh, U. (1960) The Defense Mechanism Test: A new method for diagnosis and personnel selection. *Journal of Applied Psychology, 44,* 303–309.

Kragh, U. (1962) Prediction of success of Danish attack divers by the Defense Mechanism Test (DMT). *Perceptual and Motor Skills, 15,* 103–106.

120   G.J.W. Smith and U. Hentschel

Kragh, U. (1969) *Manual till DMT* [DMT Manual: Defense mechanism test]. Stockholm: Skandinaviska Testförlaget.

Kragh, U. (1970) Pathogenesis in dipsomania. In U. Kragh & G. Smith (Eds.), *Percept-genetic analysis* (pp. 160– 178). Lund: Gleerup.

Kragh, U. (1980) Rekonstruktion verschiedener Aspekte einer Persönlichkeits-entwicklung mit dem Defense-Mechanism-Test: Eine Fallbeschreibung [Reconstruction of different aspects of a personality development with the Defense Mechanism Test: A case study]. In U. Hentschel & G. Smith (Eds.), *Experimentelle Persönlichkeitspsychologie* [Experimental personality psychology] (pp. 107–131). Wiesbaden: Akademische Verlagsgesellschaft.

Kragh, U. (1984) Studying effects of psychotherapy by the Defense Mechanism Test—Two case illustrations. In G.J.W. Smith, W.D. Fröhlich, & U. Hentschel (Eds.), *From private to public reality: Meaning and adaptation in perceptual processing* (pp. 73–84). Bonn: Bouvier.

Kragh, U. (1985) *Defense Mechanism Test—DMT Manual*. Stockholm: Persona.

Kragh, U. & Smith, G. (Eds.) (1970) *Percept-genetic analysis*. Lund: Gleerup.

Lilja, Å., Smith, G.J.W., & Salford, L.G. (1992) Micro-processes in perception and personality. *Journal of Nervous and Mental Disease, 180*, 82–88.

Lindgren, M. (1992) Neuropsychological studies of patients with organic solvent induced chronic toxic encephalopathy. Lund: University of Lund.

Neuman, T. (1978) *Dimensionering och validering av perceptgenesens försvarsmekanismer. En hierarkisk analys mot pilotens stressbeteende* [Dimensions and validation of percept-genetic mechanisms. An hierarchical analysis of the stress behavior of pilots]. FOA rapport C 55020-H6, Stockholm: Försvarets Forskningsanstalt.

Olff, M. (1991) The DMT method in Europe: State of the art. In M. Olff, G. Godaert, & H. Ursin (Eds.), *Quantification of human defense mechanisms* (pp. 148–171). Berlin: Springer.

Rubino, A., Pezzarossa, B., & Grasso, S. (1991) DMT defenses in neurotic and somatically ill patients. In M. Olff, G. Godaert, & H. Ursin (Eds.), *Quantification of human defense mechanisms* (pp. 207–221). Berlin: Springer.

Ryde-Brandt, B. (1992) Defence strategies and anxiety in mothers of disabled children. *European Journal of Personality, 5*, 367–377.

Sharma, V.H.P. (1977) *Application of a percept-genetic test in a clinical setting*. Department of Psychology, Lund University (unpublished).

Sjöbäck, H. (1991) *The Defence Mechanism Test. What pictures do you use?* Lund: Desmahago.

Sjöbäck, H. & Bäckström, M. (1990) *The Defence Mechanism Test. A bibliography*. Lund University, mimeographed.

Smith, G.J.W., Almgren, P.-E., Andersson, A.L., Englesson, I., Smith, M., & Uddenberg, G. (1980) The Mother–Child Picture Test: Presentation of a new method for the evaluation of mother–child relations. *International Journal of Behavioral Development, 3*, 365–380.

Smith, G.J.W., Almgren, P.-E., Andersson, A.L., Englesson, I., Smith, M., & Uddenberg, G. (1981) Mothers and their 7–8-year-old children: A follow-up study of mother–child relations. *Psychiatry and Social Science, 1*, 17–27.

Smith, G., Almgren, P.-E., Andersson, A., Englesson, I., Smith, M., & Uddenberg, G. (1984) Der Einfluß negativer Einstellungen und Fehlanpassungen von Müttern auf das Verhalten ihrer sieben- bis achtjährigen Kinder

[The effect of negative attitudes and maladaptation of the mothers on the behavior of their 7–8-year-old children]. In U. Hentschel & A. Wigand (Eds.), *Persönlichkeitsmerkmale und Familienstruktur* [Personality characteristics and family structure] (pp. 25–46). Munich: Weixler.

Smith, G.J.W. & Carlsson, I. (1990) The creative process. *Psychological Issues, Monogr. 57.* Madison, CT: International Universities Press.

Smith, G.J.W. & Danielsson, A. (1982) Anxiety and defensive strategies in childhood and adolescence. *Psychological Issues, Monogr. 52.* Madison, CT: International Universities Press.

Smith, G., Johnson, G., & Almgren P.-E. (1989) *MCT—The Meta-Contrast Technique.* Stockholm: Psykologiförlaget.

Stoker, P. (1982) An empirical investigation of the predictive validity of the Defence Mechanism Test in the screening of fast-jet pilots for the Royal Air Force. *Projective Psychology, 27,* 7–12.

Stoll, F. (1990) *Has the DMT passed the test?* Paper presented at the conference "Quantification of parameters for the study of breakdown in human adaptation: Psychological defense mechanisms." Copenhagen, April 1990.

Sundbom, E. (1992) *Borderline psychopathology and the Defense Mechanism Test.* University of Umeå, unpublished doctoral thesis.

Suppes, P. & Warren, H. (1975) On the generation and classification of defense mechanisms. *International Journal of Psychoanalysis, 56,* 405–414.

Terjestam, Y.C. (1989) The Body Self Test: A percept-genetic method for the study of psychological abortion reactions. *Psychological Research Bulletin, Lund University, 29,* no. 8.

Ursin, H., Baade, E., & Levine, S. (Eds.) (1978) *Psychobiology of stress. A study of coping men.* New York: Academic Press.

Vaillant, G.E. (1971) Theoretical hierarchy of adaptive ego mechanisms. *Archives of General Psychiatry, 24,* 107–118.

Westerlundh, B. & Sjöbäck, H. (1986) Activation of intrapsychic conflict and defense: The amauroscopic technique. In U. Hentschel, G. Smith, & J.G. Draguns (Eds.), *The roots of perception* (pp. 161–215). Amsterdam: North-Holland.

8
The Study of Defenses in Psychotherapy Using the Defense Mechanism Rating Scales (DMRS)

J. Christopher Perry, Marianne E. Kardos, and Christopher J. Pagano

The Defense Mechanism Rating Scales (DMRS), fifth edition, is a system for guiding clinical inference in the identification of specific defense mechanisms (Perry, 1990a). The author (JCP), created the first version in 1981 and revised it based on subsequent studies. The most recent, fifth edition included editorial suggestions by other members of the Subcommittee on Defense Mechanisms (reporting to the Multiaxial Committee of the Task Force for DSM-IV of the American Psychiatric Association), including Drs. Michael Bond, Steven H. Cooper, Marianne E. Kardos, and George E. Vaillant. The DMRS has benefited from the perspective and consensus of these researchers on definitions, functions, and examples of individual defenses. This chapter reviews issues pertinent to studying defenses in psychotherapy sessions. It describes the DMRS rating procedures and reliability, suggests an optimal program for selecting and training raters, and offers a discussion of the implications of using different data sources. The chapter ends with a brief discussion of the potential value of studying defenses in psychotherapy. The Reference section constitutes a bibliography of the DMRS.

Description of the Defense Mechanism Rating Scales

The DMRS is a manual describing how to identify 28 individual defense mechanisms. The introduction includes general directions for the qualitative and quantitative identification of defenses, along with suggestions about handling problems presented by different data sources. The body of the manual consists of directions for identifying the 28 individual defenses. These include a definition of each defense, a description of how the defense functions, a section on how to discriminate each defense from near-neighbor defenses (e.g., suppression vs. repression vs. denial), and a three-point scale. Each scale is anchored with specific examples of the probable use of the defense and the definite use of the defense. The examples offer prototypical instances of the defense, thereby providing some ostensive definition of each defense construct. Unfortunately an exhaustive catalog of all instances of each defense is impossible. Therefore, some degree of inference in rating defenses will always be required, a task that is more difficult at the conceptual boundaries of each construct.

Qualitative Scoring

The scales were originally devised for rating the qualitative presence of a defense in a 50-minute dynamically oriented interview. Qualitative assessment yields information for the current time period, answering the categorical question: "Does the subject use this defense?" Information like this can be used for a "defense diagnosis" but does not yield data on the frequency of use of individual mechanisms. Data may be rated based on events occurring in the interview itself or reported on from outside the interview. In the latter case, data are included for rating only if the event has occurred within the past 2 years, unless there is additional evidence that the defense probably is still present. This arbitrary rule decreases the problem of rating defenses as current when they were delimited to a subject's distant past. When teaching the DMRS for the first time, the author has found that the original qualitative method is more accessible.

Quantitative Scoring

The DMRS can be used for quantitative assessment when interview transcripts are used. Using this scoring method, the rater identifies each use of the defense as it occurs, bracketing that part of the text over which it operates. The distinction between probable and definite use is ignored, and all examples are treated as equal. After the completion of the ratings, the number of times each defense was rated present is divided by the total instances of all defenses to yield a percentage. The resulting profile is the percentage of defensive functioning due to each defense. Statistical uses of these scores are described below.

The Importance of Consensus Ratings

Because defenses are rated on the basis of inference from observations, there is room for disagreement. The defense definitions and scales provide guides for justifying a rating, but not firm inference rules, which are not possible. The process of having two raters score the interview independently, then discuss their ratings and form a consensus, provides several advantages. First, using two raters rather than one improves the likelihood of identifying more defensive phenomena. Second, when transcripts are not available, there occasionally may be factual questions about what occurred, and one rater may have a more vivid recollection than another, thereby providing a check on the veridicality of observation.

Third, the rater who infers from certain observations that a defense was operating must justify this inference to the other rater by reference to the defense scale. This justification process, going back and forth from observational data to the defense definition and scale, diminishes insupportable speculation. When the raters must agree about both the observations and the basis for the defense rating, only stronger inferences are supported, thereby improving validity. This also effectively calibrates the raters and improves reliability, as they develop a consensual interpretation of how to use the manual in rating less prototypical examples. Participating in consensus ratings is valuable even for experienced raters. The authors still find that two heads are better than one, even when one rater is less experienced.

A study using the DMRS, third version, estimated the gain in reliability when comparing the ratings of individuals against those of a consensus process (Perry & Cooper, 1989). Two groups of three baccalaureate level raters independently viewed 46 videotaped 50-minute initial dynamic interviews. Each rater made independent ratings blind to others' ratings. Then three raters met in each of the two consensus groups, discussed their ratings, and formed consensus ratings. The median intraclass R reliability for the six individual raters was .36, whereas for the two consensus group ratings it was .57, accounting for 58% more variance. When the scores of empirically and conceptually related defenses were summed (e.g., intellectualization + isolation + undoing = obsessional defenses), the median reliability of the resulting defense summary scores rose to .53 for the individual raters, and .74 for the consensus ratings, a gain of 40% more variance for the consensus ratings. Whether individual defenses or the combined defense summary scores were used, consensus ratings were consistently more reliable than individual ratings.

The Selection of Raters

The authors have found that certain characteristics associated with rater proficiency are worth noting. First, a certain intelligence is desirable, to ensure the ability to scan clinical material and discern a pattern connecting motivationally related data. While this requires one or two levels of inference below the raw data, the rater must be restrained from deep theorizing (i.e., justifying a defense rating by reference to a complex formulation of the patient). The opposite is the individual who avoids looking for underlying patterns, often remarking "The patient just said that; it doesn't mean anything." A second desirable characteristic for raters is some clinical experience. Training will be prolonged if raters need to be trained to observe and think dynamically, that is, to look for patterns of defense and related motives. A third characteristic is an open mind toward defenses, along with the ability to think in new ways. Potential raters with extensive preconceptions about defenses, whether based on other training or on a preference for another psychological model, have more difficulty modifying previous concepts to rate according to the manual. A worst case of this is the rater who agrees with the training but reverts to previous conceptions during subsequent ratings. This can usually be ascertained by diminishing interrater reliability. Passive–aggressive individuals should be counseled out of serving as raters. A fourth characteristic, work style, affects the consensus process. Raters who form judgments too quickly, closing their mind to additional disconfirming evidence or to articulating the data in different ways, are difficult to work with. They prove especially difficult under rushed conditions. Rather, an attitude of cooperation and give and take is necessary in the absence of an absolute criterion of valid assessment. Raters must strike compromises when a situation is somewhat ambiguous, with the rater who has the least evidence conceding. In irreconcilable disputes, raters often engage in horse trading, with the rater who feels most strongly winning, while agreeing to a future concession in the other's favor.

Rater Training

The authors have found that the following procedures optimize rater training. Prior to training, the rater should read the DMRS manual, concentrating on the definition and function sections. One should not try to learn everything, because the manual is better learned through use. Second, in training with clinical material, it is best to begin with videotapes. Transcripts alone are hard to learn from because novice raters find the auditory and visual cues very helpful. Third, raters watch a videotaped interview, make their notes (or use an accompanying transcript if available), and rate, learning the scales and other manual material as they go. During training, the rater should justify each rating by reference to the appropriate defense scale items (1b, or 2c&d, etc.). Fourth, it is best to have expert ratings available for the practice session as a gold standard, against which raters can compare and discuss their ratings. Fifth, teaching in small groups is better than one to one, because learning benefits from a variety of comments beyond one's own whether right or wrong. Four to six is an optimal number. In larger training groups, individuals do not get enough chance to talk and therefore actively learn. Finally, raters usually need to rate five practice tapes, then rate five to ten more, and either form a consensus in pairs or get expert corrective feedback. At this point most raters are quite reliable, although increasing experience results leads to increments in validity.

Methods of Comparing DMRS Defense Scores

It is possible to make cross-sectional group comparisons using either the qualitative or quantitative scoring methods. However, for detecting change over time within subjects, only the quantitative scoring method is recommended because it is much more sensitive than the qualitative method. The descriptive scores described below are all capable of detecting change.

Individual Defense Score

Subjects or groups can be compared by examining the score for any individual defense. An example of such a comparison might be to test the following hypothesis about the dynamics of obsessive–compulsive symptoms: "Do patients with obsessive–compulsive disorder score higher than depressives on the presence of isolation of affect, reaction formation, and displacement?" Another example might be to use individual defenses at intake to predict some occurrence in a subsequent psychotherapy such as: "Does the presence of acting out or passive aggression predict premature termination?"

Defense Summary Scores

Comparison of subjects or groups by the defense summary scores is statistically more powerful because summing three or four defenses produces longer scales, which are more sensitive to group differences, and higher reliability. Analyses of this type demonstrated that (a) borderline psychopathology correlated with action and major image-distorting (formerly borderline level) defenses, (b) antisocial psychopathology correlated with disavowal and minor image-distorting (formerly narcissistic) defenses, and (c) bipolar type II affective disorder correlated with obsessional defenses (Perry & Cooper, 1986).

Overall Defense Maturity Score and the Hierarchy of Adaptation

All the defense scores can be summarized by an Overall Defense Maturity score. This is calculated by multiplying each defense by a weight according to its place in the overall seven-point hierarchy of defenses [see

TABLE 8.1. The DMRS hierarchy of adaptation: defense and defense levels.

7 High adaptive level (mature)	Affilliation, altruism, anticipation, humor, self-assertion, self-observation, sublimation, suppression
6 Obsessional level	Intellectualization, isolation of affect, undoing
5 Other neurotic level	(a) Repression, dissociation
	(b) Reaction formation, displacement
4 Minor image-distorting level	Devaluation, idealization, omnipotence
3 Disavowal level	Denial, projection, rationalization
	Although not a disavowal defense, autistic fantasy is scored at this level
2 Major image-distorting level (borderline)	Splitting of other's images, splitting of self-images, projective identification
1 Action level	Acting out, hypochondriasis, passive aggression

below] and taking the weighted average of all the defenses rated in the session. Based on experience with the DMRS (Perry, 1990b; Perry & Cooper, 1989) and on reviews of existing studies (Perry & Cooper, 1987), the defenses can be grouped into seven levels, reflecting their place in the hierarchical relationship to measures of adaptiveness. The defense levels and weights and their individual defenses are shown in Table 8.1. Although the theoretical limits of the overall defense maturity score are 1 to 7, in clinical samples scores based on whole interviews usually range between 2.5 and 6.0, using either qualitative or quantitative scoring methods.

Important Considerations Regarding Different Data Sources

We have found that different data sources provide information biases that affect the identification of defenses. We describe six source conditions and their apparent effects below, moving from more to less optimal.

Videotaped Interview Plus Transcript

In observing a videotaped interview, having a remote control makes it easier to stop and review parts of the session; without it one is less likely to take the time to review difficult sections. The major advantage of the videotaped playback of the interview is the relative completeness of the data. The rater can see affect expressed, behavior, body language, and interaction between the patient and interviewer. Silences are more interpretable if you can see what is occurring, such as in the case of behavior indicating displacement (e.g., a patient appears anxious, then takes one minute to light a cigarette). Certain behaviors might be missed altogether. In one example the transcript displayed only the therapist's remark: "May I sit down?" whereas the videotape record showed the patient starting the session by putting her feet up on the therapist's chair before he sat down, which was clearly scorable as acting out (acting in the transference). Tone of voice, which is captured on audiotape, may need further interpretation supplied by seeing the facial expression. This is especially important for identifying isolation of affect in individuals without a very expressive voice. Furthermore, behavior showing changes in concentration (facial features, body attitude) may punctuate changes in topics and defenses, which are harder to discern without the visual record. The availability of a transcript of the interview material allows the rater to concentrate more fully on the interview at hand. Otherwise, having to record speech verbatim or other observations distracts from the tasks of observing and identifying defenses. Fewer defenses are missed when transcripts are available. The lack of a transcript increases the error among raters, especially in making quantitative ratings. The identification of certain defenses is improved by an accurate transcript. When considering displacement, for instance, material earlier or later in the interview may need to be reviewed to identify a conflictual person or issue away from whom affect is being directed. Finally, a transcript may allow other potential ratings, such as rating the therapist's interventions as to which defenses they address, or examining the defensive response to the interventions.

Audiotape Plus Transcript

While missing the visual information, an audio recording allows one to hear many nonlexical aspects of speech, including intonation, pauses in speech, and prolonged silences. Given a transcript, the information loss moving from video to audio recording appears less deleterious than if

TABLE 8.2. Effects of rating defense from a transcript without audio recording.

Humor	One needs to hear the delivery to discern the meaning. Reading a joke is not the same as hearing one told, and hearing may help to differentiate whether a subject is trashing him- or herself or laughing at personal foibles.
Isolation of affect	One may hear evidence of feelings when the transcript is devoid of emotionally laden words. Alternately, without listening to the audio portion, one may incorrectly infer the presence of affect whenever the subject uses words with emotional meaning, whereas the audio recording would show that no feeling were expressed.
Undoing	Repeated expressions, such as "I don't know," can be difficult to interpret without the voice quality, which would indicate whether an expression was meant to negate the preceding statement or whether it is used as filler like "ummh . . ."
Repression versus denial	Nonlexical aspects of speech help in determining whether the person is searching for an idea that cannot be found or is convinced that the idea is not present, as evidenced by a vehement tone of voice.
Dissociation	The onset of dissociation is often accompanied by a change in tone of voice to a wispy, quiet, or distant tone of voice.
Reaction formation	Tone of voice helps in discerning whether an affect has really been turned into its opposite.
Devaluation	The tone of voice helps differentiate whether certain common phrases are meant to disparage or merely to punctuate speech in a colorful way.
Idealization	Idealization may be missed if the text contains few superlatives, whereas it is highlighted by an enthusiastic tone of voice.
Rationalization	A conning or histrionic tone of voice can be very helpful in discerning an attempt to disguise a motive.
Passive aggression	Whenever in response to a therapist's question or comment, a patient says "no" or ignores something said, the tone of voice and manner of speaking indicates whether anger is indirectly conveyed.
Hypochondriasis	Help-rejecting, complaining, or whining tones of voice help underline the defensive expression of covert aggression alongside helplessness.

transcripts are used alone. Table 8.2 displays the adverse effects of absence of the sound portion.

Videotape Alone

Without a transcript, too much of the rater's attention is diverted into notetaking. This slows down the rating process and results in inevitable loss of data. While using multiple raters somewhat mitigates the information loss, raters fail to end up with the same verbatim transcripts, resulting in rating somewhat different interviews. In particular, defenses more likely to be missed are those that are better discerned by juxtaposing disparate parts of the session, something readily done when reviewing a transcript. Examples of this are splitting (e.g., describing an "all good" self-image at one point, then an "all bad" object image later) and reaction formation (e.g., expressing the wish for a girlfriend at one point but later claiming to hate women). Reviewing the transcript protects against getting caught up in the momentary story but missing the bigger picture. When transcripts are not available, there is a slight advantage to rating videotapes over audiotapes.

Audiotape Alone

The considerations noted for videotape alone apply.

Transcript Alone

If a transcript contains only several instances of humor, isolation, hypochondriasis, and the like, the lower sensitivity of a text-based data source may result in missing them altogether. However, this source will still capture some instances of those defenses if they occur at high prevalence. Thus the disadvantages of this condition have greatest effect on defenses that are better identified with their affective and behavioral cues intact.

Interviewer Alone

When the individual doing the interviewing also rates the session later without the aid of a transcript or recording, information loss and bias are most serious. In this case, the interviewer–rater's attention is divided initially into interviewing and observing tasks and later into reconstructing the session and rating tasks. However, if provided with either a transcript or audio recording, the interviewer can rate as efficiently as in any condition, using the aid to reconstruct the interview more fully. Overall, ratings from different data sources are not strictly comparable, because loss of information biases the sensitivity with which raters can identify individual defenses. While this is qualitatively clear, the exact amount of bias is yet to be determined for each defense.

Reliability of Rating Psychotherapy Sessions

The authors and colleagues rated one or two consecutive sessions early in the course of psychotherapy from eight patients who gave permission to have their sessions audiotaped and studied. Two raters listened to the audiotaped session and followed a written transcript, blind to subject identity and session number. Sessions were presented in random order. Raters independently marked each defense on the transcript and tallied each occurrence for each defense to yield a quantitative profile of defenses. The Overall Defense Maturity score was then calculated for the session, using the seven-point weighting system of the overall hierarchy of defenses. Raters subsequently discussed and arrived at consensus ratings for each session. The interrater reliability of the individual defense scores (prior to consensus discussion) based on 11 sessions yielded a median intraclass R of .70 (range .43–.83). The figures for the last seven sessions rated all exceeded .70, demonstrating effects of increasing rater experience. The Overall Defense Maturity scores across the 11 sessions demonstrated an intraclass $R = .89$. Neither figure represents the gain in reliability that would accrue from using consensus ratings. An estimate of the stability of Overall Defense Maturity score was obtained by comparing two sequential sessions from each individual. This yielded a Pearson's $r = .90$, suggesting a high one-week stability for this summary statistic of defensive functioning.

A second reliability study was conducted using transcripts only from six therapy sessions from another sample of individuals. All but one of the raters had participated in the reliability study above. Ratings were made by two raters independently. Four trained raters scored one or two sessions each, while the fifth rater (CJP) scored each session. Interrater reliability was calculated prior to the consensus. The median intraclass R was .75 (range .58–.92). In the two studies above, reliabilities were comparable whether transcript plus audio recording or transcript alone had been used. The slight gain in the second study probably reflected greater rater experience.

Potential Significance of Studying Defenses in Psychotherapy

An intriguing consequence of studying defenses as basic psychological mechanisms is that they can be viewed either as outcome or as process phenomena in psychotherapy. Defenses can be assessed at the outset of therapy and periodically reassessed as a measure of dynamic functioning. Because of the empirical support for the hierarchy of adaptation, improvement in the Overall Defense Maturity score or its constituent defenses represents improved underlying dynamic functioning. However, taking a microanalytic perspective, the individual use of a defense can be examined as an appropriate unit of psychological functioning to elucidate the process of change in psychotherapy. We suggest several areas to pursue.

1. A common complaint about descriptive diagnosis is that it does not offer useful predictions for treatment considerations. By contrast, defense mechanisms have the potential to offer a good dynamic diagnosis relevant for treatment (Bloch, Shear, Markowitz, Leon, & Perry, in press). Studies are needed that examine defenses at the outset of therapy and what they predict in the treatment. For instance, whenever the least adaptive defenses predominate (e.g., action and major image distorting), such findings should predict regressive and impulsive phenomena that require very different therapeutic interventions from those that are appropriate when obsessional or repressive–dissociative defenses predominate. These predictive relationships should be systematically studied.

2. There is a need to address questions about the lawful relationships between external stressors, affects, and salient motives (wishes and fears) and the patterns of defensive functioning. For instance, when repression–dissociation defenses predominate, there may be greater than chance associations to past sexual trauma and to current stressful triggering experiences that have sexual meanings. Given that a patient may be unaware of the current relevance of such past and current experiences, therapy would be aided by knowing what has proven empirically to be related to certain defenses. The therapist would have guideposts as to what to look for.

3. Research can also describe the associations between a patient's defensive responses and the preceding and subsequent therapist's intervention. Dynamic hypotheses about successful and unsuccessful interventions can be tested, given that defenses are a meaningful focus for assessing the patient's psychology in action. One dynamic hypothesis suggests that therapists focus interventions on defensive operations as a precursor to addressing the conflictual content triggering the defenses. This hypothesis is readily accessible to testing by, first, identifying the patient's defensive responses, and second, categorizing the therapist's intervention as to whether they address the defense and do so accurately, or whether they address something else, such as an affective response or an underlying conflict. The efficacy of the different types of intervention can be judged by subsequent improvements or decrements in the patient's overall defensive functioning either inside or outside the session. This is only one intriguing approach the authors have been exploring.

Because defenses can be viewed both as process phenomena (psychological mechanisms in action) and at the same time, when aggregated, as an outcome measure, the study of defenses may have great clinical relevance. As a result, the scientific and clinical value of assessing defenses appears to be very promising and exciting.

References

Bloch, A.L., Shear, M.K., Markowitz, J.C., Leon, A.C., & Perry, J.C. (in press) An empirical study of defense mechanisms in dysthymia. *American Journal of Psychiatry*.

Bond, M., Perry, J.C., Gautier, M., Goldenberg, M., Oppenheimer, J., & Simand, J. (1989) Validating the self-report of defense styles. *Journal of Personality Disorders, 3*, 101–112.

Perry, J.C. (1988) A prospective study of life stress, defenses, psychotic symptoms and depression in borderline and antisocial personality disorders and bipolar type II affective disorder. *Journal of Personality Disorders, 2*, 49–59.

Perry, J.C. (1990a) *The Defense Mechanism Rating Scales manual* (5th ed.). Copyright by J.C. Perry, M.D., Cambridge, MA.

Perry, J.C. (1990b) Psychological defense mechanisms in the study of affective and anxiety disorders. In J. Maser & C.R. Cloninger (Eds.), *Co-morbidity in anxiety and mood disorders* (pp. 545–562). Washington, DC: American Psychiatric Press.

Perry, J.C. & Cooper, S.H. (1986) A preliminary report on defenses and conflicts associated with borderline personality disorder. *Journal of the American Psychoanalytical Association, 34*, 865–895.

Perry, J.C. & Cooper, S.H. (1987) Empirical studies of psychological defense mechanisms. In R. Michels & J.O. Cavenar (Eds.), *Psychiatry: Vol. I* (pp. 1–19). New York: Basic Books.

Perry, J.C. & Cooper, S.H. (1989) An empirical study of defense mechanisms. I. Clinical interview and life vignette ratings. *Archives of General Psychiatry, 46*, 444–452.

Part III
Personality and Applied Psychology

9
Causal Attributions of Disease as Related to Dynamic Personality Variables

GUDMUND J.W. SMITH and GUNILLA VAN DER MEER

What do we believe to be the cause of failure and success, of illness and health? Weiner et al. (1971) were among the first in a succession of theorists to systematically analyze causal attributions, characterizing them with respect to stability, locus, control, etc., and relating them to such factors as academic achievement and future expectations. Most studies were confined to the laboratory. Causal thinking in illness situations had been studied even before that (e.g., Mabry, 1964). This interest bred speculations about how knowledge about an individual's causal attributions could possibly increase the accuracy of predictions of his success or failure in coping with future life events. A study by Lowery and Jacobsen (1985) particularly investigated the association between causal attributions of disease and the course of illness in different patient groups. Neither here nor in other studies of this kind was the outcome particularly clear-cut. A general feature of most studies of the causal attributions of disease has been the reference to the subjects' own illness. Much less effort has been invested in finding out how people generally picture the causes of health and illness, and particularly the problem of how causal attributions relate to a subject's personality characteristics. The present study is a first, unassuming attempt to address this topic.

The subjects have been elderly, normal people, most of them engaged in another study (Smith & van der Meer, 1990). The personality description is based on a projective, so-called Percept-Genetic (PG) test particularly suited to the analysis of anxiety and defensive strategies. The subjects' choice of health–illness attributions was defined by two case descriptions. The formulation of tentative hypotheses must have to wait until we have presented our test instruments.

Method

The Meta-Contrast Technique (MCT) was developed based on experiments with subliminal perception (e.g., Smith & Henriksson, 1955). The percept-genetic model forming the theoretical background of the test has been presented elsewhere (e.g., Kragh & Smith, 1970).

In the present context the following outline of the model would be most relevant. An individual confronted with a new situation is apt to react with a general state of readiness or arousal, implying mobilization of accumulated adaptive resources. When, after reiterated fixations, the person has received more information, the mobilization is gradually, often rapidly, relaxed and more specialized functions are delegated to take care of the adaptive task. Or, to view the process from a bottom-up perspective (cf. Brown, 1988): the initial stages (P-stages) of a percept-genesis are characterized by a very varied spectrum of contents, often dominated by primitive levels in the experiential hierarchy and only to a small extent restricted by sensorial constraints. During the ultrashort percept-genesis, however, irrelevant and person-proximal contents are "peeled off," leaving a gradually more prominent nucleus of stimulus–proximal contents. In other words, as the percept-genesis proceeds it becomes less marked by "subcortical" functions and more by "cortical" ones.

Experiments with subliminal perception proved that a supraliminal percept can be affected by a temporally proximal subliminal process. Hence, this technique offered a way to indirectly gain access to early stages in a perceptual process. By combining a subliminal methodology with the percept-genetic one, it would be possible to find out how a new perceptual process might influence the individual's established perceptual frame of reference. If, as in Kragh's (1985) Defense Mechanism Test (DMT), the "new" stimulation implied a threat to the established percept, particularly interesting information might be gained about the viewer.

Procedure

The MCT implies repeated tachistoscopic presentations of pairs of stimuli, one of them exposed immediately before the other. (see Chapter 7 for an extensive description of the MCT).

There are two MCT series. Only one of them was used here. The A stimulus depicts a threatening face, the B stimulus a lonely young person with whom the viewer is supposed to identify (the "hero").

The subject was instructed as follows:

Pictures will be shown on the screen in front of you. They will be presented at very short exposure times. I'll say "now" before each exposure. Be prepared to look at the screen and then tell me what you saw. Please, make special note of any changes from one exposure to the next.

Scoring

The scoring refers to changes in reports of B and interpretations of A. The sequential aspect is always important. What is scored late in a series is supposed to represent more manifest tendencies than what is reported early, the reason being that late phases are closer to the individual's habitual level of experiencing.

There are two main groups of signs: signs of anxiety and signs of defense against anxiety (cf. Chapter 7). These were the most frequent sign groups:

The group of anxiety signs. Most signs in this group represented light anxiety: nonhuman structures at the place of A are reported as disintegrating; black structures appear before the last third of the series; vague structures are seen (e.g., a rain-streaked window). Only in a few subjects were signs of more accentuated anxiety scored, like darkness late in the test series.

The group of repressive signs. These consisted of (a) typical histrionic signs (e.g., the threat is reported as a statue, a doll, or some other stiff but stimulus-proximal object) or is dressed up or masked and (b) the reports are stimulus-distant (e.g., a house, a tree, a projector).

The group of isolation signs. In the majority of cases the threat was covered by a white spot, a screen, curtains, etc. Other signs implied denial of the threat or reports of a threat turning his neck to the viewer.

Standardization Data

Details of standardization data can be found in the most recent manual (Smith, Johnson, & Almgren, 1989) (see also Chapter 7).

Reliability of the Present Scoring

Interrater reliability is mostly a question of distinct categories and training. The scoring of one part of our subjects (the selenium group) was done by three scorers with a high degree of agreement as reported in Johanson et al. (1990). The next group (the pensioners' group) was scored by the present authors; the scoring was practically unanimous (Smith & van der Meer, 1990). The remaining 16 subjects were scored by van der Meer alone.

The Cases

The subjects were asked to read the following case stories of Martha and Erna, written by Hentschel and Kießling (1989). Two 65-year-old ladies are chatting about their health. *Martha* finds no reason to complain. She broke her leg last year, an incident still causing some inconvenience, but apart from that she has no ailments. In contrast, *Erna* does not feel well: for 20 years she has suffered from stomach troubles. During that period she has been operated on three times for gastric ulcer. She must pay careful attention to what and how much she eats and be very punctual with her meals. In spite of her careful choice of food, she cannot give up medication and risk making her symptoms worse. She is constantly anxious about losing weight, feels relatively weak and brittle, and avoids strain as far as possible.

During their talk it becomes apparent that Martha had gastric ulcer 20 years ago. But her symptoms lasted only a few weeks before the ulcer healed completely. Thereafter she has not felt any symptoms. Both ladies ask themselves why Martha's ulcer healed so quickly while Erna's became chronic.

After having read the stories and the alternatives, the subjects were asked to choose four statements to explain why Martha had remained reasonably healthy and Erna was less fortunate in regaining her health: They were told to mark the most important one with 1, the next with 2, etc.

Martha examines a number of alternatives:

126. I was always a very healthy child.
127. I have always gone in for athletics and been in good physical shape.
128. I come of a decidedly sound family; in our home illness was very rare.
129. When I fell ill I had lived through a critical period, but on the whole I have an equanimous mood without abrupt ups-and-downs and no depressive periods.
130. I have always been very active and have a strong will. That is apt to make illness disappear quickly.
131. It has always been important to me not to let myself be dulled but instead to retain my sensitivity. In my job, moreover, I could use a great deal of fantasy and that helps one to conquer illness.
132. My marriage was very harmonious; my husband was of great help during that time.
133. I also asked my friends for advice when things have got into a mess. Good advice helps one to keep well.
134. I did not want to miss my work, where I was needed. Anyhow, I wanted to return, fit for work, as soon as possible to the project where I was engaged and which afforded me great joy.
135. As long as I was still sick I spared myself, in spite of everything; not until the ulcer symptoms had disappeared completely did I go back to work.
136. One of the doctors I consulted wanted to operate at once, but I declined and I believe that was a wise decision.
137. The internist who treated me wrote out a prescription for a fantastic medicine and then the symptoms quickly faded away.

Subjects were asked to identify the four most important reasons why Martha got well so quickly and remained well.

Erna also examines a number of alternatives to explain her chronic course of illness.

138. I was always sickly as a child.
139. In my mother's family there were some members with stomach troubles.

140. Physically, I was not particularly hardy.
141. Even mentally I was quite unstable.
142. I was always very dependent: my mother used to say that Erna cannot do anything all by herself.
143. I could never properly enjoy anything or feel genuine grief.
144. I cannot describe my marriage as really disharmonious, but we seem to have lived side by side without close contact.
145. Strictly speaking, I have never had any friends whom I could ask for advice or who were willing to support me.
146. My work was never particularly exciting but made me dissatisfied in the long run.
147. When my first symptoms of gastric ulcer appeared I had just taken a new job and did not want to report sick at the risk of losing it.
148. After a few months, when my health had deteriorated, my doctor wanted to operate as soon as possible in order to bring about a quick improvement. I do not think that was a good idea.
149. When the stomach troubles recurred it was a long time before the doctor could find a medicine which was at least of some help.

Subjects were asked to identify the four most important reasons why Erna, after her first stomach ulcer, developed a chronic illness and were instructed to number their selections as before.

Subjects

There were three groups of subjects in the main study. One group included 32 subjects (13 men, 19 women), aged 70–72 years and originally tested in a selenium project at the Gerontology Research Center in Lund. The next group came from a pensioners' association. There were 26 subjects (8 men, 18 women), aged 67–86 years (median 70 years). In a third group of 16 (4 men, 12 women) the age range was 57–78 (median 73) years. The first two groups were predominantly middle class, about half of them with an education beyond secondary school. The third group was entirely working class.

For the purpose of cross-validating the results, we used a group of 25 subjects (6 men and 19 women) with a median age of 41 and an age span of 25–59 years. They suffered from Crohn's disease.

Hypotheses

In an earlier study that involved part of the present sample (Smith & van der Meer, 1990), we found an association between creativity and active self-involvement in the responses to the two cases. For creative people, one's own efforts at mastering symptoms were the best way to health.

Creativity was not included in this study, partly because all subjects could not take the creativity test and partly because we did not want to limit our study to a creativity perspective but to include a broader spectrum of personality characteristics. Still, we have some knowledge about how creativity is related to various types of defense as defined by the MCT (Smith & Carlsson, 1990).

Judging from research (e.g., Weiner et al., 1971), we ought to consider the importance of the locus of causal attributions (e.g., outside or inside the individual himself). Outside causes could refer either to deterministic alternatives, like being born in a healthy family, or to reliance on authority, like the doctor's prescriptions.

Our hypotheses could not be chiseled in detail. Instead we formulated some more general assumptions.

1. People scoring for anxiety in the MCT ought to be more dependent on trusted authority figures.

2. People with stimulus-distant reinterpretations of the threat, a scoring category shown to be positively associated with creativity, could be assumed to place their locus of control inside themselves (i.e., to prefer psychologizing alternatives to explain Martha's way to health and Erna's to continued illness).

3. People with more primitive or histrionic signs of repression would probably choose alternatives in a category similar to those above, but on a more superficial level, involving more external fuss.

4. The use of isolating (obsessive) types of defense in the MCT is likely to correlate with an external locus of control. Isolation has been shown to correlate negatively with creativity, and isolation implies exclusion of subjective–emotional factors from the causal context. Among possible alternatives for isolating subjects are those in which control is placed in the hands of others and those referring to deterministic, nonpsychological factors, perhaps with a preponderance of the latter.

Results

Cluster Analyses

To bring more order among the 24 alternatives and their correlations with the MCT scoring groups, we performed a series of cluster analyses of the Ward type, a method designed to optimize the minimum variance within clusters (Aldenfelder & Blashfield, 1984). Based on squared Euclidean distances, the Ward analysis provides valid estimates of the connections in fourfold tables. The first analysis (I) included all single MCT variables but no group sums, the second analysis (II) included these variables in double dose; that is, in II we gave MCT more power. Five clusters were described in each analysis. In the I clusters there were 12, 19, 14, 7, 27 subjects, and in the II clusters 15, 27, 12, 13, 7. These two cluster solutions are described in some detail below and summarized in Table 9.1.

TABLE 9.1. Schematic overview of the cluster analyses.

Cluster	MCT signs	Case alternatives[a]
	First analysis	
I:1	Stimulus-distant transformations	Psychological (131, 134, 142, 144, 146)
I:3	Isolation	Deterministic (126, 128, 138, 139, 140)
I:4	Isolation	Deterministic (126, 129, 135, 142)
I:5	Anxiety	Doctor's orders (135, 137, 147, 149)
		Other (129)
	Second analysis	
II:1	Histrionic repression	Surface psychological (130, 142)
II:2	Anxiety	Doctor's orders (137, 147)

[a] Figures in parentheses correspond to the preformulated alternatives in the Martha and Erna cases given in the text.

In cluster I:1 stimulus-distant transformations of the threat were significantly (which here generally refers to the .01 or .001 p level) associated with alternatives 131, 134, 142, and 144, together forming a psychological index. No. 146 is also associated with this cluster but has a more stereotyped tinge, chosen by 43% of the subjects. No. 132, the most popular of all alternatives (51%) failed to appear here.

In cluster II:1 a stiffened threat is associated with 130 and 142, the former referring to a strong will, the latter also being part of the psychological index. Since both types of MCT signs belong to the greater repression group, a certain overlap between the scales was expected. Still, 130 and 142 concern more outside signs of psychological autonomy than 131, 134, and 144, where engagement in a task or with other people seems more important.

Clusters I:3 and 4 are both characterized by the most typical sign of isolation (the threat is covered up) and by the case Martha alternative 126. In I:3, 126 is accompanied by the natural associates 128, 138, 139, and 140. In I:4, 129, 135, and 142 are added. But they are, first of all, different from the foregoing ones and, moreover, also belong to other clusters.

Clusters I:5 and II:2 are both characterized by anxiety. In cluster I:5 the case alternatives are 129, 135, 137, 147, and 149, of which the four latter ones naturally combine to a "doctor's orders" scale. Nos. 137 and 147 also appear in II:2.

On the basis of these findings we constructed four indices.

1. Psychology, including alternatives 131, 134, 142, and 144 (±146).
2. Biological determinism, including alternatives 126, 128, 138, 139, and 140.
3. Doctor's orders, including alternatives 135, 137, 147, and 149.
4. Surface psychology, including alternatives 130 and 142.

Two additional cluster analyses were then performed. In III, the indices above were included. A stiffened threat in MCT appeared in two clusters, where it significantly covaried with index 4. Anxiety appeared in two other clusters, where it significantly covaried with index 3. In analysis IV, the MCT signs were summed up as anxiety, repression, isolation, and sensitivity. Isolation and anxiety correlated in two clusters significantly with index 2 and index 3. It was obvious that the ranking of alternatives was of subordinate importance.

Comparisons with the MCT

To further highlight what the cluster analyses have just demonstrated in a general way, we present a few direct comparisons between the indices and the MCT results. Table 9.2 compares stimulus-distant repression with index 1. When 146 is included in the scale, we get the results within parentheses. A median cutting yields a χ^2 of 6.22 ($p < .02$, df = 1). With the trisection shown in the table, we get $\chi^2 = 9.11$ ($p < .01$, df = 2). If 146 is included, the χ^2 increases to 12.45. The result is not quite unequivocal. But it is still obvious that stimulus-distant repression is associated with strong preference for psychological attributions. The more primitive or histrionic signs of repression (a stiffened or masked threat), on the other hand, are most closely associated with index 4 ($p < .01$).

The dominant group of defenses besides stimulus-distant repression was isolation. If we select two groups of subjects, one with stimulus-distant signs of repression but no signs of isolation, the other with isolation but no signs of repression, we get significant differences between them, both with respect to index 1 and index 2, the contrast being particularly marked with respect to the former ($\chi^2 = 10.77$, $p = .001$, df = 1).

Adding all signs of isolation and including the entire sample (Table 9.3) we find a highly significant correlation with the deterministic index 2 ($\chi^2 = 10.89$, $p < .001$, df = 1).

TABLE 9.2. Stimulus-distant transformations in the MCT and the psychological index.

MCT	Number of psychological alternative (131, 134, 142, 144) chosen from the Marthe and Erna cases				
	4	3	2	1	0
Stimulus-distant transformation	1 (3)	4 (8)	6 (1)	5 (6)	2 (0)
No such transformations	0 (2)	3 (9)	13 (19)	24 (17)	16 (9)

NOTE: Numbers within parentheses: alternative 146 included. Vertical line identifies the median.

TABLE 9.3. All signs of isolation in the MCT and the deterministic index.

MCT	Number of deterministic alternatives (126, 128, 138, 139, 140) chosen from the Martha and Erna cases	
	3–4	0–2
Isolation	13	16
No isolation	5	40

Finally, anxiety (all kinds added) is correlated with index 3 in Table 9.4. The correlation is not impressive, but significant ($\chi^2 = 6.38$, $p < .02$, df = 1).

A Cross-Validation

Since our introductory hypotheses were relatively vague, it would seem reasonable to ask whether we have unduly capitalized on chance. It is possible, however, to offer some cross-validation using the Crohn's disease group described above.

Among these subjects only three were scored for certain signs of isolation; three additional subjects were scored for isolation tendencies. None of them had the key sign of "threat covered." The fact that only one patient chose more than one deterministic alternative supports our earlier results. Moreover, among elderly subjects with isolation, 17% chose more than one psychological alternative; in the patient group, 60%.

It is difficult to make comparisons involving repression because the specific alternatives exploited above were very rare in the patient group. However, 56% of them were scored for types of repression considered to be more primitive than the stimulus-distant variety. The corresponding figure representing stimulus-proximal repression among the elderly was 35%. It is thus noteworthy that 40% of the patients choosing more than one psychological alternative preferred to include item 142, one of

TABLE 9.4. Anxiety in the MCT and the doctor's orders index.

MCT	Number of doctor's orders alternatives (135, 137, 147, 149) chosen from the Martha and Erna cases	
	≥2	0–1
Anxiety	21	14
No anxiety	12	27

the pseudopsychological alternatives typical of subjects with histrionic varieties of repression. Among the elderly, only 20% made such a choice (a chi-squared calculation yielding $p = .05$).

The doctor's orders group of alternatives constitutes a special problem among patients who depend very much on contact with a specialist. As many as 76% of them used at least one alternative involving a doctor's advice; only 54% among the elderly ($p = .05$). Here theoretical attributions of causal factors are influenced by harsh reality.

Discussion

In spite of the supporting tendencies just presented, we must interpret our results with caution. What is generalizable about them is that causal attributions are not a purely cognitive affair but are colored by personality factors. However, the personality factors are not exhausted by the groups of MCT signs isolated here. Nor are the possible alternatives limited to the present groupings of indices. In one study (Smith & van der Meer, 1990), the most "active and self-involved" alternatives in the case of Martha (126, 127, 130, 131, 132, 133, 136) were particularly typical of creative individuals. Other cases and alternatives other than those formulated here may also yield positive results.

Let us, then, consider the present MCT groups in combination with the relevant indices. Stimulus-distant or transformed interpretations imply that the MCT threat is handled with a certain degree of freedom and flexibility, on a symbolic level. It is instructive that these signs are often found in the protocols of creative people, of whom a typical characteristic is the tendency to construct their world from inside out. The psychological alternatives preferred by this MCT group focus on sensitivity and fantasy (131), delight at work (134, 146), dependency (142), and close matrimonial contact (144) as central factors in conquering illness. In other words, the person himself is made responsible for the course of illness.

The histrionic, stimulus-proximal interpretations belong to the same overall category of MCT signs but do not correlate with creativity. Histrionic subjects are usually considered to be rather more concerned with appearances than with inner substance and are likely to be tempted to use opportunistic slogans. The pseudopsychological alternatives preferred by them include importance of a strong will (130) and again the negative role of dependency. The first of these explanations is typically shallow. The second one differs from the other psychological alternatives in that it is the least specific, not relating to an interesting task or a life partner, but very generally to character weakness, the very opposite of a strong will. Thus, item 142 may fit both index 1 and index 4.

Signs of isolation clearly relate to obsessive–compulsive symptoms or character traits. Isolation means that inside, emotional factors are replaced by outside ones. The deterministic alternatives include a healthy childhood or family (126, 128), a sickly childhood or family (138, 139), or physical weakness as a permanent, fateful trait (140). Illness and health are thus explained with reference to a permanent disposition, something for which the person is not responsible.

Anxious people are inclined to rely on the help of others. The doctor's orders alternatives, which are specifically related to them, include reliance on medical prescription defined as medicine (137, 149) or rest (135, 147). Like the group 2 index, these alternatives place the cause of illness outside the person, but in the hands of a benign authority figure, the doctor, rather than impersonal fate.

Looking at the tables one will find considerable overlap in the causal attributions of health and illness between the MCT categories. The remarkable thing is that choices are still not made wholly at random but are to some extent steered by how the individual is used to handling a threatening situation, his degree of anxiety, and his defensive style. It cannot be maintained that factors other than these dynamic personality variables do not influence the choice of causal attributions, factors related to factual knowledge and real personal experience. But dynamic variables remain crucial, particularly when the choice is mainly theoretical.

References

Aldenfelder, M.S. & Blashfield, R.K. (1984) *Cluster analysis*. Beverly Hills, CA: Sage.

Brown, J.W. (1988) *Life of the mind. Selected papers*. Englewood Cliffs, NJ: Prentice Hall.

Hentschel, W. & Ricßling (1989) Interviewen: Krankheit und Gesundheit [Interview: Illness and health]. University of Mainz, mimeographed.

Johanson, A., Gustafson, L., Smith, G.J.W., Risberg, J., Hagberg, B., & Nilsson, B. (1990) Adaptation in different types of dementia in normal and elderly subjects. *Dementia, 1*, 95–101.

Kragh, U. (1985) *Defense Mechanism Test-DMT Manual*. Stockholm: Persona.

Kragh, U. & Smith, G.J.W. (Eds.) (1970) *Percept-genetic analysis*. Lund: Gleerup.

Lowery, B.J. & Jacobsen, B.S. (1985) Attributional analysis of chronic illness outcomes. *Nursing Research, 34*, 82–88.

Mabry, J.H. (1964) Lay concepts of etiology. *Journal of Chronic Diseases, 17*, 371–386.

Smith, G.J.W. & Carlsson, I. (1990) The creative process. *Psychological Issues, Monogr. 57*. Madison, CT: International Universities Press.

Smith, G.J.W. & Henriksson, M. (1955) The effect on an established percept of a perceptual process beyond awareness. *Acta Psychologica, 11*, 346–355.

Smith, G.J.W., Johnson, G., & Almgren, P.E. (1989) *MCT—The Meta-Contrast Technique*. Stockholm: Psykologiförlaget.

Smith, G.J.W. & van der Meer, G. (1990) Creativity in old age. *Creativity Research Journal, 3*, 249–264.

Weiner, B., Frieze, D., Kukla, A., Reed, L., Rest, S., & Rosenbaum, R. (1971) *Perceiving the causes of success and failure*. Morristown, NJ: General Learning Press.

10
Exploration of the Relationship Between Anxiety and Defense: Semantic Differential Ratings of Defense Mechanism Test Stimuli

Juris G. Draguns

This chapter presents the preliminary account of a series of studies designed to test empirically the interplay of anxiety and defense in the process of gradual recognition of personally arousing or threatening stimuli. Even though all the findings from this research program are not yet available, the justification for this interim report lies in the possible heuristic value in stimulating further study of the relationship between anxiety and defenses.

Such a relationship is basic for the classical psychoanalytic formulation of defense. As Rangell (1978) has pointed out, all defenses are preceded by anxiety. The original link, articulated by Freud (1963, 1964), posited the anxiety-reducing function of defense. Based on clinical observation and inference, this hypothesized relationship has seen little investigation under controlled, experimental conditions. The development of the Defense Mechanism Test (DMT) (Kragh, 1985) has opened the way for the investigation of defenses in response to gradually emerging personally arousing or threatening stimuli. Their valence is established on the basis of theoretical considerations and empirical observations. It is assumed that the representation of parental disapproval (e.g., scowling face of a father or mother figure) or the prospect of physical violence or attack (a powerful, threatening man ready to pounce on his female victim) is experienced as aversive anywhere by anyone. Yet the actual feelings aroused are not recorded or measured, but are plausibly inferred from the subsequent defensive responses elicited by these stimuli. Operationally, defenses in the DMT are defined as distortions of the peripheral threatening stimulus prior to its veridical recognition. Thus anxiety assumes the status of a hypothetical construct that bridges the gap between the visually presented threat and the verbal, defensive response to it.

The Experiment

The present series of studies was undertaken to convert anxiety from a hypothetical construct to empirical stimulus. To this end, the question is asked: How does the person experience the allegedly threatening stimulus? Possible ways of recording such responses include psychophysiological indicators of autonomic arousal which, however, stand in a complex and imperfect relationship to the psychological experience of anxiety (cf. Fröhlich, 1982). Because of that, the decision in the present research was made in favor of psychological signs. The semantic differential (Osgood, Suci, & Tannenbaum, 1957) provides such an avenue of measurement. As is well known, factor analyses have repeatedly identified the triad of Evaluation (E), Activity (A), and Potency (P) factors. Draguns (1967) provisionally equated the conjunction of low E, and high A and P with the manifestation of anxiety. This operational definition is particularly germane to the objectives of the present research. For the purpose of these studies, anxiety is construed as an aversive state which a person goes to great lengths to terminate or reduce. Major means of bringing about this end are the defense mechanisms. Therefore, the following predictions were ventured in initiating this research:

1. The DMT stimuli are rated low in E and high in P and A.
2. There is a curvilinear relationship between exposure time and E, P, and A ratings, with intermediate exposure speeds being associated with the highest P and A and the lowest E ratings.
3. More defensive responses are found at the intermediate exposure speeds rather than at the early and late stages of stimulus presentation.
4. Defensive responses to DMT stimuli are followed by a reduction in A and P and an increase in E.

In the foregoing predictions, the aversive and arousing valence of the DMT stimuli was ascribed to their anxiety-inducing properties. A competing explanation, however, would attribute the combination of increased A and P and lowered E ratings to the ambiguity of tachistoscopically presented pictures, not to their personally threatening or conflict-inducing function. Moreover, there is some evidence (e.g., Beyn, Zhirmunskaya, & Volkov, 1967; Draguns, 1967; Fröhlich & Laux, 1969) that incomplete, unclear, or ambiguous stimuli elicit various psychophysiological or psychological expressions of arousal and that uncertainty reduction has a reinforcing effect on human subjects (Nicki, 1970). To resolve these competing hypotheses, stimuli parallel to the DMT slides are necessary, but without personally arousing or threatening properties. The DMT, however, does not provide such control stimuli. They were not necessary as long as the DMT was used primarily as a springboard for the elicitation of a person's characteristic mechanisms. In the present series of studies, various steps were taken to include comparison stimuli, similar in all essential respects to DMT except for the absence of the threatening human figure in the background. With the addition of these stimuli, more hypotheses could be formulated and tested:

5. Stimuli at high levels of ambiguity (i.e., short exposure time) are rated higher in A and P and lower in E than stimuli at low levels of ambiguity.
6. The relationship between ambiguity (or exposure time) and E, A, and P ratings is curvilinear, with the highest A and P ratings and lowest E ratings at the intermediate levels of ambiguity (as indexed by exposure time).
7. Fewer defensive responses are observed in response to the control stimuli than the original DMT stimuli.

Of course, the possibility can be envisaged that all the preceding predictions would receive support, with both ambiguity and personal threat engendering the combination of aversion and arousal, which for purposes of the present research was equated with anxiety. In such a case, the question of interaction between these two antecedent conditions would have to be raised. Does threat exercise an additive or perhaps even a multiplicative effect on anxiety or arousal triggered by ambiguous stimuli?

Method

The foregoing predictions were first tested in a group of 31 undergraduate students at Pennsylvania State University who volunteered their participation in this experiment. Both men and women were represented in the research sample. Gender-appropriate DMT stimuli were used; post hoc analyses revealed no differences between male and female subjects. The two neutral stimuli were usable with both genders. One of them was a photograph of a middle-aged woman talking with a younger man in the doorway of a house. The other picture was a drawing of a picnic scene of a young woman with a toddler (who looks more like a boy than a girl). Both descriptions of the stimuli at all stages of presentation and their semantic differential ratings on three E scales (good−bad; clean−dirty; beautiful−ugly), two A scales (active−passive; fast−slow), and two P scales (strong−weak, big−small) were solicited at each exposure speed. The terminal points of the semantic differential scales were counterbalanced to prevent the formation of response sets.

The standard method of presenting DMT stimuli by means of a tachistoscope was followed, beginning with the shortest exposure speeds. The exposure speeds closely corresponded to those recommended by Kragh (1985) except that a total of 12 rather than 22 exposure speeds were used. They spanned the range from 5 to 1000 ms, with a concentration of exposure levels near the short end of the continuum.

Results

To provide a brief and global presentation of the results, one-way analyses of variance provided strong confirmation of hypothesis 1 for all of the three E scales; much weaker support was registered for one of the two A scales (active–passive), while the results for both P scales were negative. Trend analyses provided evidence of quadratic trends for all three of the E scales, and one A scale (active–passive). However, linear and cubic trends were also significant. Thus some support for hypothesis 2 was obtained. While there were significant effects for defensive responses for the DMT stimuli, closer examination of the findings did not corroborate the expectation of the greatest number of defenses at intermediate levels of presentation, thereby failing to corroborate hypothesis 3. As far as the anxiety-reducing effect of the defenses on DMT semantic differential ratings is concerned, the results were highly complex and can best be described as inconclusive. As yet, hypothesis 4 has not received substantial support. In reference to hypothesis 5, there was a significant effect of exposure time as predicted on E semantic differential ratings. Upon closer inspection it appeared to be considerably weaker than the effect of threatening stimuli. Only borderline results were obtained on one A scale (active–passive) and one P scale (strong–weak). There was no substantial confirmation of the expected curvilinear effect, leading to the rejection of hypothesis 6 at this stage. Finally, there was a significantly greater number of defensive responses to the DMT than to the newer stimuli, but this finding cannot be accepted as definitive for reasons to be presented below.

Discussion

The results at this point must be considered to be provisional. Several features of the procedure and instrumentation stood in the way of implementing a conclusive test of the predictions advanced. Perhaps the most obvious of these were the discrepancies between the neutral and the DMT stimuli. The DMT stimuli consist of drawings executed in the same style, presumably by the same artist. One of the neutral pictures, however, is a photograph. It has proved to be much more easily recognizable, thereby confounding its affectively neutral valence with the impact of its physical properties. Therefore, the apparent confirmation of hypothesis 6 cannot at this point be allowed to stand. It requires confirmation by means of comparable stimuli. Such stimuli have since been prepared and are being tested.

Second, the use of the semantic differential to obtain the anxiety-relevant stimuli has brought to the fore problems which were not yet resolved at the time the research presented here was conducted. As Petrenko and Vasilenko (1977) in Russia discovered, connotative meaning of the stimuli under conditions of percept-genetic presentation is not always in synchrony with denotative meaning. More important, semantic differential ratings may affect the descriptions of the stimuli. In the follow-up research currently being conducted, the order of the ratings and descriptions was counterbalanced, and this source of error presumably was eliminated.

Third, it is not clear whether the inconclusive findings, pertaining especially to A and P, were, in part, at least, the function of the particular adjectives selected to represent these dimensions. Choosing appropriate semantic differential scales is a subtle art. To be meaningful, they must be metaphorically applicable to the object being rated. In the case of the terms used, several of the participants found them irrelevant for the ratings of the DMT and control stimuli and rated them neutral. The negative or ambiguous results obtained may not generalize to other A and P axes of appraisal. In any case, it may be worthwhile to do pilot work with other scales within these two factors.

Fourth, a somewhat speculative argument could be advanced. A possible determinant of anxiety, common to both the DMT and the neutral stimuli, could be their social content. All these pictures feature human beings, and, as many theorists would contend, all human encounters provoke anxiety. If so, the consistently low E ratings for both classes of stimuli may have been caused not by their ambiguity but by their interpersonal content.

Fifth, a major limitation of the study was the reliance on a single method of eliciting the ratings. Moreover, the ratings were verbal and thus may have been confounded by the individual differences in readiness to put into words very mild degrees of personal discomfort to miniature pictorial stimuli in an artificial laboratory situation. The semantic differential method is subject to major limitations for the task to which it was put. Since other approaches (e.g., the psychophysiological ones), are also less than optimal, for different reasons, the situation calls for a multimethod strategy. Since the elicitation of a variety of indices would be burdensome for participants, this objective could be realized in a sequential manner, either in several sessions within the same research design or in a series of parallel but independent studies.

Despite these limitations, what, if anything, has been learned in the preliminary phases of this research product? The general conclusion that is likely to hold up upon the gathering of more substantial data is that the stimuli that engender defenses also provoke anxiety. What is not at all clear at the present stage of the available evidence is how this anxiety is related to the imposition of various defenses. However, the amount of suggestive findings obtained in the course of this investigation holds out the promise that the empirical study of the anxiety–defense relationship is an undertaking that is worth pursuing.

References

Beyn, E.S., Zhirmunskaya, E.A., & Volkov, V.N. (1967) Electroencephalographic investigation of the process of recognizing images of objects during their tachistoscopic presentation. I. *Neuropsychologia*, *5*, 203–217.

Draguns, J.G. (1967) Affective meaning of reduced stimulus input: A study by means of the semantic differential. *Canadian Journal of Psychology*, *21*, 321–241.

Freud, S. (1963) Inhibitions, symptoms, and anxiety. In *The standard edition of the complete psychological works of Sigmund Freud: Vol. 20*. London: Hogarth Press.

Freud, S. (1964) The neuro-psychoses of defense. In *The standard edition of the complete psychological works of Sigmund Freud: Vol. 3* (pp. 45–61). London: Hogarth Press.

Fröhlich, W.D. (1982) *Angst: Gefahrensignale und ihre psychologische Bedeutung*. [Anxiety: Danger signals and their psychological meaning]. Munich: DTV.

Fröhlich, W.D. & Laux, L. (1969) Serielles Wahrnehmen, Aktualgenese, Informantionsintegration und Orientierungsreaktion. [Serial perception, microgenesis, information integration and reflex of orientation]. *Zeitschrift für experimentelle und angewandte Psychologie*, *16*, 250–277.

Kragh, U. (1985) *The Defense Mechanism Test*. Stockholm: Persona.

Nicki, R.M. (1970) The reinforcing effect of uncertainty reduction on a human operant. *Canadian Journal of Psychology*, *24*, 389–400.

Osgood, C.E., Suci, G.J., & Tannenbaum, P.H. (1957) *The measurement of meaning*. Urbana: University of Illinois Press.

Petrenko, V.F. & Vasilenko, S.V. (1977) O pertsevtivnoi kategorizatsii [On perceptual categorization]. *Vestnik Moskovskogo Universiteta. Seriya Psikhologiya*, *14*(1), 26–34.

Rangell, L. (1978) Defense and resistance in psychoanalysis and life. In H.P. Blum (Ed.), *Defense and resistance: Historical perspectives and current concepts* (pp. 147–174). Madison, CT: International Universities Press.

11
The Cognitive Determinants of Defense Mechanisms

SHULAMITH KREITLER and HANS KREITLER

Defense Mechanisms (DMs) are a unique set of mental operations, first described by Freud (1923/1961, 1896/1962, 1933/1964), elaborated by Anna Freud (1966), and further developed in recent decades (e.g., Cramer, 1988; Kline, 1987; Marton, 1988; Schafer, 1987; Singer, 1990). Yet, despite their popularity, little has been learned about their acquisition as strategies for conflict resolution, their selection, cognitive roots, impact on overt behavior, and relation to personality traits.

This chapter is designed to fill in some of these gaps. We start by clarifying the close relations of DMs to cognitive strategies. We will then proceed to discuss in the framework of the cognitive orientation theory their role in the input–output chain. This will lead to a new conceptualization of DMs and their relation to belief systems, which will be followed by the description of four studies predicting the occurrence of specific DMs on the basis of belief measures. Next we focus on clarifying in the framework of the meaning system the cognitive determinants of the dynamic-operational aspect of DMs and their relations to personality traits. A study describing the prediction of DMs on the basis of both beliefs and meaning variables is then presented. Finally, we refer to some ethical, therapeutic, and cultural aspects of DMs and their modification.

Cognitive Precursors of Defense Mechanisms

In most general terms, DMs are cognitive strategies for the resolution of conflicts, which in psychoanalytic terms may be characterized as conflicts between the strivings of the id and the demands of the ego or the superego. These strategies are not specific to a particular type of conflict, which implies that a conflict, such as between a homosexual wish and the ego's striving to comply with the moral and social rules against it, may be projected, or sublimated, or modified by way of regression into childlike submission to a father figure. The intrapsychic function of DMs, emphasized by the psychoanalytic approaches, serves the following purposes: to resolve the original conflict in some form, to provide at least partial discharge to the involved tensions, to prevent the emergence of the threatening drives or wishes into consciousness (in the form of ideas or emotions) (Freud, 1915/1957; 1936), to control unacceptable id impulses, to avoid the pain of constant conflict (Munroe, 1956, p. 243), to keep emotions within tolerable limits, to restore equilibrium disrupted by sudden drive increases, to gain time for mastering changes in "life image" that cannot be easily integrated, and to deal with unresolved conflicts with important figures in one's life (Vaillant, 1983, p. 344).

However, it is evident that beyond their application for resolving conflicts between the ego or superego and the id, DMs are widely used in everyday life as strategies for the successful performance of simple or complex cognitive tasks. Most DMs are likely to remind us of highly similar procedures occurring in contexts that are unrelated to ego defense. Thus, some resemble strategies applied by children before they are assumed to have an ego that may stand in need of defense, for example, ignoring and immediately forgetting a parental restriction (i.e., repression), or assuming that a beloved doll is hungry and trying to feed it (i.e., projection). Indeed, projection remains for a long time an important means for understanding of engines and other appliances (e.g., "Look, the fireplace must be hungry, it eats the wood so fast."). It is, however, complemented by introjection that also figures often in children's attempts to comprehend how things work: Piaget (1951) described a child who understood the matchbox mechanism only after opening and closing its mouth a few times.

Most impressive are the examples demonstrating the frequent use of defenselike strategies in different domains, far removed from psychoanalysis. For example, methods for solving mathematical problems include decomposing the complex problem into its constituent parts and working on isolated parts one at a time (i.e., isolation), or focusing first on a simpler problem (i.e., regression or displacement) (Polya, 1954, 1957; Wickelgren, 1974). Also in working on nonmathematical problems it is often necessary "to repress" habitual strategies so as to overcome functional fixedness; "to isolate" strategies previously applied for solving problems of another kind, and "to project" them onto the presently given situation; "to regress" to an earlier stage, perhaps "undoing" something of what has already been done; to raise the problem onto a more theoretical, hence higher level, thus exercising sublimation; and even to engage in reversal by trying the contrary of that which has been attempted. In logic we may encounter the procedures of disproving a thesis by driving it ad absurdum (i.e., exaggeration) or by reversing it and showing that this reversal ends up in a contradiction (i.e., reversal). In geometry we deal with projection into other dimensions (i.e., projection), reversals (e.g., of symmetry), and rotations (i.e., displacement). More familiar examples concern everyday life. Thus, we often expect others to behave as we do (i.e., projection). Or, we may have become so proficient at ignoring disturbing stimuli that we no longer hear the usual traffic noise from the street (i.e., repression). Again, if irritated by recurrent misunderstanding on the part of journal editors, we may decide to write a book (i.e., reaction formation). Or, when Beethoven lost some coins he wrote "Die Wut über den verlorenen Groschen" ("Anger over the lost nickel"), which exemplifies sublimation, and perhaps acting out too.

These examples demonstrate that DMs are essentially basic and common cognitive strategies. Yet there are evident differences between the use of these strategies as DMs and in general. For example, as DMs they are much less amenable to conscious control, hence are also far less flexible and less situation-relevant. Accordingly, we suggest that DMs are cognitive strategies that have undergone a transformation as a result of their specialized use. Thus, they become DMs under three major inter-related conditions: (a) when their function is limited mainly to subserve intrapsychic needs in general or to resolving conflicts between the super-ego or ego and the id in particular; (b) when they are used without conscious control; and (c) when they have undergone schematization resulting in reduced flexibility and variation.

Belief Constellations Conducive to Defense Mechanisms

Defense Mechanisms in the Input–Output Chain

As a result of their theoretical concern with a very particular set of internal processes and their pathogenic impacts and because they were focusing on psychotherapeutic methods, psychoanalysts failed to make a systematic effort to clarify the position and role of defense mechanisms in the chain of events intervening between perceptual input and behavioral output. On the other hand, experimental investigators focused primarily on studying the effects of DMs in perception (Assor, Aronoff, & Messe, 1986; Dixon, 1981; Kragh, 1984) and output behavior, such as addictions or gambling (Ellsworth, Strain, Strain, & Vaillant, 1986; Griffin, 1986; Rosenthal, 1986; Winegar, Stephens, & Varney, 1987). It seems that no systematic attempt has been made to fill the gap between defensively distorted inputs and outputs. We have tried to fill this gap by applying to the issue of DMs the Cognitive Orientation (CO) theory (Kreitler & Kreitler, 1982).

The Cognitive Orientation (CO) Theory

The CO theory was developed originally for the prediction and modifi-cation of human overt behavior. Its major thesis is that cognitive contents and processes—meanings, beliefs, attitudes—guide human behavior. Contrary to other models (e.g., Ajzen & Fishbein, 1980), it does not confound cognition with rationality and voluntary control: rather than assuming that behavior is the product of rational decision or carefully reasoned weighing of benefits and losses, it specifies the underlying cognitive dynamics and shows how behavior proceeds from meanings and clustered orientative beliefs. Up to now it has been applied successfully for predicting in different samples (adults, children, adolescents, schizophrenics, retarded persons) a great variety of overt behaviors, such as coming on time, achievement, reactions to success and failure, exploration, smoking, quitting smoking, planning, coping with danger, self-disclosure, and undergoing examinations for the early detection of breast cancer (Kreitler & Kreitler, 1976, 1982, 1987, 1988a, in press b; Kreitler, Schwartz, & Kreitler, 1987; Tipton & Riebsame, 1987; Westhoff & Halbach-Suarez, 1989). While behavior predictions rest on correlations between specific belief constellations and overt behaviors, positing a causal impact of beliefs on behaviors requires demonstrating that modifying beliefs leads to specific changes in behavior. This was shown in studies that dealt, for example, with changing pain tolerance, raising curiosity level in children, or reducing impulsiveness and rigidity behaviors (Kreitler & Kreitler, 1976, 1988a, in press b; Zakay, Bar-El, & Kreitler, 1984).

The CO theory seemed to provide an adequate framework for examining the nature of DMs and especially their role in the different stages of behavior evocation, first because it is a comprehensive and empirically grounded theory whose major tenets were validated by research; and second, because it enabled uncovering the role of cognitions in phenomena such as menstrual disorders, sexual dysfunctions, genital infections, eating problems, chronic pain, and medical symptoms (Kreitler & Chemerinski, 1988; Kreitler & Kreitler, 1990c, 1991, in press a, Kreitler, Kreitler, & Carasso, 1987; Kreitler, Kreitler, & Schwartz, 1991) that are often considered to be affected by DMs. The detailed descriptions the CO theory provides of the processes intervening between input and output (Kreitler & Kreitler, 1976, 1982) can be grouped into four stages, each characterized by metaphorical questions and answers. The first stage is initiated by an external or internal input and is focused on the question "What is it?" It consists in assigning meaning to the input ("initial meaning") and may result in identifying the input (a) as a signal for defensive, adaptive, or conditioned response, (b) as a signal for molar action, (c) as irrelevant in the given situation, or (d) as new or especially significant, hence as a signal for an orienting response.

The second stage deals with the question "What does it mean to me and for me?" It is initiated by an input that has not been identified sufficiently to inhibit the orienting response, by a meaning signaling the need to consider molar action, or by feedback indicating failure of the conditioned or unconditioned responses to cope with the situation. By means of enriched meaning generation, it enables specifying whether action is required.

A positive answer initiates the third stage, which is focused on the question "What will I do?" The answer is sought by means of relevant beliefs of four types: (a) beliefs about goals, expressing actions or states desired or undesired by the individual (e.g., "I want to know everything people think about me."); (b) beliefs about rules and norms, expressing ethical, aesthetic, social, and other rules and standards (e.g., "One should trust no one."); (c) beliefs about self, expressing information about oneself, such as one's habits, actions, feelings, and abilities (e.g., "I often get very excited"; "As a child I was often punished by my parents"); and (d) general beliefs, expressing information concerning others and the environment (e.g., "Most people try to get the better of you."). The meaning elaboration involves matchings and interactions between beliefs ("belief clustering"), based on clarifying the "orientativeness" of the beliefs (namely, the extent to which they support or do not support the indicated course of action). If the majority of beliefs of a certain type support the action, that belief type is considered to be positively orienting in regard to that action. Alternatively, it may be negatively orienting or may lack "orientativeness". If all four belief types point in the direction of some behavior, or when three belief types support it and the fourth is neutral, a cluster of beliefs (CO cluster) orienting toward a particular act will result. Thus, a unified tendency orienting toward the performance of the action is formed. It is called behavioral intent and may answer the question "What will I do?" In other cases, when two belief types point in one direction and two in another, there may be conflict reflected in the formation of two CO clusters and two behavioral intents. There are further alternatives to the formation of a full-fledged CO cluster: the retrieval of an almost complete CO cluster that has been formed in the past in a series of similar recurrent situations (e.g., a CO cluster orienting toward achievement) and has merely to be completed and slightly adapted to a current situation; the emergence of an incomplete CO cluster due for example to the paucity of beliefs in one belief type; or the formation of an inoperable cluster due for example to the inclusion of "as if" beliefs in one or more belief types so that the cluster may orient toward daydreaming.

The fourth stage is focused on the question "How will I do it?" The answer is in the form of a program, which is a hierarchically structured sequence of instructions governing the performance of some act. It may often be analyzed profitably in terms of two kinds of levels: the level of the more general instructions or strategy ("program scheme") and the level of the more specific instructions or tactics ("operational program"). Different programs are involved in executing an overt molar act (performance programs), an act of fantasy, a cognitive act, conflict resolution, etc. It is convenient to classify programs in line with their origin: (a) innately determined programs, such as those controlling reflexes or tropisms; (b) programs determined both innately and through learning, such as those controlling instinctive sequences or linguistic behaviors; (c) programs determined only through learning, such as those controlling culturally shaped behaviors (e.g., running political elections) and personally formed habits (e.g., modes of preparing for an exam or relaxing); and (d) programs that have been constructed by the individual ad hoc, in view of the requirements of a specific situation. Implementing a behavioral intent by a program requires selecting a program, retrieving it, and often adapting it to prevailing circumstances before it can be set into operation. Sometimes the need arises to resolve a program conflict, when two different programs appear to be equally adequate for implementing the same behavioral intent or when a present program cannot be set in operation as long as another program is being enacted.

The brief account of the CO theory indicates that the major constructs to be considered in studies of predicting and changing behavior are the meaning assigned by the subject to the situation, the CO cluster concerning the particular act, and the availability of a program for performing the act. Since in many cases the meaning likely to be assigned to the situation and the availability of the program can be assumed with high probability, one may predict that an individual will show the expected behavior if there are enough relevant beliefs orienting toward that behavior in all four belief types, or at least three if the fourth does not point in a contrary direction. Beliefs are identified as relevant for a certain behavior if they represent important aspects of the meaning of that behavior, as identified by means of a standard procedure generated by the CO theory (Kreitler & Kreitler, 1982).

Defense Mechanisms as a Specific Kind of Programs

Within the framework of the CO theory DMs may be readily identified as programs. DMs are however stored programs of a specific kind. They have a special function, which is to resolve conflicts between two CO clusters, at least one of which is barred from consciousness. Such conflicts often correspond to conflicts between the id and ego or superego, in psychoanalytic terminology, and their occurrence engenders anxiety. The defensive program resolves the conflict by producing a new behavioral intent. This intent differs from those that constituted the original conflicting intents, but it is related to them, in a form specific to each DM (e.g., through displacement or reversal). Moreover, it does not impair the unconsciousness of one or both of the original conflicting behavioral intents. Furthermore, the application of the DM itself is not conscious. The new behavioral intent may become conscious, though not necessarily so. It elicits a behavioral program that may be manifested in any domain, such as motor, emotional, verbal, perceptual, or cognitive behavior. Strictly speaking, these manifestations are products of the application of the DM but are not an actual part of it. Hence, we may call them defense-based responses.

The claim that at least one of the conflicting behavioral intents is not conscious needs elaboration. Behavioral intents in general are not conscious but may become so, for example, when awareness of the intent serves a special function, such as providing the individual orientation for the future, guaranteeing the implementation of intents involving delayed action (e.g., the intent is "to go to China next year") or actions spreading over longer time periods, hence subject to interruptions and interferences (e.g., the intent is "to go to graduate school and get a doctorate"). To repeat, consciousness is not a necessary condition for the formation of behavioral intents, but many or even most intents may become conscious for shorter or longer time periods. Yet some intents are barred from consciousness. In psychoanalytic terms, this happens because the intents are repressed. In terms of the CO theory, this may happen when the intents are threatening: that is, they oppose the majority of the individual's *basic* beliefs about self and/or beliefs about rules and norms and/or beliefs about goals and/or general beliefs. Examples of basic beliefs include the following: I want to live, There exists a world outside me, Human beings are basically good (or evil), and I am capable of feeling love. Basic beliefs are permanently stored beliefs that constitute the individual's orientative core in the external and internal environments and provide the raw materials out of which other and often more temporary beliefs are formed. Because of its great importance for the individual's well-being, the core of basic beliefs is defended when endangered (Grzegolowska-Klarkowska & Zolnierczyk, 1988, showed DMs' involvement in defending, e.g., self-esteem).

Let us illustrate the processes described above. The chain of events starts with an input identified (in stage 1) by the observer (a man) as "a young man." Meaning generation (stage 2) leads to the evocation of the goal belief "I want to have sex with him." The emergence of "having sex with him" as a possible course of action initiates the third stage, in which it is subjected to meaning elaboration in terms of further beliefs, which include representatives of all four belief types. Some of the beliefs support "having sex"; others do not. A strong set of opposing beliefs may be grouped around the focus of norm beliefs of the kind "One should not have a homosexual relation." Each of the two sets includes many beliefs and beliefs of the four types. Thus, two CO clusters are formed, generating two opposing behavioral intents, say, "to have sex with the young man" and "to avoid having sex with the young man." Let us assume that the intent "to have sex with the young man" is barred from consciousness because it has been repressed or because it opposes most of the individual's basic beliefs about self. Thus, we have the situation that triggers the application of a defense mechanism as a conflict-resolving program. If "reaction formation" is applied, it may generate the behavioral intent "to reject or alienate the young man," which may be implemented by behavioral programs, such as humiliating the young man, or offending him; if "sublimation" is applied, it may generate the behavioral intent "to help young people," which may be implemented by behavioral programs, such as working as a volunteer helping young male drug addicts or donating money to schools.

To emphasize the special character of DMs, it may be useful to distinguish between them and two apparently similar kinds of programs. One type consists of different *resolution modes of cognitive inconsistencies* that have been studied primarily in the domain of cognitive dissonance and include mechanisms, such as denial, distortion, derogation of source, restructuring, changing one of the two clashing cognitions, rationalization, transcendence, and compartmentalization (Abelson, 1968; Adams, 1968; Hardyck & Kardush, 1968; Kelman & Baron, 1968). According to the original investigators of these mechanisms, the resolution modes are designed to deal with inconsistencies, dissonances, and clashes between single cognitions, mostly two. In terms of the CO theory it seems likely that these mechanisms are designed to deal with inconsistencies, dissonances, and clashes between beliefs in the stage of CO clustering (the third stage), in an attempt to avoid the formation of two CO clusters that engender a conflict. Hence, these mechanisms resemble DMs in being applied internally for cognitive manipulations and transformations. But they differ from DMs in two points: (a) they deal with clashes between different beliefs and not between behavioral intents, and (b) they are designed to prevent the formation of a conflict between behavioral intents rather than resolving it once it has formed.

The other set of mechanisms is usually known as *coping strategies*. They have been studied primarily in the framework of the domain of stress, disease, and trauma, and they include strategies such as avoidance, repression, denial, humor, problem solving, displacement, and resigned acceptance. The common definitions of coping strategies emphasize that they are designed to deal with threat, stress, life demands and goals, debilitating or chronic sickness, life threat, "very difficult conditions," "external life strains," or demands that are appraised as exceeding the person's resources (Caplan, 1981; Lazarus & Folkman, 1984; Lipowski, 1970–1971; McCrae & Costa, 1986; Moos, 1984; Pearlin & Schooler, 1978; Weisman, 1979; White, 1974). The major functions of coping are usually identified as managing the problem causing the distress by eliminating or modifying the conditions giving rise to it, altering the meaning of the distressing conditions so as to neutralize their impact, and regulating the emotional distress (Pearlin & Schooler, 1978). In terms of the CO theory, it is evident that coping strategies are programs. They differ from defense mechanisms in four points: (a) they are performance programs rather than conflict resolution programs, (b) they may be, and often are, enacted overtly rather than internally, (c) they may be applied consciously, and (d) they deal with major defined threat or stress that endangers the individual's physical or psychological survival or both.

Since coping strategies are behavioral programs, they may be expected to be amenable to prediction by CO scores, as other behaviors proved to be. An interesting example is provided by Breier's (1980) study. It showed that CO scores predicted significantly which coping strategy a person adopted under conditions of physical danger: the one designed to cope with the external source of danger (danger control), or the one designed to cope with one's internal reaction of fear (fear control).

Notably, all three sets of programs—DMs, dissonance resolution modes, and coping strategies—share a large group of apparently similar mechanisms, such as denial, displacement, and rationalization. As noted above, the same principles underlie an even broader range of programs (of thinking, interpersonal relations, etc.) than those included in mechanisms of defense, dissonance resolution, and coping. Hence, it is justified to assume that the three sets of mechanisms utilize several principles that are very basic and common in human action. Since they recur in different domains (e.g., behavioral, cognitive), we may conclude that in regard to programs they constitute the level of the overall strategy (designated in the CO theory as "program scheme") rather than the level of detailed instructions controlling the performance and operation of the program (designated as "operational program").

Predicting the Application of Defense Mechanisms

The conception that DMs are a special set of programs gave rise to the idea that elicitation of a DM depends on activation of specific beliefs of four types forming a CO cluster. Hence, we expected that the CO theory would enable predicting the application of DMs just as was done in regard to other behaviors that are program-dependent responses. Testing this expectation empirically was of particular interest in view of the paucity of theoretical and empirical material about the determinants of selecting specific DMs. Success in the prediction would lend support to our conception about DMs. The relation of defenses to belief constellations was examined in four studies.

The *first study* (Kreitler & Kreitler, 1969, study 1) was devoted to constructing a CO Questionnaire of DMs and validating it. We focused on rationalization, denial, and projection because they represent DMs differing in manifestations and elaboration, are manifested in the different domains of interpersonal, personal, and general behavior (Colby & Gilbert, 1964; DeNike & Tiber, 1968), are highly common, and may be assumed to be readily elicited under experimental conditions. After pretesting and item analyses, the CO questionnaire included beliefs of the four types referring to themes, such as control over actions and impulses, accuracy in perception, the role of adopting an ideology, or the implications of violating common morality. Thus, the beliefs did not refer directly or indirectly to the DMs to be predicted or their manifestations (in line with clinical judgments) but to contents assumed to orient toward the adoption of one or another of the DMs.

The questionnaire had four parts, one for each type of belief. The items were of the multiple-choice kind and included two or three response alternatives (representing different DMs), of which the subject was to check only one. For example, "A person should guide his or her behavior according to logical rules that can be justified" (a norm belief; rationalization), "I usually try to maintain internal calm and do not let small things upset it" (a belief about self; denial). Beliefs orienting toward denial included, for example, emphasis on preserving one's peace of mind, concentrating on one's own well-being, rising above the trivialities of everyday life, disregarding small details, and cultivating optimism and hope. Beliefs orienting toward rationalization included, for example, emphasis on promoting the public well-being, improving others, developing one's rationality and clarity of thinking, depending only on oneself, and striving for self-control. Finally, beliefs orienting toward projection included, for example, emphasis on attending to the smallest details in any event and especially in the behavior of others, preserving one's safety, getting one's due, and behaving to others as they behave to you. Each part of the questionnaire included an equal number of responses relevant to the three DMs. The subject got scores for the four belief types in regard to each of the three DMs. The four belief scores were transformed into CO scores representing the support of the four belief types for each of the three DMs.

A sample of 45 subjects was administered the CO questionnaire as well as two scales assessing aggression and hostility: the Buss–Durkee inventory and the authors' scale of Personal Aggression, assessing readiness to admit anger in highly frustrating situations. The results showed that the scores of the four belief types had satisfactory reliability and were not significantly interrelated with one another, but each was significantly related to the overall CO score. Furthermore, the questionnaire's validity was confirmed by findings in regard to the aggression scales. As expected, on the Buss–Durkee inventory, highest aggression scores characterized subjects with the pattern of CO scores Projection > Rationalization > Denial and the lowest those with the pattern Denial > Rationalization > Projection. Similarly, on the Personal Aggression scale subjects with CO scores supporting Projection more than Rationalization admitted the highest degrees of anger.

The *second study* (Kreitler & Kreitler, 1972) was devoted to predicting on the basis of the CO Questionnaire of DMs which defensive response a subject would preferentially manifest: rationalization, denial, or projection. The subjects (24 undergraduates of both genders) participated in two independent sessions, 4–6 weeks apart, in one of which they were administered the CO questionnaire and in the other they were exposed individually to several frustrating incidents designed to evoke anger or aggression under conditions that do not promote direct emotional expression. The most frustrating aspect of the situation was that the subjects, who were led to believe that their clinical intuition and sensitivity were being tested, had to cooperate with another subject (an accomplice) who contributed very little but presented to the experimenter the products of the cooperation as if they were his or her alone. The subject's DMs (the dependent variables) were assessed by the subject's evaluation of the accomplice, responses to pictures portraying aggression and violence, and responses to a questionnaire assessing DMs (DMs Questionnaire). All three measures were based on precoded response alternatives and provided scores of the frequency with which the subject used each of the three DMs in each measure and in all together (= weighted behavior index).

The results showed that the ranking of beliefs orienting toward rationalization, denial, and projection according to CO scores is related positively and significantly to the ranking of the behavioral manifestations of these DMs according to each of the dependent measures separately and together. In line with the theory, all four belief types or at least three were involved in the relation of the CO measure with the behaviors. The validity of the results is further increased by the fact that the matching was equally good for each of the three ranks and for each of the three DMs; indeed, in many subjects it was perfect.

Also the *third study* (Zemet, 1976) dealt with predicting defense-based responses on the basis of CO scores, but it extended the scope of the former study: first, the sample included schizophrenics in addition to normals; second, a broader range of eliciting conflict situations was used; third, a broader range of response types was assessed; and fourth, the responses were assessed by a different method. Hospitalized schizophrenics ($N = 30$) and normal subjects ($N = 34$) of both genders were administered a modified version of the CO Questionnaire of DMs (shortened and extended to include items referring to two further common responses: coping, and doing nothing). The questionnaire provided CO scores (index scores representing the four belief types) concerning each of the five responses: denial, rationalization, projection, coping, and doing nothing. The reactions to conflict were assessed by the subjects' role playing in 14 predetermined scenes, each of which included some problem as its major theme (e.g., faithfulness and obligation toward one's parents versus the desire to be independent in a scene dealing with leaving the home of one's parents to live on one's own). In line with the procedure developed in the Psychodramatic Role Test (Kreitler &

Kreitler, 1964, 1968), the subjects enacted the role of themselves as well as of the other "persons" in the scenes. All behavioral and verbal responses were recorded and classified into one of the five categories (e.g., denial, coping), in line with predetermined criteria. The results showed that in both schizophrenics and normals CO scores were related significantly and in the expected direction to four of the five response categories. That is, high scorers on the CO of denial used denial significantly more often in their responses to the conflicts than low scorers. The only deviations from the expected were (a) concerning "projection" in normals (the responses were in the expected direction but the difference between high and low scorers was nonsignificant, probably because these responses were very infrequent in normals) and (b) concerning "coping" in schizophrenics (the relation was significant but reversed, probably because for schizophrenics the program bound to coping is projection!).

In the *fourth study* (Eldar, 1976), the original CO Questionnaire of DMs was applied for predicting the responses of subjects in a situation presenting incongruities between messages conveyed concurrently through different communication channels. Clarifying the determinants of selectivity in such situations is important because incongruous communications are common and play a role in interpersonal relations in general and psychopathology in particular (e.g., Bugenthal, 1974; Bugenthal, Love, Kaswan, & April, 1971; Watzlawik, Beavin, & Jackson, 1967). The hypotheses were that high scorers on CO of rationalization would focus on the verbally conveyed content of the communications (because they seem more "rational" and definite), disregarding the nonverbal communications; high scorers on the CO of projection would focus on the nonverbally conveyed communications (because they are more indirect and fuzzy), disregarding the verbally expressed content; whereas high scorers on the CO of denial would focus on the positive aspects of the communications, regardless of channel, disregarding the negative aspects.

The 51 subjects (27 men, 24 women) were selected from a sample of 197 tested individuals according to their scores on the CO questionnaire and belonged to one of three subgroups: (a) subjects scoring high on the CO of denial and low on the COs of rationalization and projection; (b) subjects scoring high on the CO of rationalization and low on the COs of denial and projection; and (c) subjects scoring high on the CO of projection and low on the COs of denial and rationalization. They were exposed to evaluative communications (positive or negative) of one person to another that were conveyed simultaneously through three channels: verbal, visual, and auditory. The communications were structured so that the evaluative aspects conveyed through the different channels were contradictory: for example, the verbal content "You have done an absolutely wonderful job" was conveyed by a person with a rejecting facial expression and in a rejecting tone of voice. All combinations of evaluations in the three channels were used (after extensive pretesting of the credibility and intensity of effects in each channel). Half the communications were presented by men and half by women (all professional actors). The subjects were exposed to the communications, which were presented as videotaped excerpts of conversations between students, and were asked to consider each as if it had been addressed to them personally. Their task was to evaluate the degree of positiveness or negativeness of each communication on a nine-point scale. The results confirmed the three hypotheses in the sample of men, and the hypothesis about projection in the sample of women too. There were however unexpected results in the female sample: the high scorers on the CO of rationalization focused more than the others on all channels rather than on the verbal alone (as if rationalization necessitated consideration of as much information as was available); and the high scorers on the CO of denial focused on the positive content but especially if it was conveyed nonverbally. In sum, even though we have no explanation for the different patterns of results in the two genders, the point to emphasize is that individuals with different CO scores on the CO Questionnaire of Defense Mechanisms respond differentially to incongruous inputs.

Cognitive Dynamics Underlying Defense Mechanisms

In a Search for the Determinants of Defense-Implementing Programs

According to the CO theory, the occurrence of defense-based responses depends on (a) a sufficiently high number of beliefs of the four types, relevant for a specific DM, to permit the formation of a behavioral intent orienting toward that DM and (b) a program implementing the behavioral intent. The last section dealt with the first condition; the present section focuses on the second. How do individuals acquire the specific conflict resolution programs we call DMs? Why do some individuals adopt consistently the program we call projection and others programs we call denial or rationalization? Anna Freud (1966, p. 62) is of no help in this respect because she claimed that DMs are "as old as the instincts . . . or at least . . . as the conflict." So far, little is known about the determinants of the actual programs. The dynamic approaches, including psychoanalysis, would tend to emphasize identification with the preferred parent as the source of an individual's beliefs. Yet, there are no empirical data supporting this claim by showing, for instance, congruence in the preferred defenses of parents and offspring (e.g., Cermak & Rosenfeld, 1987). The learning approaches would emphasize the impact of learning from adults and peers, in formal and informal contexts, whereas the social approaches would emphasize the sociocultural impacts on program acquisition and application (e.g., Gibbs, 1987; Sahoo, Sia, & Panda, 1987). Yet so far there are only few data supporting these approaches. Furthermore, they do not account for individual differences in the availability of programs.

In this context we will present evidence about the role of cognitive determinants in accounting for individual differences in DMs. The determinants we discuss can be considered to constitute the micro level of cognitive functioning, for they deal with units and processes underlying larger units, such as beliefs or programs, constituting the macro level. They consist of meanings and meaning properties as outlined in the framework of the theory of meaning (Kreitler & Kreitler, 1990a; see below). Our concept of meaning differs markedly from that adopted in the framework of the information processing model of cognition, according to which meaning consists of inactive content items to be inserted, for example, into the empty slots of grammatical structures. The narrow limits of this approach to meaning become evident in Chomsky's (1972) example of a grammatically perfect but nonetheless completely meaningless sentence, such as "Colorless green ideas sleep furiously." In contrast to this approach, which distinguishes sharply between meaning and cognition, we define cognition as the meaning processing system whose functioning is codetermined by meaning characteristics in general as well as by the meanings it is currently processing. Hence, cognition and meaning are complementary terms in the sense that one cannot be exhaustively defined and understood without the other. Each meaning operation is a cognitive act, whereas each cognitive function has aspects that can be understood satisfactorily only by considering meaning characteristics. Nonetheless cognition is the more comprehensive term because often it operates on levels and produces units that can be described more efficiently without invoking the meaning system. Constructs such as beliefs and DMs depend on cognitive processes that may best be described in terms of the meaning system, but it would be cumbersome and misleading to describe the major processes of the CO theory in terms of meaning variables. This would produce results as adequate as describing whisky in terms of molecules, atoms, or worst of all, subatomic particles. Thus, to examine the processes underlying the operation of specific DMs, we would first describe the meaning system.

The Meaning System

The system of meaning was developed for characterizing and assessing human meanings of different kinds (e.g., Kreitler & Kreitler, 1976, 1982, 1986, 1988b,c, 1990a,b). It was designed to be broader in coverage and to have higher validity than the available measures of meaning. The only aspects of the system presented are those necessary for describing the studies about the meaning-anchored determinants of DMs.

The major assumptions underlying the system are that meaning is a complex phenomenon with a multiplicity of aspects, that it is essentially communicable, that it may be expressed through verbal and different nonverbal means, and that it comes in two varieties—the lexical-interpersonally shared meaning and the subjective–personal one. These assumptions have enabled collecting and coding a great amount of empirical data in regard to a rich variety of inputs, from thousands of subjects differing in age, education, gender, and cultural background.

On the basis of this material we define meaning as a referent-centered pattern of content items. The referent denotes the representation of the input to which meaning is assigned, for example, a word, an image, an object, or a situation. The content items, called meaning values, denote particular cognitive contents, expressed verbally or nonverbally (e.g., red, dangerous, made of wood), which are assigned to the referent and express or communicate its meaning. The referent and the meaning value together form the meaning unit. Four kinds of meaning variables are used for characterizing the meaning values and their relations to referents (Tables 11.1): (a) meaning dimensions, which characterize the contents of the meaning values in terms of general kinds of information about the referent (e.g., Sensory Qualities, Material, or Structure); (b) types of relation, which characterize the relation of the meaning value to the referent in terms of its immediacy or directness (e.g., attributive or metaphoric–symbolic); (c) forms of relation, which characterize the relation of the meaning value to the referent in formal–logical terms (e.g., positive or conjunctive); and (d) referent shifts, which characterize the sequential shifts in the referent in the course of meaning assignment (e.g., a modified or associated referent).

Our concept of meaning is double-faced in that, on the one hand—in the static application—it serves for coding, characterizing, quantifying, and evaluating cognitive contents or the results of cognitive performance, and, on the other hand—in the dynamic application—it serves as a set of interrelated strategies that explain major aspects of cognitive functioning.

The assessment of meaning is done by coding in terms of the meaning variables units of contents in the cognitive product (e.g., a dialogue, a text, a solution to a problem, jokes, questions, or the meaning communications of individuals). The subject's meaning assignment tendencies are assessed by the Meaning Test. This test requires the subjects to communicate to an imaginary other person the meaning (general and/or personal) of a standard set of 11 stimuli. Coding the responses consists of assigning to each response unit four scores, one of each type of meaning variables (i.e., one meaning dimension, one type of relation, etc.). Thus, the response "blue" to the stimulus "ocean" is coded in terms of the meaning dimension Sensory Qualities, the attributive type of relation, the positive form of relation, and no referent shift. Summing these scores across all response units yields the subject's meaning profile, namely, the

TABLE 11.1a. Major variables of the meaning system.

I.	Meaning dimensions		
Dim.	1. Contextual allocation	Dim.	14. Quantity and number
Dim.	2. Range of inclusion	Dim.	15. Locational qualities
	2a. Subclasses	Dim.	16. Temporal qualities
	2b. Parts of	Dim.	17. Possession
			17a By referent
			17b Of referent
			(Belongingness)
Dim.	3. Function, purpose, and role		17b. And belongingness
Dim.	4. Actions and potentialities for action	Dim.	18. Development
			19. Sensory qualities
	4a. By referent	Dim.	19a. Of referent
	4b. To/with referents		19b. Perceived by referent
Dim.	5. Manner of occurrence or opereration	Dim	20. Feelings and emotions
			20a. Evoked by referent
Dim	6. Antecedents and causes		20b. Experienced by referent
Dim.	7. Consequences and results	Dim.	21. Judgments and evaluations
Dim.	8. Domain of application		21a. About referent
	8a. Referent as subject		21b. Of referent
	8b. Referent as object	Dim.	22. Cognitive qualities
Dim.	9. Material		22a. Evoked by referent
Dim.	10. Structure		22b. Of referent
Dim.	11. State and changes in state		
Dim.	12. Weight and mass		
II.	Types of relation*	TR	3. Exemplifying—illustrative
TR	1. Attributive		3a. Exemplifying instance
	1a. Qualities to substance		3b. Exemplifying situation
	1b. Actions to agent		3c. Exemplifying scene
TR	2. Comparative	TR	4. Metaphoric–symbolic
	2a. Similarity		4a. Interpretation
	2b. Difference		4b. Conventional metaphor
	2c. Complementariness		4c. Original metaphor
	2d. Relationality		4d. Symbol
III.	Froms of relation		
FR	1. Positive	FR	6. Not negative but positive
FR	2. Negative	FR	7. Double negation
FR	3. Mixed positive and negative	FR	8. Obligatory
FR	4. Conjunctive	FR	9. Question
FR	5. Disjunctive		
IV.	Shifts of referent**		
SR	1. Identical	SR	6. Higher level referent
SR	2. Opposite	SR	7. Associative
SR	3. Partial	SR	8. Grammatical variation
SR	4. Former meaning value	SR	9. Linguistic label
SR	5. Modified	SR	10. Unrelated

* Modes of meaning: lexical mode [TR 1 + TR 2]; personal mode [TR 3 + TR 4].
**Close SR, 1 + 8 + 9; Medium SR, 3 + 4 + 5 + 6; Far SR, 2 + 7 + 10.

distribution of the subject's frequencies of responses in each meaning variable. These frequencies were found to be characteristic of the individual; hence we call them meaning assignment tendencies. Various studies showed that the meaning assignment tendencies are related to different cognitive activities, such as planning, memory, analogical thinking, or conceptualizations (Arnon & Kreitler, 1984; Kreitler & Kreitler, 1986, 1987, 1988b, 1990b). For example, high scorers on the meaning dimension Locational Qualities perform better than low scorers on problems requiring consideration of spatial properties such as mazes. Findings of this kind demonstrate the cognitive function of meaning assignment tendencies. These tendencies also play a role in personality, because it was shown that each of over 100 common personality traits corresponds to a unique pattern of meaning assignment tendencies (Kreitler & Kreitler, 1990a).

Patterns of Meaning Variables and Defense Mechanisms

The study (Kreitler & Kreitler, 1990e) was devoted to exploring the interrelations between meaning variables and DMs. We expected such an interrelation because we conceive of DMs as essentially basic means of cognitive manipulations and transformations (see Cognitive Precursors of Defense Mechanisms). As such, they are to be expected to depend on processes of meaning, which constitute the basic dynamic core of cognition.

The subjects were 129 undergraduates of both genders who were administered in random order in two group sessions, 6–8 weeks apart, the standard Meaning Test and the CO Questionnaire of DMs. The Meaning Test was designed to provide information about the subject's meaning assignment tendencies (the meaning profile), the CO Questionnaire about the subject's predispositions (viz., behavioral intents) toward rationalization, denial, and projection. Assessing the predispositions seemed to us to provide more reliable and stable measures of DMs than assessing specific manifestations of these DMs in one or another domain. The significant intercorrelations presented in Tables 11.2 demonstrate that each DM is correlated with a specific set of meaning variables. This indicates the possibility that an individual adopts preferentially that DM which matches most closely his or her characteristic meaning assignment tendencies. Furthermore, analyzing the meaning variables in the sets corresponding to the three DMs shows that each set consists of the kind of cognitive processes that enable implementing the performance of the DM.

Let us illustrate the latter conclusion. For example, high scorers on the CO of denial (Table 11.2a) tend to refer to the size, to the quantity and possessions of inputs, and to their superordinate and subordinate classes, but not to emotions, internal sensations, judgments and evaluations, and cognitive qualities (see positive and negative correlations with meaning dimensions, respectively). Notably, the aspects to which they refer are relatively "objective" whereas those they disregard are "subjective" and potentially emotionally loaded. Furthermore, the deniers tend to shift away from the presented inputs, but not too far away (see positive correlation with shifts to near referents and negative with far associations) and usually focus on aspects of the referent that they themselves have brought up, a tendency that would enable dwelling preferentially on the "safe" aspects. In case a threatening aspect does emerge, the deniers can still rely on their tendency to emphasize differences and thus explain away the apparent similarity to a threat; or they may apply their tendency toward metaphorization and grasp the input in a metaphorical way, which diminishes the threat.

Furthermore, high scorers on the CO of rationalization (Table 11.2b) have a rich store of cognitive tendencies: they tend to refer to actions,

TABLE 11.2a. Meaning variables correlated significantly with the three defense mechanisms: Denial.

Meaning dimensions		Types of relation		Referent shifts	
Contextual allocation	.28**	Comparative: difference	.31***	Sticking to presented referent (identical)	−.25**
		Metaphoric-symbolic:			
Range of inclusion (subtypes)	.36***	Original metaphor	.40***	Shift to former meaning value	.38***
Consequences and results	.29**			Shift to referent related only by association	−.27**
Structure	−.25**			Shift to grammatical variation of referent	−.26**
Size and dimensionality	.37***			Close shifts	.35***
Quantity and number	.31***				
Sensory qualities (internal)	−.42***				
Feelings and emotions (by referent)	−.27**				
Judgments and evaluations (by referent)	−.42***				
Cognitive qualities (evoked by referent)	−.37***				

NOTE: *$p < .05$, **$p < .01$, ***$p < .001$.

TABLE 11.2b. Meaning variables correlated significantly with the three defense mechanisms: Rationalization.

Meaning dimensions		Types of relation		Froms of relation		Referent shifts	
Function, purpose, and role	.31**	Attributive: qualities to subject	.26**	Negative	.41***	Sticking to presented referent (identical)	.26**
Action (by referent)	.26**	Attributive: actions to agent	.31***	Mixed positive and negative	.40***	Shift to former meaning value	−.38***
Action (to/with referent)	.28**	Attributive: qualities and actions	.32***	Double negation	.40***	Shift to referent related only by association	.42***
Manner of occurrence or operation	.39***	Comparative: similarity	−.37***			Shift to linguistic label	−.38***
Domain of application (referent as object)	.37***	Comparative: complementariness	.33***			Close shifts	−.45***
Consequences and results	−.46***	Exemplifying-illustrative: Exemplifying instance	.38***			Far shifts	.41***
Structure	.37***	Metaphoric-symbolic: interpretation	−.27**			Number of different shifts	.35***
Quantity and number	−.27**	Metaphoric-symbolic: Original metaphor	.34**				
Belongingness	−.25***						
Judgments and evaluations (about referent)	.36***						
Judgments and evaluations (about and of referent)	.42***						
Cognitive qualities (evoked by and of referent)	.49***						

NOTE: $* \ p < .05$, $** \ p < .01$, $*** \ p < .001$.

TABLE 11.2c. Meaning variables correlated significantly with the three defense mechanisms: Projection.

Meaning dimensions		Types of relation		Froms of relation		Referent shifts	
Range of inclusion (parts)	-.33***	Attributive: qualities and actions	-.52***	Positive	-.33***	Shift to part	-.41***
Antecedents and causes	-.48***	Exemplifying-illustrative: Exemplifying instance	.37***	Conjunctive	-.42***	Shift to linguistic label	-.36***
Consequences and results	-.54***	Metaphoric-symbolic: interpretation	.52***	Not negative but positive	-.26**	Far shifts	.55***
Domain of application (referent as subject and as object)	.51***	Metaphoric-symbolic: all subtypes	-.28**	Obligatory	-.30***		
Structure	.48***						
State	-.39***						
Locational qualities	-.31***						
Belongingness	-.42***						
Development	-.36***						
Feelings and emotions (evoked)	-.36***						
Feelings and emotions (evoked and experienced by referent)	-.35***						
Judgments and evaluations (about and by referent)	-.32***						

NOTE: $*p < .05$, $**p < .01$, $***p < .001$.

how actions occur, who or what is involved in an event or situation, and to functions, structures, evaluations, and cognitive properties, while they disregard aspects such as quantity, belongingness, and results. They tend to grasp relations either in a straightforward way (i.e., attributive) or metaphorically; they present examples but do not dwell on similarities. They use preferentially negations or modulated connections (e.g., "sometimes") and tend to shift away from the given inputs, mostly to distant referents. Notably, they have a rich stock of referent-modulating mechanisms and of contents (meaning values) that enables them to present an issue to themselves and others in an acceptable "rational" form (see also the finding about the richness of information acquired by women, high scorers on rationalization in study 4, above; Eldar, 1976).

Finally, high scorers on the CO of projection (Table 11.2c) tend not to refer to the causes of inputs, their constituent parts, their state, size, location, belongingness, and development, or to emotional and evaluative aspects, while they do refer to structure, and who or what is involved in the situation. It is likely that disregarding so many aspects of inputs may subserve the tendency of these subjects to replace the perceived with the conceived or desired. This tendency may be further subserved by the disregard for interpersonally shared reality (see negative correlation with the attributive type of relation), and preferences for subjective interpretations and shifting away from the presented inputs to far referents. Notably, the concern with structure and with whole referents (see negative correlation with shifting to partial referent) could contribute to implementing the potential for paranoia sometimes related to projection.

The examples given above illustrate how the cognitive processes and contents assessed by the meaning variables may implement the operation of the defenses. If one assumes that meaning dimensions reflect to a greater extent a focus on contents, whereas the other kinds of meaning variables reflect rather a focus on cognitive processes, it is possible to examine whether the patterns of meaning variables corresponding to DMs are biased more in the direction of contents or processes. As programs they may be expected to be fairly content free. However, comparing the distribution of meaning variables in the patterns (dimensions vs. other kinds) with that expected in view of the structure of the meaning system shows that in no case were the deviations significant (the chi-square values for Denial, Rationalization, and Projection were .215, .0002, and .005, respectively). Hence, it seems that DMs rely on both cognitive contents and processes.

The relatively large number of meaning variables in the patterns should not be surprising. Previous studies (Kreitler & Kreitler, 1990a) showed that the patterns provide a variety of means for implementing the program's overall strategy. These means are alternatives that may be applied selectively according to the demand characteristics of the situation or the problem at hand, one at a time, or several in a sequence in case former conflict resolution attempts have failed. Thus, denial may be implemented by referring to aspects of the input such as size and quantity, which do not suggest emotions, or by dwelling on the general superordinate category suggested by the input (e.g., human suffering in general, if input is painful), or by metaphorization, which enables changing the meaning of the perceived. The variety of means guarantees the flexibility, hence the pervasiveness, of a DM once it has been adopted by an individual.

As may be expected, each of the patterns of meaning variables corresponding to the three DMs has unique characteristics. The richest pattern is the one corresponding to rationalization, perhaps because of its commonness in a normal population and its emphasis on a cognitively acceptable façade. The highest number of negative constituents is found in the pattern corresponding to projection (76%) as compared with 40% in rationalization and 25% in denial (the percentage for projection differs significantly from those for rationalization, $z = 3.802$, $p < .001$, and for denial, $z = 2.466$, $p < .01$). Previous studies (Kreitler & Kreitler, 1990a) showed that negative correlations are indicative of active disregard for the cognitive operation or content domain represented by that meaning variable. Accordingly, the frequencies of negative elements in the patterns correspond to the prevalent psychoanalytic conception that projection involves the highest degree of repression and cognitive transformation, and denial the least (A. Freud, 1966). Comparing the three patterns shows that they share only five meaning variables: the meaning dimensions results, belongingness, and evaluations, and the types of relation exemplifying instance and metaphor. This is a relatively narrow common core. Moreover, the direction of the correlations across patterns is not the same for any of the variables. Hence, the data for the three defenses do not support the hypothesis of a general tendency for defensiveness that transcends the specific defense mechanisms (e.g., see Weinberger, Schwartz, & Davidson, 1979).

As noted above, personality traits were found to correspond each to a pattern of meaning variables. These patterns have specific characteristics (Kreitler & Kreitler, 1990a). Is it justified to conclude that the three DMs are personality traits? To answer this question, it is necessary to examine whether the patterns corresponding to the DMs resemble those corresponding to personality traits in terms of five major empirically based criteria (Table 11.3). Table 11.3 shows that the patterns for denial and rationalization do not deviate from those for personality traits in more than one of the criteria. This degree of deviation is considered to be acceptable, so that the patterns corresponding to these two DMs fall within the boundaries of variation of personality traits. Hence, denial and rationalization can be considered as personality traits. In contrast, projection cannot be considered to be a personality trait (the pattern of meaning variables corresponding to it deviates from personality traits

TABLE 11.3. Comparing the patterns of meaning variables corresponding to the three defense mechanisms with the patterns corresponding to personality traits.

Criteria of comparison		Rationalization	Denial	Projection
1. Number of different kinds of meaning variables in pattern [3 or 4]		4 [no dev.]	3 [no dev.]	4 [no dev.]
2. Proportion of different kinds of meaning variables in pattern:				
Meaning Dimensions	54.75%	45.16%	55.00%	52.00%
Types of Relation	25.75%	25.80%	20.00%	20.00%
Forms of Relation	5.90%	9.38%	0.00%	16.00%
Referent Shifts	12.57%	19.35%	5.00%	12.00%
Chi^2 of differences		7.76 [no dev.]	19.48*** [no dev.]	18.74*** [dev.]
3. Proportion of negative correlations [.38]		.26 $z = 1.30$ [no dev.]	.40 $z = .35$ [no dev.]	.76 $z = 3.45$*** [dev.]
4. Number of meaning variables in pattern [range 7–20]		31 [dev.]	20 [no dev.]	25 [dev.]
5. Proportion of general to specific meaning variables in pattern [.44]		.41 $z = .37$ [no dev.]	.40 $z = .40$ [no dev.]	.61 $z = .90$ [no dev.]
Total number of deviations		1	1	3

NOTES: The standard values of the criteria are presented in brackets. For a more complete presentation and illustration of the produre for checking the similarity to personality traits, see Kreitler & Kreitler (1990a, pp. 303–310).
dev. = deviation from the pattern of personality traits.
***$p < .001$.

according to three criteria). Denial and rationalization resemble traits perhaps because they are common in a normal population, or at least more common than projection, which reflects to a greater extent psychopathological tendencies. Be it as it may, the findings in regard to denial and rationalization support the psychoanalytic claim that DMs may affect character so that character itself turns into a DM (Munroe, 1956, pp. 264–266).

Beliefs and Meaning Variables as Predictors of Defenses

In view of the presented evidence that belief constellations predict which of three DMs an individual will adopt, whereas meaning variables clarify the underlying cognitive dynamics of the operation of the DMs, it is likely that combining CO scores and meaning variables would provide a better prediction than either alone. This expectation was confirmed in such other fields of study as planning and curiosity (Kreitler & Kreitler, 1987, in press-b). Accordingly, in the last stage of our work in the domain of DMs (Kreitler & Kreitler, 1990e), we assessed in a group of 159 subjects of both genders (85 high school students, 17–18.2 years old, and 74 undergraduates, 22–31 years old) the CO for each of the three DMs (by the CO Questionnaire of DMs), the meaning profile (by the Meaning Test), and two kinds of defense-based response: The DMs Questionnaire (see second study, above) and a slightly modified version of the Hopkins Symptom Checklist (Derogatis, Lipman, Rickels, Uhlenhuth, & Covi, 1974), which requested rating on a four-point scale the degree of distress caused by 72 items and provided a measure of neurotic symptoms. The questionnaires were administered in two group sessions in random order. Each subject got (a) three CO scores, one for each defense, indicating the number of belief types supporting the DM (range 0–4); (b) three meaning variables indices, one for each DM, that summarized the number of meaning variables in the subject's meaning profile matching those in the pattern corresponding to the DM (matching was defined as a variable's frequency above the group's mean when the variable in the pattern has a positive sign, and below the group's mean when the variable has a negative sign); (c) three scores, one for each DM, on the basis of responses in frustrating situations (DMs Questionnaire); and (d) one score reflecting the overall self-reported distress of neurotic symptoms. Scores a and b served as predictors, whereas scores c and d served as dependent variables.

Table 11.4 shows that the CO scores and meaning variable indices predicted significantly the defense-based responses obtained on the DMs Questionnaire. Together they accounted on the average for 39.1% of the variance in the responses, ranging from 33.64% for rationalization to 47.61% for projection. The prediction for projection was significantly highest (it differed from that for denial, CR = 2.10, and for rational-

TABLE 11.4. The results of multiple stepwise regression analyses with CO scores and indices of meaning variables as predictors and responses on the Defense Mechanisms Questionnaire and neurotic symptoms as dependent variables.

	Multiple correlation coefficients	
Predictors	DM Questionnaire	Neurotic symptoms
CO of Rationalization	.40***	.18*
CO of Rationalization + Meaning Index of Rationalization	.58***	.29**
Meaning Index of Denial	.54***	.35**
Meaning Index of Denial + CO of Denial	.60***	.54***
Meaning Index of Projection	.56***	.17*
Meaning Index of Projection + CO of Projection	.69***	.22*

NOTES: In the column headed DM Questionnaire, the dependent variable in the first two rows is Rationalization, in the next two rows it is Denial, in the last two rows it is Projection. The predictors are listed in the order in which they were entered into the prediction equation.
* $p < .05$, ** $p < .01$, *** $p < .001$.

ization, CR = 2.53, $p < .01$). In one case CO scores were entered first into the prediction equation; in two cases they were entered second (the same order was obtained for neurotic symptoms). The mean improvement in the prediction due to the addition of the second predictor was 13.58% (ranging from 6.84% for denial to 17.64% for rationalization).

The prediction was lower in regard to the neurotic symptoms (14.13% mean variance accounted for as compared with 39.1% in the case of the DMs Questionnaire, CR = 5.03, $p < .001$). This was to be expected, first, because DMs are only one of the determinants of neurotic symptoms, possibly not even the major one; and second, because the predictors were not adapted specifically for the prediction of the dependent variable. The highest rate of accounted-for variance was obtained when the predictors were the CO and meaning index of denial (29.16% of the variance was accounted for) but it was low when the predictors were the CO and meaning index of rationalization (8.41%) or projection (4.84%). These findings are in accord with the psychoanalytic claim (Fenichel, 1945) that neurotic symptoms are based on repression and denial more than on the other two assessed DMs.

Modifying Defense Mechanisms

Modifying Defenses in the Framework of Psychoanalysis

The goal of psychoanalytic treatment has often been considered to be the elimination or at least modification of DMs. The major psychoanalytic means applied for this purpose are (a) providing insight into the harmful DMs and (b) transference-supported suggestions for a more realistic and healthier approach to one's internal processes. These means are more often than not frustrated by the patients' resistance or, in the best case, require years of therapeutic work. The resistance may become so intense that Freud (1937/1964) was doubtful whether the venture can at all be successful. The main difficulty encountered by psychoanalysts derives from their attempt to combat the consciousness-distorting DMs by rendering their functioning conscious. It would be advisable to circumvent this vicious circle by modifying the conscious processes and entities that underlie DMs, namely, modifying the beliefs conducive to DMs and the meaning assignment tendencies that implement them.

Modifying CO Clusters and Meaning Variables

Modifying CO clusters has been done successfully in an experimental framework in different domains, including impulsive behavior in children, rigidity, pain tolerance, and curiosity (Kreitler & Kreitler, 1976, 1988a, in press; Zakay et al., 1984). The basic methods for modifying beliefs consist of working systematically through each aspect of the belief's meaning, proceeding from one belief type to another, until all four have been covered. The techniques of change use means such as exposing inconsistencies between beliefs or between beliefs and behavior, changing the meaning of the major terms of the belief, or narrowing down the belief's meaning (Kreitler & Kreitler, 1990d). The major thrust of the effort is directed at mobilizing sufficient support of relevant beliefs for the desired course of operation, without however dealing with the action itself by way of persuasion, training, or reinforcement. Our results show that providing for the formation of the adequate CO cluster produces the motivationally supported disposition for the specific action. Also the individual's meaning variables can be modified, as shown by successful attempts in the domains of anxiety, creativity, problem solving, and cognitive enrichment of retarded persons (Arnon & Kreitler, 1984; Kreitler & Kreitler, 1977, 1988c, 1990b,d, in press-c). For example, a study of special interest in this context showed that modifying specific sets of meaning variables changed the Rorschach responses of schizophrenics in the direction of normality and of normals in the direction of pathology (Kreitler, Kreitler, & Wanounou, 1987–1988). Thus, it is very likely that it would be possible to modify successfully also CO clusters and patterns of meaning variables conducive to particular DMs. However, for ethical reasons this did not seem to us justifiable: weakening DMs may involve subjects in sudden exposure to repressed wishes or motivations that could precipitate a breakdown at least in some individuals, especially when experimenters work with subjects they hardly know, whereas strengthening DMs could set people on the course of developing neurotic symptoms, if not worse.

But what may be dangerous for a researcher may be safe for the psychotherapist, who has enough time and opportunity to form a reliable estimate of the client's ego strength and personality resources. Weakening a given DM can be done, for example, by weakening beliefs relevant for that DM or by strengthening beliefs and meaning variables involved in some other response likely to inhibit the DM or replace it. Also it is possible to try to resolve the conflict underlying the use of a DM by modifying the CO clusters that gave rise to the two clashing behavioral intents. Finally, the CO conception of DMs as special programs of conflict resolution raises the possibility that many individuals may have at their disposal too few means for coping with problems. In such cases an attempt could be made to combat DMs by alerting the individual to the conflict and teaching him or her new ways of resolving conflicts.

Summing Up and Some Afterthoughts

We started from the conception that DMs are a special type of program, designed to subserve the intrapsychic function of resolving a conflict between two behavioral intents, at least one of which is sufficiently threatening to be barred from consciousness. A DM's application results in forming a new behavioral intent that differs from the conflicting intents but is related to them and is manifested in some defense-based response, for example, in the behavioral, emotional, or perceptual field. The DMs are basic cognitive strategies, used also in other domains, which have undergone schematization and are applied without conscious control. We described briefly six studies showing that both the constellation of beliefs assessed through CO scores and a set of meaning variables assessed through the Meaning Test contribute to selecting a particular DM rather than another. The beliefs and meaning variables are specific for each DM. It is likely that the beliefs orient toward a particular DM, thus producing a motivational disposition toward a specific DM, whereas the meaning variables constitute the cognitive means through which the DM may be implemented. Analysis of the means suggests that they may be applied as alternative means, hence may be selected in line with the requirements and possibilities of specific situations. In view of successful modifications of CO clusters and meaning variables, it is likely that the change of those involved in DMs is possible, as well.

Thus, our project has led DMs from their psychoanalytic birthplace to a new location within a cognitive theory of behavior and personality. This new context may make many wonder whether there is still much left for DMs to defend in a world in which sexual and aggressive wishes are discussed with more frankness than the corruption of governments. It seems to us however that the objects of defense are not necessarily limited to superego-banned wishes and drives. From the viewpoint of a cognitively based personality theory, defense-worthy objects would include basic beliefs about oneself, basic rules and norms, basic wishes and goals, and basic beliefs about the world and others that form the core of orientation in the internal and external environments. These beliefs address issues such as: What kind of person am I? Does life in general and my life in particular make sense, and if yes, what sense? Is there justice in the world? Are people basically good or evil? and Should I behave in a moral way? Also from the viewpoint of a more emotionally and motivationally based theory of personality, there are enough issues that may provoke anxieties sufficiently serious for triggering DMs. These include the morbidity and loneliness of old age, the unanswered questions of the "why" and "what" of existence and death, the progressive loss of wishes due to their fulfillment, the certainty of unavoidable uncertainty, and last but not least, the need for limitations and restrictions and the unconquerable wish to cross them (see also Snyder, 1988). Confronting such problems is not a cause for shame, hence is not likely to promote repression. Denying them and still maintaining a workable contact with common reality would be almost impossible. Yet denying their immediate and personal relevance by projecting them into the postpersonal future is already rather common. So is partial regression, often called learned helplessness (Seligman, 1975). Rationalization adorned by sublimated presentation is the preferred answer of many existentialist and humanistic therapists or philosophers, while future-denial made many of the "flower children" very happy until the present hit them through harsh confrontation.

In sum, it seems likely that defenses are used and will continue to be used beyond the realm of superego-banned contents and domains. It is however beyond the scope of this chapter to deal with questions such as whether human beings would be happier if they were helped to live without using any DMs and whether this is at all possible and desirable.

References

Abelson, R.P. (1968) A summary of hypotheses on modes of resolution. In R.P. Abelson, E. Aronson, W.J. McGuire, T.M. Newcomb, M.J. Rosenberg, & P.H. Tannenbaum (Eds.), *Theories of cognitive consistency: A sourcebook* (pp. 716–720). Skokie, IL: Rand McNally.

Adams, J.S. (1968) A framework for the study of modes of resolving inconsistency. In R.P. Abelson, E. Aronson, W.J. McGuire, T.M. Newcomb, M.J. Rosenberg, & P.H. Tannenbaum (Eds.), *Theories of cognitive consistency: A sourcebook* (pp. 655–669). Skokie, IL: Rand McNally.

Ajzen, I. & Fishbein, M. (1980) *Understanding attitudes and predicting social behavior*. Englewood Cliffs, NJ: Prentice Hall.

Arnon, R. & Kreitler, S. (1984) Effects of meaning training on overcoming functional fixedness. *Current Psychological Research and Review*, *3*, 11–24.

Assor, A., Aronoff, J., & Messe, L.A. (1986) An experimental test of defensive processes in impression formation. *Journal of Personality and Social Psychology*, *50*, 644–650.

Breier, G. (1980) *Effects of cognitive orientation on behavior under threat.* Master's thesis, Department of Psychology, Tel Aviv University (summarized in Kreitler & Kreitler, 1982, pp. 137–140).

Bugenthal, D.E. (1974) Interpretation of naturally occurring discrepancies between words and intonation: Modes of inconsistency resolution. *Journal of Personality and Social Psychology*, *30*, 125–133.

Bugenthal, D.E., Love, L.R., Kaswan, J.W., & April, C. (1971) Verbal–nonverbal conflict in parental messages to normal and disturbed children. *Journal of Abnormal Psychology*, *77*, 6–10.

Caplan, G. (1981) Mastery of stress. *American Journal of Psychiatry*, *138*, 413–420.

Cermale, T.L. & Rosenfeld, A.A. (1987) Therapeutic considerations with adult children of alcoholics. *Advances in Alcoholism and Substance Abuse*, *6*, 17–32.

Chomsky, N. (1972) *Language and mind* (enlarged ed.). New York: Harcourt Brace Jouanouich.

Colby, K.M. & Gilbert, J.P. (1964) Programming a computer model of neurosis. *Journal of Mathematical Psychology*, *1*, 405–417.

Cramer, P. (1988) The Defense Mechanism Inventory: A review of research and discussion of the scales. *Journal of Personality Assessment*, *52*, 142–164.

DeNike, L.D. & Tiber, N. (1968) Neurotic behavior. In P. London & D. Rosenhan (Eds.), *Foundations of abnormal psychology*. New York: Holt, Rinehart and Winston.

Derogatis, L.R., Lipman, R.S., Rickels, K., Ulenhuth, E.H., & Covi, L. (1974) The Hopkins Symptom Checklist (HSCL): A measure of primary symptom dimensions. In P. Pichot (Ed.), *Psychological measurements in psychopharmacology: Modern problems in pharmacopsychiatry: Vol. 7* (pp. 79–110). Basel: Karger.

Dixon, N.F. (1981) *Preconscious processing*. Chichester, England: Wiley.

Eldar, S. (1976) *Cognitive orientation and the perception of incongruent communication*. Master's thesis, Department of Psychology, Tel Aviv University.

Ellsworth, G.A., Strain, G.W., Strain, J.J., & Vaillant, G.E. (1986) Defensive maturity ratings and sustained weight loss in obesity. *Psychosomatics, 27*, 772–781.

Fenichel, O. (1945) *The psychoanalytic theory of neurosis*. New York: Norton.

Freud, A. (1966) *The ego and the mechanisms of defense* (rev. ed). Madison, CT: International Universities Press.

Freud, S. (1936) The problem of anxiety. New York: Norton.

Freud, S. (1957) Repression. In J. Strachey (Ed.), *The standard edition of the complete psychological works of S. Freud: Vol. 14* (pp. 141–158). London: Hogarth Press. (Originally published in 1915)

Freud, S. (1961) The ego and the id. In J. Strachey (Ed.), *The standard edition of the complete psychological works of S. Freud: Vol. 19* (pp. 3–66). London: Hogarth Press. (Originally published in 1923)

Freud, S. (1962) Further remarks on the neuro-psychoses of defense. In J. Strachey (Ed.), *The standard edition of the complete psychological works of S. Freud: Vol. 3* (pp. 162–185). London: The Hogarth Press. (Originally published in 1896)

Freud, S. (1964) New introductory lectures on psychoanalysis. In J. Strachey (Ed.), *The standard edition of the complete psychological works of S. Freud: Vol. 22* (pp. 3–182). London: Hogarth Press. (Originally published in 1933)

Freud, S. (1964) Analysis terminable and interminable. In J. Strachey (Ed.), *The standard edition of the complete psychological works of S. Freud: Vol. 23* (pp. 211–253). London: Hogarth Press. (Originally published in 1937)

Gibbs, J.T. (1987) Identity and marginality issues in the treatment of biracial adolescents. *American Journal of Orthopsychiatry, 57*, 265–278.

Griffin, S.E. (1986) Sex roles in addiction: Defense or deficit? *International Journal of the Addictions, 21*, 1307–1312.

Grzegolowska-Klarkowska, H. & Zolnierczyk, D. (1988) Defense of self-esteem, defense of self-consistency: A new voice in an old controversy. *Journal of Social and Clinical Psychology, 6*, 171–179.

Hardyck, J.A. & Kardush, M. (1968) A modest model for dissonance reduction. In R.P. Abelson, E. Aronson, W.J. McGuire, T.M. Newcomb, M.J. Rosenberg, & P.H. Tannenbaum (Eds.), *Theories of cognitive consistency: A sourcebook* (pp. 684–692). Skokie, IL: Rand McNally.

Kelman, H.C. & Baron, R.M. (1968) Determinants of modes of resolving inconsistency dilemmas: A functional analysis. In R.P. Abelson, E. Aronson, W.J. McGuire, T.M. Newcomb, M.J. Rosenberg, & P.H. Tannenbaum (Eds.),

Theories of cognitive consistency: A sourcebook (pp. 670–683). Skokie, IL: Rand McNally.

Kline, P. (1987) The scientific status of the DMT [Defense Mechanism Test]. *British Journal of Medical Psychology*, *60*, 53–59.

Kragh, U. (1984) Defense mechanisms manifested in perceptgenesis. In W.D. Fröhlich, G. Smith, J.G. Draguns, & U. Hentschel (Eds.), *Psychological processes in cognition and personality* (pp. 165–170). Washington, DC: Hemisphere.

Kreitler, S. & Chemerinski, A. (1988) The cognitive orientation of obesity. *International Journal of Obesity*, *12*, 403–412.

Kreitler, H. & Kreitler, S. (1964) Modes of action in the psychodramatic role test. *International Journal of Sociometry and Sociatry*, *4*, 10–15.

Kreitler, H. & Kreitler, S. (1968) The validation of psychodramatic behavior against behavior in life. *British Journal of Medical Psychology*, *41*, 185–192.

Kreitler, H. & Kreitler, S. (1969) Cognitive orientation and defense mechanisms. *Research Bulletin* (RB-69-23), Princeton, NJ: Educational Testing Service.

Kreitler, H. & Kreitler, S. (1972) The cognitive determinants of defensive behavior. *British Journal of Social and Clinical Psychology*, *11*, 359–372.

Kreitler, H. & Kreitler, S. (1976) *Cognitive orientation and behavior*. New York: Springer.

Kreitler, H. & Kreitler, S. (1977) *Cognitive habilitation-by-meaning of aphasic patients and imbecile children*. Invited address, celebrations of the 500th anniversary of the Johannes Gutenberg University, Mainz, Germany.

Kreitler, H. & Kreitler, S. (1982) The theory of cognitive orientation: Widening the scope of behavior prediction. In B. Maher & W.B. Maher (Eds.), *Progress in experimental personality research: Vol. 11* (pp. 101–169). New York: Academic Press.

Kreitler, S. & Kreitler, H. (1986) Types of curiosity behaviors and their cognitive determinants. *Archives of Psychology*, *138*, 233–251.

Kreitler, S. & Kreitler, H. (1987) The motivational and cognitive determinants of individual planning. *Genetic, Social and General Psychology Monographs*, *113*, 81–107.

Kreitler, S. & Kreitler, H. (1988a) The cognitive approach to motivation in retarded individuals. In N.W. Bray (Ed.), *International review of research in mental retardation: Vol. 15* (pp. 81–123). San Diego, CA: Academic Press.

Kreitler, S. & Kreitler, H. (1988b) Horizontal decalage: A problem and its resolution. *Cognitive Development*, *4*, 89–119.

Kreitler, S. & Kreitler, H. (1988c) Trauma and anxiety: The cognitive approach. *Journal of Traumatic Stress*, *1*, 35–56.

Kreitler, S. & Kreitler, H. (1990a) *The cognitive foundations of personality traits*. New York: Plenum.

Kreitler, H. & Kreitler, S. (1990b) Psychosemantic foundations of creativity. In K.J. Gilhooly, M. Keane, R. Logie, & G. Erdos (Eds.), *Lines of thought: Reflections on the psychology of thinking: Vol. 1* (pp. 15–28). Chichester, England: Wiley.

Kreitler, S. & Kreitler, H. (1990c) Cognitive orientation and sexual dysfunctions in women. *Annals of Sex Research*, *3*, 75–104.

Kreitler, H. & Kreitler, S. (1990d) Cognitive primacy, cognitive behavior guidance, and their implications for cognitive therapy. *Journal of Cognitive Psychotherapy*, *4*, 151–169.

Kreitler, S. & Kreitler, H. (1990e) *The cognitive approach to personality*. Unpublished book manuscript. Tel Aviv University.

Kreitler, S. & Kreitler, H. (1991) Cognitive orientation and physical disease or health. *European Journal of Personality*, *5*, 109–129.

Kreitler, S. & Kreitler, H. (in press-a) Cognitive orientation and disorders of the menstrual cycle. *Archives of Psychology*.

Kreitler, S. & Kreitler, H. (in press-b) Motivational and cognitive determinants of exploration. In H. Keller & K. Schneider (Eds.), *Curiosity and exploration: Theoretical perspectives, research fields and applications*. New York: Springer.

Kreitler, S. & Kreitler, H. (in press-c) *The cognitive rehabilitation of severely retarded children*. New York: Plenum.

Kreitler, S., Kreitler, H., & Carasso, R. (1987) Cognitive orientation as predictor of pain relief following acupuncture. *Pain*, *28*, 323–341.

Kreitler, S., Kreitler, H., & Schwartz, R. (1991) Cognitive orientation and genital infections in young women. *Women and Health*, *17*, 49–85.

Kreitler, S., Kreitler, H., & Wanounou, V. (1987–1988) Cognitive modification of test performance in schizophrenics and normals. *Imagination, Cognition, and Personality*, *7*, 227–249.

Kreitler, S., Schwartz, R., & Kreitler, H. (1987) The cognitive orientation of expressive communicability in schizophrenics and normals. *Journal of Communication Disorders*, *24*, 73–91.

Lazarus, R.S. & Folkman, S. (1984) *Stress, appraisal, and coping*. New York: Springer.

Lipowski, Z.J. (1970–1971) Physical illness, the individual and the coping process. *International Journal of Psychiatry in Medicine*, *1*, 91–102.

McCrae, R.R. & Costa, P.T. (1986) Personality, coping and coping effectiveness in an adult sample. *Journal of Personality and Social Psychology*, *54*, 385–405.

Marton, F.K. (1988) Defenses: Invincible and vincible. *Clinical Social Work Journal*, *16*, 143–155.

Moos, R.H. (Ed.) (1977) *Coping with physical illness: Vol. 1*. New York: Plenum.

Moos, R.H. (Ed.) (1984) *Coping with physical illness: Vol. 2, New perspectives*. New York: Plenum.

Munroe, R.L. (1956) *Schools of psychoanalytic thought* (3rd printing). New York: Dryden Press.

Pearlin, L.I. & Schooler, C. (1978) The structure of coping. *Journal of Health and Social Behavior*, *19*, 2–21.

Piaget, J. (1951) *Play, dreams, and imitation in childhood*. New York: Norton.

Polya, G. (1954) *Induction and analogy in mathematics: Vol. 1*. Princeton, NJ: Princeton University Press.

Polya, G. (1957) *How to solve it*. Garden City, NY: Doubleday.

Rosenthal, R.J. (1986) The pathological gambler's system for self-deception. *Journal of Gambling Behavior*, *2*, 108–120.

Sahoo, F.M., Sia N., & Panada, E. (1987) Individualism, collectivism and coping styles. *Journal of Psychological Researches*, *31*, 77–81.

Schafer, R. (1987) Self-deception, defense, and narration. *Psychoanalysis and Contemporary Thought*, *10*, 319–346.

Seligman, M. (1975) *Helplessness*. San Francisco: Freeman.

Singer, J.L. (Ed.) (1990) *Repression and dissociation*. Chicago: University of Chicago Press.

Snyder, C.R. (1988) From defenses to self-protection: An evolutionary perspective. *Journal of Social and Clinical Psychology*, *6*, 155–158.

Tipton, R.M. & Riebsame, W.E. (1987) Beliefs about smoking and health: Their measurement and relationship to smoking behavior. *Addictive Behaviors*, *12*, 217–223.

Vaillant, G.E. (1983) Childhood environment and maturity of defense mechanisms. In D. Magnusson & V.L. Allen (Eds.), *Human development: An interactional perspective* (pp. 343–352). San Diego, CA: Academic Press.

Watzlawick, P., Beavin, J.H., & Jackson, D.D. (1967) *Pragmatics of human communication*. Palo Alto, CA: Norton.

Weinberger, D.A., Schwartz, G.E., & Davidson, R.J. (1979) Low anxious, high anxious, and repressive coping styles: Psychometric patterns and behavioral and physiological responses to stress. *Journal of Abnormal Psychology*, *88*, 369–380.

Weisman, A.D. (1979) *Coping with cancer*. New York: McGraw-Hill.

Westhoff, K. & Halbach-Suarez, C. (1989) Cognitive orientation and the prediction of decisions in a medical examination context. *European Journal of Personality*, *3*, 61–71.

White, R.W. (1974) Strategies of adaptation: An attempt at systematic description. In G.V. Coelho, D.A. Hamburg, & J.E. Adams (Eds.), *Coping and adaptation* (pp. 47–48). New York: Basic Books.

Wickelgren, W.A. (1974) *How to solve problems*. San Francisco: Freeman.

Winegar, N., Stephens, T.A., & Varney, E.D. (1987) Alcoholics Anonymous and the alcoholic defense structure. *Social Case Work*, *68*, 223–228.

Zakay, D., Bar-El, Z., & Kreitler, S. (1984) Cognitive orientation and changing the impulsivity of children. *British Journal of Educational Psychology*, *54*, 40–50.

Zemet, R. (1976) *Cognitive orientation theory and patterns of behavior in conflictual situations in schizophrenic and normal subjects*. Master's thesis, Department of Psychology, Tel Aviv University (summarized in Kreitler & Kreitler, 1982, pp. 150–153).

12
Development of the Repression-Sensitization Construct: With Special Reference to the Discrepancy Between Subjective and Physiological Stress Reactions

CARL-WALTER KOHLMANN

Research on the construct "repression-sensitization" has developed from a fusion of two traditions, one "perception oriented" and the other "clinical" (cf. Erdelyi, 1990; Krohne, in press). The perception-oriented line of development has its origins in Brunswik's functionalistic interpretations of behavior (Brunswik, 1947) and has served as the basis for a person-oriented approach in perception research (cf. Bruner, 1951; Bruner & Postman, 1947; Frenkel-Brunswik, 1949; Klein & Schlesinger, 1949). The "clinical" approach is represented by psychoanalytical approaches to "anxiety defense mechanisms" (Freud, 1936).

The expectancy or hypothesis theory of perception (Bruner, 1951), developed to be adequate for dealing with both the laboratory experiment in perception and the observation of the clinician, forms the foundation for the fusion of these different traditions. According to this theory, the progression and result of a perceptual operation are predominantly determined by the "hypotheses" an individual brings into the perceptual situation. The type and strength of these hypotheses should be determined by person-specific needs (e.g., the need for safety and order or for control over instinctive impulses). In their classical experiment on "perceptual defense," inspired by Jung's word association studies (1906/1909), Bruner and Postman (1947) could register two forms of reacting to emotionally significant stimuli. Individuals with a "defensive" orientation attempted to avoid the perception of the critical stimulus as long as possible. This contrasted a so-called sensitizing orientation, characterized by intensified vigilance in the face of emotionally significant stimuli (for overviews, methodological criticisms, and continuations cf. Blum, 1955; Dixon, 1971, 1981; Erdelyi, 1974, 1990; Goldiamond, 1958; Hentschel & Smith, 1980; Holmes, 1974, 1990; Krohne, 1978; Shevrin, 1990).

Eriksen (1951) argued that defense mechanisms could be divided into two basic forms, which are generally antagonistic with regard to their function: anxiety reduction by avoiding danger-related stimuli and anxiety reduction by intensified attention as well as sensitization to such stimuli (for an investigation cf. Lazarus, Eriksen, & Fonda, 1951). The type of mechanism a person preferably employs to cope with (i.e., perceive) anxiety-arousing circumstances can be qualified by a personality characteristic. Gordon (1957) introduced the designation "repression-sensitization" for this one-dimensional bipolar personality variable. To empirically determine this trait, a number of projective methods as well as scale combinations, based mostly on the MMPI, were proposed (cf. Byrne, 1964). The most prominent operationalization of repression-sensitization is represented by Byrne's Repression–Sensitization scale (R-S scale: Byrne, 1961; cf. also Byrne, Barry, & Nelson, 1963; Epstein & Fenz, 1967; Krohne, 1974), which is compiled from MMPI items.

In a great number of studies on the construct repression-sensitization (for overviews cf. Bell & Byrne, 1978; Byrne, 1964; Krohne, in press; Krohne & Rogner, 1982; Singer, 1990; Tucker, 1970), associations, although often weak, could be established between repression-sensitization and certain theoretically relevant behavioral indicators. An example is a relatively recent study conducted by Halperin (1986). This study examined the relationship between repression-sensitization (assessed by the revised R-S scale, Byrne et al., 1963) and the visual focusing of attention when viewing slides that arouse pleasant or unpleasant emotions (for a similar study using films, cf. Haley, 1974). While the subjects viewed neutral (i.e., landscape), sexual (i.e., men and women in different stages of undress), or nauseating (i.e., open wounds caused by injury) slides, the areas viewed the longest amount of time were registered using an eye movement camera. In pilot studies "key areas" of the sexual and nauseating slides that particularly induced emotion, as well as the interesting parts of the neutral ones, could be determined. The hypothesis that sensitizers direct their attention only to the "key areas" longer than repressors when viewing unpleasant slides could not be completely confirmed: when confronted with slides that induced emotion (i.e., nauseating as well as sexual), sensitizers generally examined the central areas prominently longer (injury theme: 41% of the viewing time; sexual theme: 37%) than a "middle group" with R-S scores in the middle section of the distribution (28%, 22%) and repressors (27%, 22%). The groups did not differ when viewing the areas of the neutral slides judged to be interesting. Halperin (1986) believes that these results fundamentally confirm the construct validity of the R-S scale. However, he also doubts the linearity of the scale, since the mean group and repressors did not differ. Moreover, the author suggests that the criteria range of the "approach–avoidance construct" should be extended from only stimuli or situations that arouse unpleasant emotions to general emotional stimuli. From the information-theoretical as well as percept-genetic view of repression-sensitization (Erdelyi, 1974; Krohne, 1978; see also Fröhlich,

1984), it would be interesting to know whether repressors, when viewing slides that induce emotion, already focus on and register the emotionally relevant areas in a very early phase of the perceptual process and then turn away from them (in a relatively permanent manner). Halperin's data, however, have not been analyzed according to this perspective yet.

Regarding the operationalization of repression-sensitization, a series of objections has been formulated. According to Krohne (in press), the objections can be summarized into two central points:

1. The R-S scale correlates with anxiety scales in the area of good reliability coefficients (cf. Abbott, 1972; Bell & Byrne, 1978; Boucsein & Freye, 1974; Krohne, 1974; Watson & Clark, 1984). The confounding of both characteristics leads to the assumptions that both constructs are associated with a common emotionality factor (cf. Watson & Clark, 1984: "negative affectivity") or that the R-S scale is merely appropriate for recording self-reported emotional and psychopathological symptoms (Budd & Clopton, 1985; cf. also Lefcourt, 1966). The second problem is directly related to this criticism.

2. A linear relationship exists between the R-S scale and different indicators of emotional adaptation, which contradicts a theoretical conceptualization of extremely high or low repression-sensitization scores as indicators of rigid and thereby frequently unadaptive forms of coping.

A curvilinear relationship would have better met expectations (cf. Bell & Byrne, 1978). Moreover, the homogeneity of that group of individuals in the middle section of the distribution of scores for the R-S scale is controversial with regard to their coping behavior (cf. Chabot, 1973). It is however not surprising that the answers to questions on the R-S scale regarding, for example, bodily symptoms, health, and depression (as "indirect" indicators of defensive style) correlate with reports and observations of the same factors (as "direct" indicators of emotional adaptation; cf. also Angleitner, 1980; Watson & Pennebaker, 1989). The disregarded "item overlapping" in the predictor and criteria operationalizations in the "life-event research" also led to an initial, methodologically contingent overestimation of the strength of the relationship between "critical" life events and the appearance of impairment to the psychic and physical well-being (cf. Schroeder & Costa, 1984).

Later developments in the theoretical and operational determination of repression-sensitization pursue an optimization of different focal points. The multiple variable approaches, which are based on the simultaneous application of anxiety and defensiveness scales, attempt to overcome the confounding of anxiety and repression-sensitization and suggest, in particular, a separation of "truly" low-anxious individuals from repressors; the intersection of high anxiety and sensitization appears, in contrast, to be viewed as less problematic. Several authors (e.g., Beck &

Clark, 1988; Carver & Scheier, 1988; Eysenck, 1988) determine anxiety using some cognitive processes assumed to be characteristic of sensitization (e.g., selective perception and processing of threatening stimuli, anticipation of negative events). In more recent, person-oriented approaches, the preferences for certain coping behavior are not "inferred," as is still done in multiple variable approaches; in contrast, persons are concretely asked about their preferred coping reactions and actions in imaginary stressful situations.

Multiple Variable Approaches with Traditional Instruments

Since both repression-sensitization and anxiety are conceptualized as one-dimensional personality characteristics, a separation of high anxiety and sensitization, as well as low anxiety and repression, is not possible due to the strong correlations between anxiety tests and the R-S scale. To overcome this difficulty, many authors (Hill & Sarason, 1966; Holroyd, 1966; Kogan & Wallach, 1964; Krohne & Rogner, 1985; Lefcourt, 1969; Weinberger, Schwartz, & Davidson, 1979) have suggested "multiple variable approaches" (cf. Krohne & Rogner, 1985) with the simultaneous application of tests for anxiety (e.g., the Manifest Anxiety Scale, MAS, J.A. Taylor, 1953), defensiveness and anxiety denial (e.g., scales for the "social desirability tendency," Crowne & Marlowe, 1960; Edwards, 1957).[1]

The anxiety test should serve to determine the tendency to judge situations as more or less threatening. In contrast, the scales for defensiveness should register the variable tendency to avoid threatening situations and their aversive character and to deny contingently evoked anxiety. Since the empirical indicators for both these tendencies are in general only very weakly correlated, the calculation of the median for both score distributions reveals four approximately equally large groups of individuals, which are characterized by different yet distinctive patterns of anxiety and defensiveness.

Individuals who exhibit comparatively low scores on both tests are designated "nondefensive" or "truly low-anxious" (e.g., Krohne & Rogner, 1985; Weinberger et al., 1979). They should judge comparatively few

---

[1] For a recent definition of coping strategies within a broader view of social emotional adjustment, see Weinberger (1990) and Weinberger and Schwartz (1990). Their typology is based on the intersection of two superordinate dimensions, also. One, a self-control dimension, is conceptualized as the suppression of egoistic desires. The other, an affective dimension, is formulated as the subjective experience of distress. Repressors, for example, are defined as individuals who report low distress but high levels of self-restraint.

situations as threatening and have little motivation to deny anxiety. Similarly low anxiety scores in combination with comparatively higher defensiveness indicate individuals who largely deny environmental threats as well as the appearance of their own emotional and cognitive anxiety reactions. This group represents the "repressors."[2] The interpretation of the other two patterns is debatable. Weinberger et al. (1979), for example, who are most concerned with the separation of "truly" low-anxious individuals and repressors, designate the pattern of high anxiety and low defensiveness "high-anxious" and that of high anxiety and high defensiveness "defensively high-anxious." The designation proposed by Weinberger et al. is also accepted by other researchers including Asendorpf and Scherer (1983), Davis (1987; cf. also Davis & Schwartz, 1987), Hansen and Hansen (1988), and Tremayne and Barry (1988).

In contrast, Krohne and Rogner (1985) have suggested considering the pattern "high anxiety/high defensiveness" to be an indicator of "unsuccessful coping" (equivalent to high anxiety). Since they admit their anxiety in spite of a general tendency to block negative emotions (cf. also Hill, 1971), individuals with high scores on both scales should, according to Krohne and Rogner, experience anxiety particularly frequently and intensely. Krohne and Rogner interpret the configuration of comparatively high anxiety and low defensiveness as "sensitization," since persons in this group do not block their anxiety although they rate many situations as threatening.

If the defensiveness scale is, however, interpreted according to Crowne and Marlowe (1964) as "the search for social acceptance," then the defensiveness interpretation favored by Weinberger et al. (1979) cannot be rejected. Intensified anxiety would then be instrumentally reported in the sense of an excuse for inadequate performance (cf. Laux & Glanzmann, 1987; for a similar functional interpretation of the lowering of the aspiration level cf. Wieland-Eckelmann & Bösel, 1987). The difference in interpretation of the desirability scale, in either the direction "defense" (Krohne & Rogner) or "search for social acceptance" (Weinberger et al.), appears to particularly underlie the different designations of the coping groups. While defensively high-anxious individuals, accord-

---

[2] The operationalization of the repressive coping style by the combination of low anxiety and high defensiveness scores shows some similarities with the psychiatric concept of "alexithymia" (Sifneos, 1973). It denotes a disturbance characterized by inadequacy in discriminating feeling states from emotional (i.e., bodily) reactions (for critical overviews, see Kohlmann, 1986; Lesser, 1981; Martin & Pihl, 1985; G.J. Taylor, 1984). Bonanno and Singer (1990) wonder whether the alexithymia concept has any independence or whether it may be reflecting a facet of the better-measured repressive style. According to Krohne and Kohlmann (1990), a possible difference between the two concepts may be that alexithymia refers to the ability to communicate feelings, whereas repression is concerned with the willingness to communicate feelings.

ing to Weinberger et al., report their anxiety because of their tendency to crave social acceptance, the high-anxious, as conceptualized by Krohne and Rogner, still report their intensified anxiety in spite of their increased defensiveness.

Investigations on the predictive validity of the two-dimensional conceptualization of coping strategies are described by Asendorpf and Wallbott (1985; Asendorpf, Wallbott, & Scherer, 1983). According to them, the approach is primarily supported by analyses of the "discrepancy hypothesis," which relates coping behaviors or coping dispositions to differential stress reactions on different levels.

The Discrepancy Hypothesis

The discrepancy hypothesis is based on the idea formulated by Lazarus (1966) that the patterns of coping reactions on the subjective–affective, physiological–biochemical, and behavioral–expressive levels can be interpreted as indicators for the employment of intrapsychic coping behavior. The following quotations represent his central premise:

The point is that we should not necessarily expect all classes of response to agree with each other. It is their combined pattern that yields the best information about the psychological processes we wish to understand. Thus, when a person says he does not feel anxious or disturbed but shows a marked physiological-stress reaction, we learn something different about the ongoing psychological processes (assuming physical demands have been ruled out) than if he reports marked anxiety along with concordant physiological responses. In the former instance, we might speak of social pressures or defensive efforts; in the latter, these are evidently not operating. The answer, therefore, is that no one of these classes of response must be considered *the* indicator of threat processes by itself. A more dependable and complete analysis can be accomplished using combinations of indicators and examining their patterning. . . . different ways of coping with threat are associated with different autonomic as well as behavioral patterns of reaction. (Lazarus, 1966, pp. 387–388, 390)[3]

Although Lazarus argues that discrepancies are indicators of actual coping behavior ("defensive efforts"), the overwhelming majority of the studies on the discrepancy hypothesis do not directly analyze the relation-

---

[3] In the meantime, however, Lazarus has taking back his assumption: ". . . when studies are done across measurement levels, what is commonly produced from one method is largely uncorrelated with findings from another method and, in effect, method variance overwhelms everything else. Our preferred solution to the problem of method variance is to persist with a single measure, in that case self-report, until findings or the lack of them are clear. . . . We believe that at this stage of our knowledge this is a more economical and practical solution than combining methods catch-as-catch-can before having established findings." (Lazarus & Folkman, 1984, p. 323)

ship between actual coping behavior and patterns of subjective and objective stress reactions (for exceptions, see Houston & Hodges, 1970; Kohlmann, Singer, & Krohne, 1989). Most of the studies follow a more "indirect" path. Under the assumption that coping dispositions determine actual coping behavior and that this behavior leads to certain reaction patterns, they primarily attempt to predict the pattern of stress reactions by using their knowledge of certain coping dispositions.

The first studies that were conducted in connection with the discrepancy hypothesis were derived from the one-dimensional operationalization of repression-sensitization. The initial research impulse was given by a study performed by Weinstein, Averill, Opton, and Lazarus (1968). Using a reanalysis of several empirical studies conducted by Lazarus' research group, the authors investigated the hypothesis that low anxiety is reported by repressors when they respond with comparatively high physiological arousal, while sensitizers report high anxiety despite exhibiting low physiological anxiety. For each of the dependent variables (i.e., mean heart rate, skin conductance, and verbal anxiety reports), z-scores were calculated and integrated into respective activation indices. Individual discrepancy scores were then calculated by subtracting the activation indices (physiological minus subjective index). According to expectations, repressors verbally admitted less anxiety than they manifested physiologically while sensitizers reacted in the opposite manner (for a replication cf. Otto & Bösel, 1978; for a further experimental study, see Scarpetti, 1973; for a clinical study, see Shipley, Butt, Horwitz, & Farbry, 1978). Weinstein et al. (1968) explicitly point out, however, that the differences between the groups were found only for the verbal anxiety report. Repressors and sensitizers did not differ in regard to heart rate or skin conductance. Asendorpf and Wallbott (1985; see also Asendorpf et al., 1983) believe that the most significant weakness of the study of Weinstein et al. lies in the fact that no control group (e.g., a repression-sensitization middle group) took part in the study along with the repressor and sensitizer groups.

Parsons, Fulgenzi, and Edelberg (1969) did conduct a comparison of repressors, sensitizers, and an R-S middle group. In group discussions, repressors rated themselves as unaggressive and dominant (experiments 1 and 2) while an observer judged them as especially aggressive (experiment 1). In addition, repressors reacted with more frequent changes in skin conductance than the other two groups (experiment 2). The observed ("genuine") discrepancies between the self-description and the observer's description as well as the physiological activation support the assumptions of the discrepancy hypothesis. Contradictory results were found, for example, in a study by Stein (1971), in which the R-S middle group reacted more strongly during sentence association tasks than the extreme groups. In a study by Boucsein and Frye (1974), repressors manifested stronger subjective than physiological reactions to criticism while sensitizers showed the opposite reaction pattern. This effect is diametrically contradictory to the theoretical expectations.

Thayer (1971, experiment 2) determined the discrepancy score for the difference between physiological and subjective measures of activation changes and correlated the discrepancy measure with, among other factors, repression-sensitization. It is not surprising that no relationship was found, since only "sleepiness," which is not anxiety related, was used as the subjective indicator of arousal.

Asendorpf et al. (1983) trace the equivocal and partly contradictory results especially back to the varied selection of extreme groups.[4] The necessity of separating repressors from "truly" low-anxious individuals is particularly represented by Asendorpf et al. The comparison of R-S extreme groups with a middle group, whose status is unclear with regard to the preferred coping behavior (cf. Chabot, 1973), is not appropriate for solving this problem.

Empirical analyses of the discrepancy hypothesis based on the two-dimensional operationalization of coping styles focus on the prediction of different reactions manifested by low-anxious individuals (i.e., low anxiety/low defensiveness) and repressors (i.e., low anxiety/high defensiveness).

Weinberger et al. (1979) did indeed introduce the designations "repressor," "low-anxious," "high-anxious," and "defensively high-anxious" for the four coping groups differentiated by an anxiety and defensiveness test, but in their investigation they took only three groups into account: repressors (i.e., anxiety < median; defensiveness > 75% ranking), low-anxious (i.e., anxiety < median; defensiveness < 75%), and "moderately" high-anxious individuals (i.e., anxiety > median, defensiveness < 75%). While freely associating to sentences with neutral, sexual, and aggressive content, these three groups were compared using different parameters. Repressors reacted, in contrast to the low-anxious, with higher increases in heart rate, the number of spontaneous changes in skin resistance and frontal muscular tension (with reference to a baseline, resp.). In addition, they manifested longer reaction times when confronted with aggressive and sexual content. In the transcribed statements, higher indices for avoidance of the affective content in the presented sentences were registered for repressors. It is worth mentioning that the reaction times of the "moderately" high-anxious group lay between those for low-anxious and repressors. They behaved like repressors with regard to increases in heart rate, while their changes in skin resistance were similar to those of low-anxious individuals. Subjective stress reactions were not recorded. Conclusions about subjective stress reactions were

---

[4] Based on a review of 38 studies on construct validity of the R-S scale, Halperin (1986) also points out the problem of falsely classifying subjects, especially when placing them in the R-S middle group.

supposedly made possible by only two applications of a shortened form of the MAS (Bendig, 1956), one 7 weeks before the investigation and the other immediately following it. While the "moderately" high-anxious reacted with an increase in anxiety, the low-anxious showed no changes and the repressors even showed a decrease of anxiety.[5]

Asendorpf et al. (1983) interpret the results of Weinberger et al. as an almost perfect confirmation of the repression-sensitization concept. However, a major disadvantage of this study is that the effects of anxiety and defensiveness were not considered to be separate factors in the analyses. If one considers not the changes but the actual levels of the Bending MAS, then primarily those differences in anxiety necessary for the group division were confirmed: persons who differ in their MAS scores 7 weeks before the investigation also had correspondingly different MAS scores immediately following the investigations ("moderately" high-anxious: $6.45 \rightarrow 8.55$; low-anxious: $2.93 \rightarrow 3.27$; repressors: $2.50 \rightarrow 1.64$; no analyses were reported by the authors with regard to the level differences). The reaction times, verbal interference, changes in spontaneous fluctuations, and frontal-EMG results appear, on the other hand, to be completely explainable as a main effect of the defensiveness scale (the Social Desirability Scale [SDS] of Crowne & Marlowe, 1960). Repressors (high SDS scores) manifest higher values than low-anxious (low SDS scores) and "moderately" high-anxious (low SDS scores) individuals for all variables. Thus the results of Weinberger et al. can be recapitulated in the following manner:

1. The level of anxiety reported after the experiment depends on the anxiety before the experiment.

---

[5] In a similar study by Newton and Contrada (1992), subjects first prepared and then delivered a speech about their most undesirable trait, while either one person (i.e., private condition) or three people (i.e., public condition) observed via closed-circuit television. Blood pressure and heart rate were monitored during a baseline period, the 3-minute preparation, and the 3-minute speech. Heart rate elevations were greatest for repressors (i.e., low anxiety/high defensiveness) in the public condition during speech delivery. Significantly lower heart rate elevations were seen in the same subjects during speech preparation. Additionally, repressors showed a substantial discrepancy between their high autonomic activity and low self-report of negative affect only while delivering a self-disclosing speech to three observers. Such a discrepancy was not in evidence while they self-disclosed to a single individual. High-anxious subjects (i.e., high anxiety/low defensiveness) in both conditions showed a reverse discrepancy (i.e., negative affect was stronger as compared to heart rate), whereas low-anxious subjects (i.e., low anxiety/low defensiveness) did not exhibit a discrepancy. According to the authors, these results replicated previous findings of dissociated autonomic and self-report indices of negative affect in repressors and further suggest that the repressive coping style may be activated by conditions likely to evoke social evaluative concerns (see also Note 2). Unfortunately, the group with the pattern "high anxiety/high defensiveness" was not included in the study.

2. Following stress, the "anxiety" of high-anxious individuals (high MAS score), rises while it remains rather constant (low-anxious) or sinks (repressors) for people with lower anxiety (low MAS scores).

3. Objective measures (i.e., longer reaction times, verbal interference, increase in spontaneous fluctuations, rises in frontal-EMG and heart rate) that record the active engagement (i.e., associations) in the experiment vary particularly in their dependence on the social desirability tendency.

Two additional studies, in which subjective and objective stress reactions were associated with anxiety and social desirability, will be considered to determine whether they can confirm the above-mentioned interpretation.

Asendorpf and Scherer's study (1983) adopted the method put forward by Weinstein et al. (1979). In addition to the low-anxious and repressor groups, two additional groups determined by extreme scores on the MAS and SDS were taken into consideration: a "high-anxious" (i.e., high MAS score/low SDS score) and a "defensively high-anxious" (i.e., high MAS score/ high SDS score) group. During a sentence association task, the subjects with high MAS scores (i.e., high-anxious and defensively high-anxious) reported more anxiety than subjects with low MAS scores (i.e., low-anxious and repressors). With regard to the objective stress indicators (i.e., heart rate adjusted to a baseline, amplitude of the finger pulse volume, mimic anxiety), only the repressors (i.e., low MAS score/ high SDS score) manifested higher reactions than the low-anxious (i.e., low MAS score/low SDS score). Analyses of possible main and interaction effects of MAS and SDS would have been possible in this study but were not conducted.

A somewhat revised approach was selected by Gudjonsson (1981). Subjects were asked questions with neutral themes (e.g., "Are you wearing black shoes?") and "lie-questions" (e.g., "Have you ever lied?"), which had to be answered with "yes" or "no." For each question, the skin conductance reactions (SCRs), spontaneous fluctuations of the electrodermal activity (NSRs), and subjective arousal estimations were recorded and then summarized for all questions (not separated by theme!). The distributions for SCRs, NSRs, and subjective arousal estimations were divided at the medians. It was then tested whether the subjective and objective data for a person lay in the same or a different half of the distribution. Individuals who were under the median for the subjective variable and above for the objective variable were designated "repressors." The group with the opposite configuration made up the "sensitizers," while subjects with both the subjective and objective arousal above or below the median, respectively, were placed into a middle group. These three groups were compared with regard to their scores on the neuroticism, extraversion, and lie scales of the Eysenck

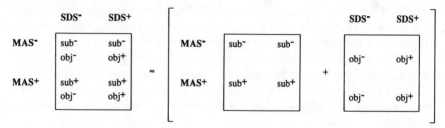

FIGURE 12.1. Subjective arousal (sub) as a function of anxiety (MAS). Objective arousal (obj) as a function of the social desirability tendency (SDS). Low and high distinctions indicated by − and +, respectively. (Figure adapted from Kohlmann, 1990b, Fig. 3, p. 42.)

Personality Inventory (EPI: Eysenck & Eysenck, 1964) as well as the SDS. Repressors manifested significantly lower neuroticism scores and higher lie and SDS scores than both the other groups. Moreover, the authors reported that the SDS was positively correlated with electro-dermal activity (SCRs: $r = .42$, NSRs: $r = .49$), but there was almost no correlation or a rather negative one with neuroticism ($r = -.20$, $r = -.39$, resp.). Associations between subjective arousal and personality variables were not reported.

Both these reported studies suggest the hypothesis that the results for discrepancy between subjective and objective measures of arousal when employing multiple variable approaches in determining coping dispositions (using MAS and SDS) can be almost completely explained by two main effects: (a) increased trait anxiety leads to a report of higher anxiety, and (b) increased social desirability leads to an intensified engagement, which is accompanied by increased physiological arousal. Schulz (1982) demonstrated that subjects who strive for social acceptance (cf. Crowne and Marlowe's original interpretation of SDS) invest an extremely high amount of time and energy (increase in psychophysiologi-cal arousal) when solving tasks. From this perspective, we can completely dispense with the R-S concept as an explanation of the discrepancies between subjective and objective indicators of arousal. "Discrepancies" then simply represent the effects of two main effects on two different classes of variables. Figure 12.1 illustrates this interpretation.

Person-Oriented Approaches

Attempts to classify coping dispositions with the instruments just men-tioned pay little attention to how people evaluate stressful situations and at best allude only indirectly to the fact that people have definite prefer-ences regarding their use of distinct coping behaviors. Thus, very little is learned about the strategies preferred by a person in a given situation. To overcome these problems, the Miller Behavioral Style Scale (MBSS: Miller, 1987), the Mainz Coping Inventory (MCI: Krohne, 1986; Krohne, Rösch, & Kürsten, 1989), and the Multidimensional Coping Scale (MCS: Cook, 1985) have been developed to assess preferred coping strategies on a dispositional level. Taking the lead from stimulus–response inventories in anxiety research (cf. Endler, Hunt, & Rosenstein, 1962), these instruments present several fictitious situations, followed by a number of statements representing vigilant or avoidant ways of dealing with the situation, with which respondents either agree or disagree. Because these instruments require subjects to report their use of coping strategies rather than their awareness of specific symptoms, they more directly assess the cognitive and behavioral referents of vigilance and avoidance. In particular, the MBSS scale "monitoring," the MCI scale "vigilance," and the MCS scale "approach" represent approachlike coping preferences, whereas the MBSS scale "blunting," the MCI scale "cognitive avoidance," and the MCS scale "avoidance" represent avoidantlike coping preferences.[6]

An assumption of two kinds of "intolerance" responsible for approachlike and avoidantlike coping preferences has been introduced by Krohne and colleagues (Kohlmann, 1990b; Krohne, 1989; Krohne & Fuchs, 1991) with respect to the dimensions vigilance and cognitive avoidance. However, provided approach and avoidance preferences are operationalized as independent of each other, this assumption can, in principle, be applied to several instruments (cf. Kohlmann, 1990b). Basic is the idea of "intolerance of uncertainty" underlying vigilantlike coping preferences, and "intolerance of emotional arousal" underlying avoidantlike preferences. In a similar way, Rothbart and Mellinger (1972) already identified the motivation to avoid harm and the ability to tolerate short-term fear arousal as the two central factors effecting coping behavior (see also Frenkel-Brunswik, 1949). They proposed that repressors differ from sensitizers on both these variables. The "model of coping modes" (Krohne, 1989) assumes fundamental differences between repressors and

---

[6] Besides the theoretical similarities of especially the approaches developed by Miller (1987) and Krohne (1986, 1989), they also overlap on an empirical level. In a recent study, applying both the MBSS (Miller, 1987; German adaptation by Schumacher, 1990) to assess monitoring and blunting and the MCI (Krohne et al., 1989) to assess vigilance and cognitive avoidance, associations between the corresponding scales could be demonstrated. After correlations had been computed between the four coping scales using the data of 72 male and female undergraduates (Kohlmann, 1990b), only two significant correlations between the four coping variables emerged: while cognitive avoidance was positively associated with blunting only ($r = .46$), vigilance correlated only with monitoring ($r = .47$). Applying a principal component analysis to the four coping scores resulted in a clear two-factor solution with vigilance and monitoring as the first factor and cognitive avoidance and blunting as the second factor.

sensitizers on the two dimensions, also. However, repression and sensitization are not the only modes of coping considered. Because of the independence of both dimensions of habitualized coping, four configurations of coping patterns (in part related to those introduced by Weinberger et al., 1979) can be distinguished:

1. A rigid vigilant mode: persons with high vigilance and low avoidance are called "sensitizers." They should primarily be stressed by experienced uncertainty in a situation of threat, hence should show an increased tendency over diverse situations of threat to seek out information about the stressor in order to construct a mental picture of the anticipated confrontation. Without taking into account coping-relevant characteristics of the stress situation, these persons should try to attain information about the situation.

2. A rigid avoidant mode: persons with high avoidance and low vigilance are named "repressors." For these subjects, the emotional arousal triggered by cues prior to a confrontation with an aversive event probably constitutes a major threat. Therefore, they should generally tend to pay little attention to threat-relevant characteristics of situations.

3. A flexible, situation-related use of coping strategies: persons with the pattern "low vigilance and low avoidance" are called "nondefensives" or "flexible copers." In a situation of threat, they should not be intolerant of either the possibility of uncertainty or negative surprise or the possibility of emotional arousal. The mode of flexible use of coping strategies is assumed to be characterized by a marked orientation toward whatever situational requirements prevail at any given time. For example, a "flexible coper" would monitor a dentist's warning signal (e.g., raising a hand before the drill comes close to a nerve) if it reliably predicts painful drilling. However, if the dentist's behavior were unreliable regarding the painfulness of the medical attendance, the "flexible coper" would no longer monitor the unreliable signal but instead would engage in distracting thoughts.

4. An inconsistent, unsuccessful coping mode: persons with the pattern "high vigilance and high avoidance" are called "anxious persons." They should be heavily stressed by both the uncertainty in aversive situations and the emotional arousal triggered by cues. This is supposed to elicit unstable coping behavior. When attempting to reduce the uncertainty that they experience as stressful by increased preoccupation with the stressor, they simultaneously should increase their emotional arousal to a level exceeding that which they can tolerate. On the other hand, when turning away from the stressor to reduce anxiety, their uncertainty should increase together with the stress resulting from it. At the dentist's, for example, the "inconsistent coper," like the "flexible coper," should exhibit a nonrigid coping behavior. However, variations in the actual coping behavior are assumed not to result in a "fit" between situational

demands (e.g., the reliability of the dentist's signals) and actual coping efforts.

Thus, according to the model outlined above, the employment of a specific coping strategy is, of course, to a certain degree dependent on situational characteristics. There is, for example, generally more vigilance in predictable situations and an increased cognitive avoidance in unpredictable situations (Krohne & Rogner, 1982; Miller, 1981). Nevertheless, there is also a strong dependence in the use of coping strategies on dispositional antecedents. This is obviously implied in the definitions of the rigidly vigilant (i.e., sensitizers) and rigidly avoidant (i.e., repressors) coping modes. But even in the case of persons who employ strategies of different quality in different situations, coping behavior can be attributed to personality dispositions: for example, to the competency in analyzing situations appropriately and in choosing that strategy of one's coping repertoire that best fits the situational requirements (cf. Mischel, 1984; for a first critical empirical evaluation of some aspects of the model, see Kohlmann, 1990b).

Applying the MBSS (Miller, 1987) or the MCI (Krohne et al., 1989), important findings regarding health-related behavior have been documented.[7] Miller, Brody, and Summerton (1988) studied patients visiting a primary care setting for acute medical problems. Monitors (i.e., high monitoring and low blunting scores) and blunters (i.e., low monitoring and high blunting scores) differed in the level of seriousness of their actual medical problem. Evaluations by the physicians showed that monitors actually had less severe medical problems than blunters. Miller (1990) concludes that monitors may have a lower threshold of scanning for internal bodily cues. This would make them more inclined to detect new or changing physical symptoms (for studies on the role of vigilantlike and avoidantlike coping preferences in interoception, see Hodapp & Knoll, 1993; Kohlmann, 1993). In a study on the anticipation of an unpleasant laboratory stressor, Kohlmann (1990a) found a generally higher heart rate (baseline-corrected scores) for subjects being characterized by high blunting scores compared to those with low blunting scores.

Krohne (1989) analyzed the influence of vigilant and avoidant coping strategies on self-reported and biochemical stress indicators as evidenced by patients facing surgery. Free Fatty Acids (FFA) and state anxiety were measured the day after admission to hospital, after the pre-op visit in the afternoon before surgery, on the morning of surgery, and prior to

---

[7] For health-related research applying the multiple variable approach introduced by Weinberger et al. (1979), see Schwartz (1990) for an overview and Jensen (1987) for an impressive study.

induction of anaesthesia. A discrepancy score between subjective and objective stress reactions was operationalized by transforming the raw data into z-scores and subtracting the FFA from anxiety scores. In the case of the pattern "high vigilance/low cognitive avoidance" (i.e., "sensitizers"), a marked positive z-score emerged, indicating that the subjective presurgical stress reactions were stronger than the physiological ones.

Concluding Remark

The idea of the repressive coping style being associated with specifically physiological responses to stress seems to be supported by a number of studies. This finding can be generalized for avoidantlike coping preferences (when formulated in a broader theoretical concept, cf. Roth & Cohen, 1986) as assessed by the R-S scale (Byrne, 1961), a combination of anxiety and defensiveness scores (e.g., Weinberger et al., 1979), or one of the stimulus–response coping inventories (e.g., Krohne et al., 1989; Miller, 1987). For future research regarding the prediction of discrepancies between subjective and physiological stress reactions, it appears useful to measure approach- and avoidantlike coping preferences by these several instruments within a single study as a means of determining their distinctive contributions.

References

Abbott, R.D. (1972) On confounding of the Repression-Sensitization and Manifest Anxiety scales. *Psychological Reports*, *30*, 392–394.

Angleitner, A. (1980) *Einführung in die Persönlichkeitspsychologie. Band 1: Nichtfaktorielle Ansätze* [Introduction to personality: Nonfactorial approaches] Bern: Huber.

Asendorpf, J.B. & Scherer, K.R. (1983) The discrepant repressor: Differentiation between low anxiety, high anxiety, and repression of anxiety by autonomic–facial–verbal patterns of behavior. *Journal of Personality and Social Psychology*, *45*, 1334–1346.

Asendorpf, J.B. & Wallbott, H.G. (1985) Formen der Angstabwehr: Zweidimensionale Operationalisierung eines Bewältigungsstils [Modes of anxiety-defense: Two-dimensional operationalization of a coping-style] In K.R. Scherer, H.G. Wallbott, F.J. Tolkmitt, & G. Bergmann (Eds.), *Die Streßreaktion: Physiologie und Verhalten* (pp. 39–49). Göttingen: Hogrefe.

Asendorpf, J.B., Wallbott, H.G., & Scherer, K.R. (1983) Der verflixte Represser: Ein empirisch begründeter Vorschlag zu einer zweidimensionalen Operationalisierung von Repression-Sensitization [The confounded repressor: An empirically based suggestion for a two-dimensional operationalization of repression-sensitization]. *Zeitschrift für Differentielle und Diagnostische Psychologie*, *4*, 113–128.

Beck, A.T. & Clark, D.A. (1988) Anxiety and depression: An information processing perspective. *Anxiety Research, 1,* 23–36.

Bell, P.A. & Byrne, D. (1978) Repression-sensitization. In H. London & J.E. Exner (Eds.), *Dimensions of personality* (pp. 449–485). New York: Wiley.

Bendig, A.W. (1956) The development of a short form of the Manifest Anxiety Scale. *Journal of Consulting Psychology, 20,* 384.

Blum, G.S. (1955) Perceptual defense revisited. *Journal of Abnormal and Social Psychology, 51,* 24–29.

Bonanno, G.A. & Singer, J.L. (1990) Repressive personality style: Theoretical and methodological implications for health and pathology. In J.L. Singer (Ed.), *Repression and dissociation: Implications for personality theory, psychopathology, and health* (pp. 435–470). Chicago: University of Chicago Press.

Boucsein, W. & Frye, M. (1974) Physiologische und psychische Wirkungen von Mißerfolgsstress unter Berücksichtigung des Merkmals Repression-Sensitization [Physiological and psychological consequences of negative feedback with reference to the repression-sensitization dimension]. *Zeitschrift für experimentelle und angewandte Psychologie, 21,* 339–366.

Bruner, J.S. (1951) Personality dynamics and the process of perceiving. In R.R. Blake & G.V. Ramsey (Eds.), *Perception: An approach to personality* (pp. 121–147). New York: Ronald.

Bruner, J.S. & Postman, L. (1947) Emotional selectivity in perception and reaction. *Journal of Personality, 16,* 69–77.

Brunswik, E. (1947) *Systematic and representative design of psychological experiments: With results in physical and social perception.* Berkeley: University of California Press.

Budd, E.C. & Clopton, J.M. (1985) Meaning of the Repression-Sensitization scale: Defensive style or self-report of symptoms of psychopathology. *Journal of Clinical Psychology, 41,* 63–68.

Byrne, D. (1961) The Repression-Sensitization scale: Rationale, reliability, and validity. *Journal of Personality, 29,* 334–349.

Byrne, D. (1964) Repression-sensitization as a dimension of personality. In B.A. Maher (Ed.), *Progress in experimental personality research: Vol. 1* (pp. 169–220). New York: Academic Press.

Byrne, D., Barry, J., & Nelson, D. (1963) Relation of the revised Repression-Sensitization scale to measures of self-description. *Psychological Reports, 13,* 323–334.

Carver, C.S. & Scheier, M.F. (1988) A control-process perspective on anxiety. *Anxiety Research, 1,* 17–22.

Chabot, J.A. (1973) Repression-sensitization: A critique of some neglected variables in the literature. *Psychological Bulletin, 80,* 375–389.

Cook, J. (1985) Repression-sensitization and approach–avoidance as predictors of response to a laboratory stressor. *Journal of Personality and Social Psychology, 49,* 759–773.

Crowne, D.P. & Marlowe, D. (1960) A new scale of social desirability independent of psychopathology. *Journal of Consulting Psychology, 24,* 349–354.

Crowne, D. & Marlowe, D. (1964) *The approval motive.* New York: Wiley.

Davis, P. (1987) Repression and the inaccessibility of affective memories. *Journal of Personality and Social Psychology, 53,* 585–593.

Davis, P. & Schwartz, G.E. (1987) Repression and the inaccessibility of affective memories. *Journal of Personality and Social Psychology, 52,* 155–162.

Dixon, N.F. (1971) *Subliminal perception: The nature of a controversy*. London: McGraw-Hill.

Dixon, N.F. (1981) *Preconscious processing*. New York: Wiley.

Edwards, A.L. (1957) *The social desirability variable in personality assessment and research*. New York: Dryden.

Endler, N.S., Hunt, J.McV., & Rosenstein, A.J. (1962) An S-R inventory of anxiousness. *Psychological Monographs*, 76, 17, whole no. 536.

Epstein, S. & Fenz, W.D. (1967) The detection of areas of emotional stress through variations in perceptual threshold and physiological arousal. *Journal of Experimental Research in Personality*, 2, 191–199.

Erdelyi, M.H. (1974) A new look at the New Look: Perceptual defense and vigilance. *Psychological Review*, 81, 1–25.

Erdelyi, M.H. (1990) Repression, reconstruction, and defense: History and integration of the psychoanalytical and experimental frameworks. In J.L. Singer (Ed.), *Repression and dissociation: Implications for personality theory, psychopathology, and health* (pp. 1–31). Chicago: University of Chicago Press.

Eriksen, C.W. (1951) Some implications for TAT interpretation arising from need and perception experiments. *Journal of Personality*, 19, 282–288.

Eysenck, H.J. & Eysenck, S.B.G. (1964) *Manual of the Eysenck Personality Inventory*. London: Hodder & Stoughton.

Eysenck, M.W. (1988) Anxiety and attention. *Anxiety Research*, 1, 9–15.

Frenkel-Brunswik, E. (1949) Intolerance of ambiguity as an emotional and perceptual personality variable. *Journal of Personality*, 18, 108–143.

Freud, A. (1936) *Das Ich und die Abwehrmechanismen* [The ego and the defense mechanisms]. Vienna: Internationaler Psychoanalytischer Verlag.

Fröhlich, W.D. (1984) Microgenesis as a functional approach to information processing through search. In W.D. Fröhlich, G. Smith, J.G. Draguns, & U. Hentschel (Eds.), *Psychological processes in cognition and personality* (pp. 19–52). Washington, DC: Hemisphere.

Goldiamond, I. (1958) Indicators of perception: I. Subliminal perception, subception, unconscious perception: An analysis in terms of psychophysical indicator methodology. *Psychological Bulletin*, 55, 373–411.

Gordon, J.E. (1957) Interpersonal predictions of repressors and sensitizers. *Journal of Personality*, 25, 686–698.

Gudjonsson, G.H. (1981) Self-reported emotional disturbance and its relation to electrodermal reactivity, defensiveness and trait anxiety. *Personality and Individual Differences*, 2, 47–52.

Haley, G.A. (1974) Eye movement responses of repressors and sensitizers to a stressful film. *Journal of Research in Personality*, 8, 88–94.

Halperin, J.M. (1986) Defensive style and direction of gaze. *Journal of Research in Personality*, 20, 327–337.

Hansen, R.D. & Hansen, C.H. (1988) Repression of emotionally tagged memories: The architecture of less complex emotions. *Journal of Personality and Social Psychology*, 55, 811–818.

Hentschel, U. & Smith, G. (Eds.) (1980) *Experimentelle Persönlichkeitspsychologie: Die Wahrnehmung als Zugang zu diagnostischen Problemen* [Experimental personality psychology: Perception as a tool for diagnostic problems]. Wiesbaden: Akademische Verlagsgesellschaft.

Hill, K.T. (1971) Anxiety in the evaluative context. *Young Children*, 27, 97–118.

Hill, K.T. & Sarason, S.B. (1966) The relation of test anxiety and defensiveness to test and school performance over the elementary school years: A further longitudinal study. *Monographs of the Society for Research in Child Development, 31* (2, serial no. 104).

Hodapp, V. & Knoll, J.F. (1993) Heartbeat perception, coping, and emotion. In H.W. Krohne (Ed.), *Attention and avoidance: Strategies in coping with aversiveness* (pp. 191–211). Seattle: Hogrefe & Huber.

Holmes, D.S. (1974) Investigation of repression: Differential recall of material experimentally or naturally associated with ego threat. *Psychological Bulletin, 81*, 632–653.

Holmes, D.S. (1990) The evidence for repression: An examination of sixty years of research. In J.L. Singer (Ed.), *Repression and dissociation: Implications for personality theory, psychopathology, and health* (pp. 85–102). Chicago: University of Chicago Press.

Holroyd, K. (1972) Repression-sensitization, Marlowe–Crowne defensiveness, and perceptual defense. *Proceedings of the 80th Annual Convention of the American Psychological Association, 7*, 401–402.

Houston, B.K. & Hodges, W.F. (1970) Situational denial and performance under stress. *Journal of Personality and Social Psychology, 16*, 726–730.

Jung, C.G. (Ed.) (1906/1909) *Diagnostische Assoziationsstudien. Beiträge zur experimentellen Psychopathologie* (2 vols.). Leipzig: Barth.

Jensen, M.R. (1987) Psychobiological factors predicting the course of breast cancer. *Journal of Personality, 55*, 317–342.

Klein, G.S. & Schlesinger, H.J. (1949) Where is the perceiver in perceptual theory? *Journal of Personality, 18*, 32–47.

Kogan, N. & Wallach, M.A. (1964) *Risk taking: A study in cognition and personality*. New York: Holt, Rinehart and Winston.

Kohlmann, C.W. (1986) *Alexithymie* [Alexithymia] (*Mainzer Berichte zur Persönlichkeitsforschung Nr. 12*). Mainz: Johannes Gutenberg-Universität, Psychologisches Institut.

Kohlmann, C.W. (1990a) *Rigid and flexible modes of coping: The role of coping preferences. (Mainzer Berichte zur Persönlichkeitsforschung Nr. 30)*. Mainz: Johannes Gutenberg-Universität, Psychologisches Institut.

Kohlmann, C.W. (1990b) *Streßbewältigung und Persönlichkeit* [Personality and coping with stress]. Bern: Huber.

Kohlmann, C.W. (1993) Strategies in blood pressure estimation: The role of vigilance, cognitive avoidance, and gender. In H.W. Krohne (Ed.), *Attention and avoidance: Strategies in coping with aversiveness* (pp. 213–238). Seattle: Hogrefe & Huber.

Kohlmann, C.W., Singer, P., & Krohne, H.W. (1989) Coping dispositions, actual coping, and the discrepancy between subjective and physiological stress reactions. In P. Lovibond & P. Wilson (Eds.), *Clinical and abnormal psychology* (pp. 67–78). Amsterdam: North-Holland.

Krohne, H.W. (1974) Untersuchungen mit einer deutschen Form der Repression-Sensitization-Skala [Investigations of a German version of the Repression-Sensitization scale]. *Zeitschrift für Klinische Psychologie, 3*, 238–260.

Krohne, H.W. (1978) Individual differences in coping with stress and anxiety. In C.D. Spielberger & I.G. Sarason (Eds.), *Stress and anxiety: Vol. 5* (pp. 233–260). Washington, DC: Hemisphere.

Krohne, H.W. (1986) Coping with stress: Dispositions, strategies, and the problem of measurement. In M.H. Appley & R. Trumbull (Eds.), *Dynamics of stress* (pp. 209–234). New York: Plenum.

Krohne, H.W. (1989) The concept of coping modes: Relating cognitive person variables to actual coping behavior. *Advances in Behavior Research and Therapy, 11*, 235–248.

Krohne, H.W. (in press) Repression-Sensitization [Repression-sensitization]. In M. Amelang (Ed.), *Enzyklopädie der Psychologie. Serie Differentielle Psychologie: Band 2*; *Bereiche/Dimensionen individueller Differenzen*. Göttingen: Hogrefe.

Krohne, H.W. & Fuchs, J. (1991) The influence of coping dispositions and danger-related information on emotional and coping reactions of individuals anticipating an aversive event. In C.D. Spielberger, I.G. Sarason, J. Strelau, & J.M.T. Brebner (Eds.), *Stress and anxiety: Vol. 13* (pp. 131–155). Washington, DC: Hemisphere.

Krohne, H.W. & Kohlmann, C.W. (1990) Persönlichkeit und Emotion [Personality and emotion]. In K.R. Scherer (Ed.), *Enzyklopädie der Psychologie. Serie Motivation und Emotion: Band 3*; *Psychologie der Emotion* (pp. 485–559). Göttingen: Hogrefe.

Krohne, H.W. & Rogner, J. (1982) Repression-sensitization as a central construct in coping research. In H.W. Krohne & L. Laux (Eds.), *Achievement, stress, and anxiety* (pp. 167–193). Washington, DC: Hemisphere.

Krohne, H.W. & Rogner, J. (1985) Mehrvariablen-Diagnostik in der Bewältigungsforschung [Multi-variable diagnostic in coping research]. In H.W. Krohne (Ed.), *Angstbewältigung in Leistungssituationen* (pp. 45–62). Weinheim: edition psychologie.

Krohne, H.W., Rösch, W., & Kürsten, F. (1989) Die Erfassung von Angstbewältigung in physisch bedrohlichen Situationen [The measurement of coping in physical threat situations]. *Zeitschrift für Klinische Psychologie, 18*, 230–242.

Laux, L. & Glanzmann, P. (1987) A self-presentational view of test anxiety. In R. Schwarzer, H.M. van der Ploeg, & C.D. Spielberger (Eds.), *Advances in test anxiety research: Vol. 5* (pp. 31–37). Lisse, Netherlands: Swets & Zeitlinger.

Lazarus, R.S. (1966) *Psychological stress and the coping process*. New York: McGraw-Hill.

Lazarus, R.S., Eriksen, C.W., & Fonda, C.P. (1951) Personality dynamics and auditory perceptual recognition. *Journal of Personality, 19*, 471–482.

Lazarus, R.S. & Folkman, S. (1984) *Stress, appraisal, and coping*. New York: Springer.

Lefcourt, H.M. (1966) Repression-sensitization: A measure of the evaluation of emotional expression. *Journal of Consulting Psychology, 30*, 444–449.

Lefcourt, H.M. (1969) Need for approval and threatened negative evaluation as determinants of expressiveness in a projective test. *Journal of Consulting and Clinical Psychology, 33*, 96–102.

Lesser, I.M. (1981) A review of the alexithymia concept. *Psychosomatic Medicine, 43*, 531–543.

Martin, J.B. & Pihl, R.O. (1985) The stress–alexithymia hypothesis: Theoretical and empirical considerations. *Psychotherapy and Psychosomatics, 43*, 169–176.

Miller, S.M. (1981) Predictability and human stress: Toward a clarification of evidence and theory. In L. Berkowitz (Ed.), *Advances in experimental social psychology: Vol. 14* (pp. 203–256). New York: Academic Press.

Miller, S.M. (1987) Monitoring and blunting: Validation of a questionnaire to assess styles of information seeking under threat. *Journal of Personality and Social Psychology*, *52*, 345–353.

Miller, S.M. (1990) To see or not to see: Cognitive informational styles in the coping process. In M. Rosenbaum (Ed.), *Learned resourcefulness: On coping skills, self-regulation, and adaptive behavior* (pp. 95–126). New York: Springer.

Miller, S.M., Brody, D.S., & Summerton, J. (1988) Styles of coping with threat: Implications for health. *Journal of Personality and Social Psychology*, *54*, 142–148.

Mischel, W. (1984) Convergences and challenges in the search for consistency. *American Psychologist*, *39*, 351–364.

Newton, T.L. & Contrada, R.J. (1992) Repressive coping and verbal-autonomic response dissociation: The influence of social context. *Journal of Personality and Social Psychology*, *62*, 159–167.

Otto, J. & Bösel, R. (1978) Angstverarbeitung und die Diskrepanz zwischen Selfreport und physiologischem Streßindikator: Eine gelungene Replikation der Weinstein-Analyse [Coping with anxiety and the discrepancy between subjective and physiological stress reactions: A positive replication of the Weinstein analysis]. *Schweizerische Zeitschrift für Psychologie*, *37*, 321–330.

Parsons, O.A., Fulgenzi, L.B., & Edelberg, R. (1969) Aggressiveness and psychophysiological responsivity in groups of repressors and sensitizers. *Journal of Personality and Social Psychology*, *12*, 235–244.

Roth, S. & Cohen, L.J. (1986) Approach, avoidance, and coping with stress. *American Psychologist*, *41*, 813–819.

Rothbart, M. & Mellinger, M. (1972) Attention and responsivity to remote dangers: A laboratory simulation for assessing reactions to threatening events. *Journal of Personality and Social Psychology*, *24*, 132–142.

Scarpetti, W. (1973) The repression-sensitization dimension in relation to impending painful stimulation. *Journal of Consulting and Clinical Psychology*, *40*, 377–382.

Schroeder, D.H. & Costa, P.T. (1984) Influence of life event stress on physical illness: Substantive effects or methodological flaws? *Journal of Personality and Social Psychology*, *46*, 853–863.

Schulz, P. (1982) Person-Unwelt-Interaktion und Streß [Person-environment interaction and stress]. In H.W. Hoefert (Ed.), *Person und Situation* (pp. 44–66). Göttingen: Hogrefe.

Schumacher, A. (1990) Die "Miller Behavioral Style Scale" (MBSS): Erste Überprüfung einer deutschen Fassung [The "Miller Behavioral Style Scale": First investigation of a German adaptation]. *Zeitschrift für Differentielle und Diagnostische Psychologie*, *11*, 243–250.

Schwartz, G.E. (1990) Psychobiology of repression and health: A systems approach. In J.L. Singer (Ed.), *Repression and dissociation: Implications for personality theory, psychopathology, and health* (pp. 405–434). Chicago: University of Chicago Press.

Shevrin, H. (1990) Subliminal perception and repression. In J.L. Singer (Ed.), *Repression and dissociation: Implications for personality theory, psychopathology, and health* (pp. 103–119). Chicago: University of Chicago Press.

Shipley, R.H., Butt, J.H., Horwitz, B., & Farbry, J.E. (1978) Preparation for a stressful medical procedure: Effect of amount of stimulus preexposure and coping style. *Journal of Consulting and Clinical Psychology*, *46*, 499–507.

Sifneos, P.E. (1973) The prevalence of "alexithymic" characteristics in psychosomatic patients. *Psychotherapy and Psychosomatics*, *22*, 255–262.

Singer, J.L. (Ed.) (1990) *Repression and dissociation: Implications for personality theory, psychopathology, and health*. Chicago: University of Chicago Press.

Stein, S.H. (1971) Arousal level in repressors and sensitizers as a function of response context. *Journal of Consulting and Clinical Psychology*, *36*, 386–394.

Taylor, G.J. (1984) Alexithymia: Concept, measurement, and implications for treatment. *American Journal of Psychiatry*, *141*, 725–732.

Taylor, J.A. (1953) A personality scale of manifest anxiety. *Journal of Abnormal and Social Psychology*, *48*, 285–290.

Thayer, R.E. (1971) Personality and discrepancies between verbal reports and physiological measures of private emotional experiences. *Journal of Personality*, *39*, 57–69.

Tremayne, P. & Barry, R.J. (1988) An application of psychophysiology in sports psychology: Heart rate responses to relevant and irrelevant stimuli as a function of anxiety and defensiveness in elite gymnasts. *International Journal of Psychophysiology*, *6*, 1–8.

Tucker, I.F. (1970) *Adjustment: Models and mechanisms*. New York: Academic Press.

Watson, D. & Clark, L.A. (1984) Negative affectivity: The disposition to experience aversive emotional states. *Psychological Bulletin*, *96*, 465–490.

Watson, D. & Pennebaker, J.W. (1989) Health complaints, stress, and distress: Exploring the central role of negative affectivity. *Psychological Review*, *96*, 234–254.

Weinberger, D.A. (1990) The construct validity of the repressive coping style. In J.L. Singer (Ed.), *Repression and dissociation: Implications for personality theory, psychopathology, and health* (pp. 337–386). Chicago: University of Chicago Press.

Weinberger, D.A. & Schwartz, G.E. (1990) Distress and restraint as superordinate dimensions of self-reported adjustment: A typological perspective. *Journal of Personality*, *58*, 381–417.

Weinberger, D.A., Schwartz, G.E., & Davidson, R.J. (1979) Low-anxious, high-anxious, and repressive coping-styles: Psychometric patterns and behavioral and physiological responses to stress. *Journal of Abnormal Psychology*, *88*, 369–380.

Weinstein, J., Averill, J.R., Opton, E.M., & Lazarus, R.S. (1968) Defensive style and discrepancy between self-report and physiological indexes of stress. *Journal of Personality and Social Psychology*, *10*, 406–413.

Wieland-Eckelmann, R. & Bösel, R. (1987) Konstruktion eines Verfahrens zur Erfassung von dispositionellen Angstbewältigungsstilen im Leistungsbereich [Development of a procedure for the assessment of coping-styles in achievement situations]. *Zeitschrift für Differentielle und Diagnostische Psychologie*, *8*, 39–56.

13
Augmenting/Reducing: A Link Between Perceptual and Emotional Aspects of Psychophysiological Individuality

Most theories of personality and temperament include statements about spontaneous and elicited behavior. We may refer to them as activity and reactivity statements. Personality theories are abstracted systems of dispositional traits that predict behavior on qualitative or quantitative bases. The type of prediction and the database vary in different theories. Some do not include statements regarding physiological indicators while others neglect social factors.

A psychophysiological theory considers from its inception behavioral, introspective, and physiological information. The inclusion of information of these types does not imply that they are isomorphic or redundant. A basic tenet underlying our research is the notion that homeostatic regulation can be achieved either physiologically (short loop regulation, internal homeostasis) or behaviorally (long loop regulation, external homeostasis). A theory of individual differences predicts that each subject possesses his own style of homeostatic awareness and concomitant behavior. In this sense, it can be said that individual patterns of defense mechanisms mirror cognitive styles mediating psychophysiological stability. Many psychometric instruments (e.g., Gleser and Ihilevich 1986) take this into account.

Classic Notions of Augmenting/Reducing

The notion that individuals respond differently to stimulation and emotion dates back at least to the humoral theories of temperament and constitutes the basis of theories proposed by writers as diverse as Pavlov, Freud, and Sherrington. In a modern version of the theory, known as stimulus intensity modulation theory, three assumptions are made. The first is that individuals differ from each other in the magnitude of their response to sensory stimulation. "Reducers" and "augmenters" differ both in the level of preferred stimulation and in overt behavioral manifestations. A second assumption is that there is some optimal level of internal or endogenous stimulation (or arousal) that is pleasurable and is sought out. A third assumption, not explicitly stated by all authors, is that the level of stimulation perceived as optimal tends to be similar across individuals. This is a point that deserves emphasis, since it defines the personality characteristic not by differences in subjective perception but by differences in the amount of objective stimulation necessary to achieve and maintain a certain level of functioning. The personal equation is a differential quantity.

Recent Work

Although classical work on the augmenter/reducer typology emphasized perceptual reactivity, it is obvious that the underlying construct need not be restricted to perception and cognition and can encompass emotional and motivational aspects as well (Larsen & Zarate, 1991). It is in this latter aspect that it overlaps with psychodynamic defense concepts. The system for stimulus modulation or regulation may be said to be programmed and reprogrammed throughout life. The idea here is that the program is read out recursively: genetic factors determine certain forms of behavior that mold the environment, which in turn poses certain demands. It cannot be ascertained whether a given outcome is cause or effect, antecedent or consequence, if context, time, and developmental factors are not taken into account.

Dating back to at least humoral theory, statements regarding spontaneous and reactive behavior refer to quality and intensity. While psychodynamic theories base predictions on the quality of behavior or affect that predominates or can be aroused by environmental demands, most physiological theories emphasize intensity and explain diversity on the basis of quantitative differentiations along continua of physiological activation. Intensity regulation can be effected by both internal and external mechanisms. In relation to behavior, writers as diverse as Pavlov, Sherrington, and Freud suggested mechanisms for controlling overstimulation: transmarginal inhibition, stimulus barrier, central inhibitory state (see Silverman, 1972). The Freudian notion of complementary series, referring to intensity aspects of organisms–environment transactions, is a forerunner to later stress theories (von Knorring, Jacobsson, Perris, & Perris, 1980). The pioneering work of Petrie (1960) kindled an interest in the biological foundations of individual differences that later developed into a growing body research on the augmenting/reducing construct. The original studies were based on the Kinesthetic Figural Aftereffect (KFA). In one of its forms of application, this procedure is based on the subjective judgment of the width of a bar before and after kinesthetic stimulation. Subjects who judge the magnitude of the stimulus as larger after a distractive stimulus were termed augmenters; reducers judged the standard as markedly reduced after distraction. In ensuing years, the relationship of this categorization to established psychometric knowledge regarding validity and reliability of the procedure were posed. KFA is a complex task involving joint position and tactile stimulation and might be influenced by dexterity, experience, and sequence effects; like other difference measures, it showed poor test–retest reliability. This led researchers to search for other ways of evaluating augmentation/reduction (A/R). Brain electrical potentials evoked by sensory stimulation have constituted the second most important source of data regarding the A/R construct (see Buchsbaum, Haier, & Johnson, 1983). In this procedure, a subject is termed an augmenter if the slope of the amplitude/intensity function is positive, that is, greater than 0, and reducer if a paradoxical reduction in amplitude ensues with increased stimulation intensity or if, comparatively, slopes are lower for a given group of subjects. It should be noted that what is measured with this procedure is not a behavioral aftereffect but the response to stimulation.

In clinical or research applications, an important issue is measurement. The augmenting/reducing construct is a descriptive label that can be applied to behavioral or physiological data. It may overlap with other descriptive labels—such as strength of the nervous system, extraversion-introversion, repression-sensitization, sensation seeking, and defense style—and shows differences depending on the assessment procedure. Regarding the nature of the underlying process, augmenters and reducers could show the characteristic features in all sensory systems, meaning that it is a general property of the central nervous system. On the other hand, predictions could be valid only within a given sensory modality (Lolas, Collin, Camposano, Etcheberrigaray, & Rees 1989). One could hypothesize, for instance, that auditory augmenters need not be visual augmenters and that a further differentiation in terms of the preferred modality for augmenting or reducing would introduce a more specific, individual factor (Lolas, 1987). This could be brought to bear on differentiations made on the basis of perceptual predispositions assumed by certain personality theories (Lolas, Camposano, & Etcheberrygaray, 1989). It might be hypothesized that not all people employ the same perceptual defenses or the same modality regulation. A/R as a general property of the CNS could be differently expressed depending on modality and recording site. This does not contradict the notion that it may represent an unspecific feature, but allows for specific perceptual reactances for each sensory system or motivational system. Different defense systems could be employed in different sensory contexts. "Sensoriostasis"—an appropriate name for sensory and informational homeostasis—would not only interact with bodily homeostasis but would also provide a clue to physiological dysfunction and its symptomatic expression (Lolas, 1991). In this regard, the search for appropriate markers of central nervous system activity and reactivity might produce information relevant to psychodynamic theory-building in the field of defense mechanisms.

References

Buchsbaum, M., Haier, R., & Johnson, J. (1983) Augmenting and reducing: Individual differences in evoked potentials. In A. Gale & J.A. Edwards (Eds.), *Physiological correlates of human behavior* (pp. 117–138). London: Academic Press.

Gleser, G.C. & Ihilevich, D. (1986) *Defense mechanisms: Their classification, correlates, and measurement with the Defense Mechanisms Inventory*. Owosso, MI: DMI Associates.

Larsen, R.J. & Zarate, M.A. (1991) Extending reducer/augmenter theory in the emotion domain: The role of affect in regulating stimulation level. *Personality and Individual Differences, 12*, 713–723.

Lolas, F. (1987) Aumento/reducción: La investigación electrofisiologicá de la reactividad sensoriál. *Anales de Salud Mental, 2*, 45–53.

Lolas, F. (1991) Attention, meaning and somatization: A psychophysiological view. *Psychopathology, 24*, 147–150.

Lolas, F., Camposano, S., & Etcheberrigaray, R. (1989) Augmenting/reducing and personality: A psychometric and evoked potential study in a Chilean sample. *Personality and Individual Differences. 10*, 1173–1176.

Lolas, F., Collin, C., Camposano, S., Etcheberrigaray, R., & Rees, R. (1989) Hemispheric asymmetry of augmenting/reducing in visual and auditory evoked potential (VEP) reducing: A vertex feature of late components. *Research Communications in Psychology, Psychiatry and Behavior, 14*, 173–176.

Petrie, A. (1960) Some psychological aspects of pain and the relief of suffering. *Annals of the New York Academy of Sciences, 86*, 13–27.

Silverman, J. (1972) Stimulus intensity modulation and psychological disease. *Psychopharmacologica, 24*, 42–80.

Von Knorring, L., Jacobsson, L., Perris, C., & Perris, H. (1980) Reactivity to incoming stimuli and the experience of life-events. *Neuropsychobiology, 6*, 297–303.

14
A Psychodynamic Activation Study of Female Oedipal Fantasies Using Subliminal and Percept-Genetic Techniques

BERT WESTERLUNDH

This chapter presents an experimental study of conflict and defense originating in the female Oedipus complex, using subliminal stimulation and a tachistoscopic percept-genetic technique. This is related to Kragh's (1985) Defense Mechanism Test (DMT) and consists of successively prolonged presentations of interpersonal stimuli, to which subjects report, verbally and with a drawing. In the experiment, factors were varied within and between subjects. All subjects saw and reported to two percept-geneses. For one of these, all percept-genetic presentations were preceded by a neutral subliminal verbal message, the words "Taking a walk." For the other, the presentations were preceded by a provoking subliminal message, "Fuck daddy." These messages were the same for all subjects. For half of the subjects, the two percept-genetic stimuli showed a girl (central figure, technically "hero") and a man, for the other half a girl and a woman. The only difference between the sets of stimuli was in the sex of the grown-up "peripheral person" (pp). The presentation order for the subliminal and the percept-genetic stimuli was balanced, and the subjects randomly assigned to the different combinations. The design was thus of a mixed type.

In classical psychoanalytic theory (e.g., Bonaparte, 1953; Fenichel, 1946; Freud, 1925/1961; Nagera, 1975), the oedipal period is the time when the difference between the sexes begins to have psychological consequences. The boy directs his phallic sexual love toward his mother, feelings that are ultimately renounced under the influence of castration fear. The boy's Oedipus complex is terminated by the castration complex. The story for the girl is different. She starts with the same phallic longings, but upon her recognition of the difference between the sexes she experiences a crucial disappointment—she has not got what it takes, her mother has let her down. Under the influence of this disappointment and maturational changes, she turns from the mother as a love object toward the father. Her sexual aim changes from phallic/active (clitoral) to a more passive mode, based on earlier (oral and anal) incorporative modes. She feels jealous rivalry toward the mother and tender sexual impulses toward the father, together with a wish to have a child by him. For the girl, the castration complex antedates and leads up to the Oedipus complex. In contrast to the anxiety-laden and abrupt end of the boy's oedipal strivings, the girl's Oedipus complex dissolves gradually, with time giving place to other forms of object choice.

As has been demonstrated by, among others, Silverman (1983; Silverman & Geisler, 1986), oedipal strivings and conflicts are common in normal adults and can be studied experimentally. In the present investigation, female students served as subjects. It is expected that a sizeable proportion will show observable reactions indicating conflict and defense, in accordance with the hypotheses of psychoanalytic theory.

Hypotheses

Henceforth, the girl-man percept-genetic stimuli will be called the "Man" and the girl-woman the "Woman" stimuli. The sexually provocative subliminal message, "Fuck daddy", will be abbreviated fd, and the neutral message, "Taking a walk" will be referred to as tw. The combinations of factors (e.g., girl-man percept-genetic stimulus preceded by the fd message) will be called Man fd, etc.

The first group of predictions concerns general indications of psychological conflict. As will soon be evident, the load of provocation in the different conditions can be conceived of in the following way (where "+" stands for provocation):

	Man	Woman
fd	++	+
tw	+	0

There are three general indications of conflict. The *later* percept-genetic signs of anxiety and defense are scored in the series, the greater the conflict. Thus, if significantly more subjects have late signs in one condition in comparison to another, the former condition has activated more conflict. The *greater* the number of such signs scored, the greater the conflict. Many subjects with many signs is an indicator of conflict. Finally, *many different scored variants* of percept-genetic signs in a protocol point to problems of adaptation. Different numbers of subjects with many different variants in separate conditions indicate more conflict activation in the condition with the greater number.

The second group of predictions concerns specific signs of impulse, anxiety, and defense. They will be discussed for the different conditions under separate headings.

Man Conditions

For women, an oedipal, erotic interpretation of the Man stimuli should be close at hand. It is not known whether the Man and fd/tw factors interact additively or whether one of the provoking factors is enough to produce the expected results in regard to the Man stimuli. Thus, no differential predictions are given for the Man fd and Man tw conditions.

Impulse

The wishes supposed to be activated by the girl-man stimuli and the fd message are oedipal sexual ones, fantasies about having sexual intercourse with the father. Such wishes are of course strongly prohibited by the incest taboo, and impulsive reports of this type are not expected.

Anxiety

The reverse of the erotic wish is the basic feminine genital anxiety of being sexually assaulted and torn, mangled, and castrated by the father in the intercourse. This type of anxiety may determine, for example, female hypochondria, mania for surgery, and certain developments of penis envy. Horney, for instance, discussed it in a number of classical papers, later collected in a book (Horney, 1973). This leads to the following predictions regarding signs of anxiety: more subjects should give reports of perceived aggression and introaggression (damage, injury, and anxiety: stimulus inadequate black parts) to the Man than to the Woman stimuli. (The basic situation is one of aggression from pp toward a damaged hero, but the location of aggression and damage may sometimes vary as a result of superimposed layers of projective and introjective mechanisms.) Both Man fd and Woman fd are provoking conditions, and no differences are expected here with regard to reports of anxiety and fear, but more subjects should give such reports in the Man tw than in the Woman tw condition.

Defense

The mechanism of choice against activated oedipal sexual impulses is repression, and that against the threat of aggression is isolation (Fenichel, 1946, pp. 522–524, and in an experimental context, e.g., Westerlundh & Sjöbäck, 1986). Thus, in comparison to the Woman stimuli, the Man stimuli should produce reports of repression and isolation in more subjects.

Woman Conditions

In contrast to the Man, there is no strongly compelling interpretation of the Woman stimuli. The subliminal messages should steer the interpretation of them and give differential conflict activation.

Impulse

The Woman fd condition should, in comparison to Woman tw, produce reports related to oedipal rivalry. More subjects in Woman fd are expected to activate aggressive impulses directed toward the mother. But more dramatic or violent signs of this activation are not expected. Presumably, these reports will concern specifically female forms of aggression. However, at this stage, this is speculative. Three such types of report— that perceived persons leave each other, that one of them is beautiful while the other is not, and that their affective communication is negative or strangulated—will be explored.

Anxiety

More subjects should give reports of anxiety and fear in the provoked Woman fd than in the Woman tw condition.

Defense

The type of report primarily seen in percept-genetic tests as a defense against one's own aggressive impulses is reaction formation against aggression. Such reports were early supposed to be related to inhibition of aggression (Kragh, 1969), an idea that was later experimentally verified (Westerlundh, 1976). Thus more subjects are expected to give such reports of reaction formation in the Woman fd than in the Woman tw condition (actually, compared to any other condition). This rather anti-commonsensical statement is the central prediction concerning defense activation with regard to these comparisons.

In addition to these questions, the effect of presentation order will be studied. In the experiment, fd and tw are equally often associated with the first and the second percept-genetic series. Some design-threatening order effects are possible.

1. Reports to a percept-genesis administered after another series with the same thematic content may show contraction as a consequence of perceptual automatization. Then fewer scorable signs of anxiety and defense will be found. In that case, fd after tw should be a less efficient provocation than fd before, and half of the protocols will be contaminated.

2. The provoking fd shown before the presentations of the first percept-genesis may initiate mental processes that reverberate into—and perhaps through—the second series. In that case, reports to tw after fd may well reflect this provocation, and the other half of the protocols will be contaminated. In both cases, the probability of finding predicted results will decrease.

Method

Subjects

Eighty female university students, volunteers who were paid for their participation, served as subjects. They were randomly assigned to the eight subgroups of the experiment (Man/Woman percept-genetic stimuli x percept-genetic stimulus A first/B first × subliminal fd first/tw first), with 10 in each. The mean age for those who saw the Man stimuli was 22.5 years, with a standard deviation of 1.5 and a range of 20–25 years. Corresponding values for those who saw the Woman stimuli were 22.4, 1.6, and 20–25 years.

Stimuli

Half the subjects saw two percept-genetic stimuli depicting a girl and a man (Man stimuli). One pair was shown in a landscape (stimulus A), the other in a townscape (stimulus B). The other half saw two such stimuli, in all respects equivalent to the Man stimuli, but with the man exchanged for a woman (Woman stimuli). Before the percept-genetic presentations, one of two subliminal stimuli were shown. These were verbal messages, printed on one line and consisting of two words:

Stimulus (Swedish/English)	Horizontal visual angle (degrees)
KNULLA PAPPA / FD	9.34
PÅ PROMENAD / TW	8.56

The messages had irregular black frames to avoid easily recognized right angles, and were presented centrally on the area of the screen where the percept-genetic pictures were seen.

Apparatus

The components of the experimental arrangement were two projectors, one with a timer and a rheostat for subliminal presentations, the other with a camera shutter for tachistoscopic ones. Both projectors were standard, with 220 V input and a 24 V, 150 W lamp. The projector for sub-liminal presentations was always fed 34 V. There were 14 tachistoscopic presentations. The presentation times (ms) were: exposure 1, 20; 2–4, 40; 5–7, 100; 8–10, 200; 11–14, 500. Placed at one end of a table, the projectors were arranged vertically to project on the same area of a screen. This screen, made from plastic-coated white linen, measuring 50 cm high × 61 cm wide was placed on the table. The projected picture was 15.0 cm high × 22.5 cm wide. The picture area was indicated by four small black points at its corners. The subject sat at the end of the table, facing the screen. When looking at it, the subject's head was fixed by a support. The screen was 65 cm from the eyes. The only source of light in the room during the experiment was a lamp, mounted behind the screen together with the projectors, and directed at the table. It gave an illuminance at the screen of 50 lux, as measured at the subject's side of the table. This value was not affected by subliminal presentations, but rose to 63 lux when a tachistoscopic picture was shown (with the tachistoscope in "constant on" position). These values were constant for all conditions.

Presentation Mode

The testing was individual. The session started with instructions to the subject to report what she saw on the screen, verbally and with a drawing. Reporting format followed the DMT standard (Kragh, 1985; Westerlundh, 1976). A trial consisted of a 7-second presentation of one of the sublimi-nal stimuli. This was immediately followed by a tachistoscopic stimulus presentation. After this presentation, the subject reported what she had seen. Fourteen trials, with the same stimuli and increasing exposure times, were run in a row. These constitute a percept-genetic series.

A control for subliminality was performed after testing (see below). During the instructions at the beginning of the session, the DMT demon-stration picture was shown at 200 ms. Before and after the experiment, the DMT distractor picture was shown once at 40 ms. Between the two series, two such presentations were given.

Blindness of Tester and Scorer

Both tester and scorer knew the design and the conditions of the experi-ment. The tester knew the percept-genetic stimuli each subject saw, and the order in which they were shown. The tester also knew that each percept-genetic stimulus presentation was paired with a subliminal one, but not which subliminal stimulus was used. The subliminal stimuli were always placed in the projector magazine in such a way that a number at their back, but nothing else, could be seen. The tester had to feed the ap-propriate stimulus into the projector in accordance with a randomization list, and was instructed never to handle them in any other way. Before each testing, the tester controlled the focusing of the subliminal projector by increasing its voltage and looking at a blank stimulus, consisting only of an irregular black frame. Then she immediately reduced the voltage to 34 V for the experiment. The scorer did not know at all what condition any experimental subject belonged to. The identification pages of the precept-genetic protocols were removed by the tester, who marked them, as well as the protocols, with a number from 1 to 80 chosen by her. The identification pages were filed out of reach from the scorer until the scoring was completed.

Subliminality

After testing, the subliminality of the verbal stimuli was investigated. The subject was (a) told that a very weak picture had been shown before each short one and (b) asked if she had seen any of them. No subject in any condition reported having seen anything structured. Then, the subject was shown the two subliminal stimuli in the same way as subliminal presentations in the experiment. She was told that these two stimuli would be shown in this way 10 times in all and was asked to guess which one it was each time. This is a variant of Silverman's (1966) discrimination task. Subjects with eight or more correct identifications were excluded from the study and immediately replaced. The number of subjects that had to be replaced was five, to be compared to a chance expectation of 4.4. This shows that the verbal stimuli fulfill criteria for subliminality.

Percept-Genetic Scoring

The reports to the tachistoscopic presentations were scored with a scoring scheme related to that of Kragh's (1985) DMT. A more extended presentation, with definitions of the separate variants, can be found, for example, in Westerlundh and Sjöbäck (1986).

The main scoring classes were as follows.

1. Repression: all reports where hero or the peripheral person (pp) is made rigid or lifeless.
2. Isolation: combines categories 21 and 22.
21. Barrier isolation: hero and pp are separated by a barrier, referred to different levels of reality, or separated by a distance.
22. Deficient reconstruction: depicted persons are not perceived, or earlier perceived person disappears, partially or completely.
3. Denial of aggression: aggression is explicitly denied with regard to hero, pp, or the situation in its totality.
4. Reaction formation: hero acts positively toward pp, pp toward hero, they have a positive relationship, or the mood in the picture is said to be positive.

51. Aggression: reports of aggression from hero toward pp, from pp toward hero, or emanating from the field.
52. Fear: hero or pp is afraid, the situation is said to be dangerous.
 6. Introaggression: hero, pp, or an object in the field is either damaged, hurt, dead, or worthless, or stimulus inadequately blackened.
 7. Faulty sex ascriptions: hero or pp either is ascribed incorrect sex or changes sex from correct to undecided or incorrect.
 8. Multiplications: more than two persons are said to be in the picture.
 9. Affect reports: positive or negative affect reported, with regard to hero or pp. (Relating to affects not otherwise scored.)
02. Pp young: pp is seen as a child or teenager, under 20 years of age.

Results

General Signs of Conflict Activation

Only significant results are given in Table 14.1. For last scored sign and number of signs, the data refer to the number of subjects showing the characteristic (late last scored sign, great number of signs) in the different groups, but for subjects/variant the data refer to the number of variants, where one group is represented by more subjects than another in the comparisons. The total number of variants scored (excepting affect and "pp young" reports) was 44.

More subjects show late last scored percept-genetic sign in the fd than in the tw condition. The difference is caused by the Man fd subjects. These have significantly later last sign than both the Man tw and the Woman fd subjects. Regarding the number of signs scored in the series,

TABLE 14.1. General signs of conflict activation: χ^2, sign, and binomial tests; one-tailed tests: 18 comparisons.

	+	−	z	$p \leqslant$
Last scored sign				
fd (+)/tw (−)	42	25	1.96	.025
Man fd (+)/Man tw (−)	23	10	2.09	.02
	Median	Subjects/total	χ^2	$p \leqslant$
Man fd/Woman fd	13.0	22/12	4.14	.025
Number of signs				
Man tw/Woman tw	7.0	24/15	3.20	.05
	+	−	z	$p \leqslant$
Subjects/variant				
Man (+)/Woman (−)	27	11	2.43	.007
Man tw (+)/Woman tw (−)	27	10	2.63	.004

there is one significant difference: Man tw subjects have more signs than Woman tw ones. Finally, more subjects have many different variants of percept-genetic signs in the Man as compared to the Woman condition. Here, the contrast between the Man tw and the Woman tw subgroups is especially strong.

Specific Signs

Tables 14.2 and 14.3 give information about specific signs of anxiety and defense. The only sign that shows significant differences between conditions in the fd/tw (with subgroups) comparisons is reaction formation. This sign is reported by more subjects in Woman fd than in any other condition. Calculated significant differences are found in the fd/tw, Woman fd/Woman tw, Man/Woman, and Man fd/Woman fd comparisons. Table 14.3 shows that the variants of reaction formation—one perceived person behaves positively toward the other, the mood in the picture is said to be positive—contribute equally to the results. Further predictions of fd/tw differences concerned a greater number of subjects with reports of fear/anxiety and female aggression in the Woman fd than in the Woman tw condition. Reports of fear/anxiety are generally few in these conditions, and no differences are found between them. Of the reports presumably showing female forms of aggression, the beautiful/ugly category was discarded, since it was difficult to score reliably. The separation and affect categories did not give any significant fd/tw contrasts but were instead of interest in Man/Woman comparisons. There is a tendency for separation reports to be given by more of those who saw the Woman as compared the Man stimuli. The Woman fd and Woman tw subgroups contribute equally to this result. The same statements are true for two types of affect report: no positive hero affect is ever mentioned and no hero affect at all is ever mentioned. Here, the results are much stronger and generally reach significance level.

With regard to the Man-Woman comparisons, the predicted greater number of subjects reporting repression and isolation in Man is found in the Man/Woman and Man fd/Woman fd comparisons. The result for repression is weak in the Man tw/Woman tw comparison, but the result for isolation reaches tendency level. Table 14.2 shows that it is not the sign subclass barrier isolation but the subclass deficient reconstruction that determines the result. Here all contrasts are significant. Table 14.3 further shows that both subgroups of deficient reconstruction, total or partial loss of earlier perceived person and no pp seen initially for one-third of the series, contribute, but that the contrasts are stronger for the latter subgroup.

The predicted greater number of subjects reporting direct aggression in Man as compared to Woman is found in all comparisons. Furthermore, denials of aggression show a tendency in the same direction in Man/Woman

TABLE 14.2. Sign classes: fd/tw and Man/Woman comparisons; χ^2, Fisher and (for fd/tw) McNemar changes tests.

Sign class	fd/tw						Man fd/Man tw						Woman fd/Woman tw					
	A	B	C	D	χ^2	$p<$	A	B	C	D	χ^2	$p<$	A	B	C	D	χ^2	$p<$
	+-	++	--	-+			+-	++	--	-+			+-	++	--	-+		
4. Reaction formation	27	27	14	12	5.03	.05	12	10	11	7	.84	—	15	17	3	5	4.05	.025*

Sign class	Man	Woman	χ^2	$p<$	Man fd	Woman fd	χ^2	$p<$	Man tw	Woman tw	χ^2	$p<$
1. Repression	21	12	3.30	.05*	15	6	4.13	.025*	9	6	.33	—*
2. Isolation	38	30	4.80	.025*	29	20	3.37	.05*	31	24	2.09	.10*
21. Barrier Isolation	30	28	.06	—*	23	19	.45	—*	22	22	.05	—*
22. Deficient reconstruction	25	11	8.54	.005*	16	6	5.08	.025*	17	6	6.10	.01*
3. Denial	13	5	3.51	.10	7	3	1.03	—	8	2	2.86	.10
4. Reaction formation	29	37	4.24	.05	22	32	4.62	.025*	17	22	.80	—
51. Aggression	20	6	9.63	.005*	12	2	7.01	.005*	13	4	4.78	.025*
52. Fear	18	6	7.20	.01	10	3	3.31	.10	12	3	5.25	.025*
6. Introaggression	19	7	6.89	.005*	7	6	0	—*	13	2	8.21	.005*
71. Incorrect sex	24	33	3.91	.05	15	23	2.46	—	14	21	1.83	—
74. Sex changes	10	13	.24	—	4	6	.11	—	7	8	0	—
8. Multiplications	17	16	0	—	11	11	.06	—	10	6	.70	—

NOTE: *, predicted contrasts, one-tailed tests.

TABLE 14.3. Results for subclasses and further results: Man/Woman comparisons; χ^2 and Fisher tests; two-tailed tests.

Subclasses of	Man	Woman	χ^2	$p <$	Man fd	Woman fd	χ^2	$p <$	Man tw	Woman tw	χ^2	$p <$
22. Deficient reconstruction												
220–232. Within the series	21	11	4.21	.05	16	6	5.08	.05	12	6	1.79	—
242b. No pp seen initially	15	0	16.08	.001	8	0		.01	8	0		.01
4. Reaction formation												
41. Activity	15	20	.81	—	11	16	.89	—	8	11	.28	—
42. Affect	25	31	1.49	—	16	23	1.80	—	16	19	.20	—
6. Introaggression												
61. Damage	13	4	4.78	.05	5	3		—	9	1	5.6	.02
62. Blackening	8	4	.88	—	3	3		—	5	1		—
71. Incorrect sex												
710–711. Both or hero	12	11	0	—	8	5	.37	—	7	8	0	—
712. Pp only	14	31	13.00	.001	7	18	5.82	.02	8	15	2.20	—
Further results												
210c. Separation	9	17	2.79	.10	5	9	2.79	—	6	11		—
931. No positive hero affect	9	25	11.52	.001	23	31		.10	20	31	5.41	.02
941. Negative hero affect	15	10		—	8	3		—	8	7		—
951. No hero affect	2	20	18.12	.001	16	28	6.11	.02	15	26	5.00	.05
02. Pp child or youthful	6	22	12.36	.001	3	12	5.25	.05	3	14	7.47	.01

and Man tw/Woman tw. Fear reports show the expected Man dominance in Man tw/Woman tw, and introaggression the same expected significance, except for the Man fd/Woman fd comparison. Of the two subclasses of introaggression, damage and blackening, significances are limited to damage reports for the Man/Woman and Man tw/Woman tw comparisons.

There are two unpredicted significances. Faulty sex ascriptions are reported by more subjects in the Woman than in to the Man condition. Table 14.3 reveals that this result concerns only the peripheral person. The trend is the same in all conditions, and significances reached in Man/Woman and Man fd/Woman fd. Furthermore, more subjects report a young peripheral person in Woman than in Man. The result is significant in all comparisons. These two categories correlated positively, with a significance in the Woman tw condition ($p < .01$).

Order Effects

The only significant presentation order differences were found for sign 7, faulty sex ascriptions. The general trend of the results is in the direction of fewer subjects attributing wrong or undecided sex to the perceived persons in the second series.

Discussion

The use of subliminal stimuli raises a number of questions. The use of verbal subliminal stimuli was discussed by Spence in a path-breaking paper (Spence, Klein, & Fernandez, 1986). His conclusions, while complex, were quite negative for the subliminal psychodynamic activation paradigm. My own studies (Westerlundh, 1986) show that Spence is partly correct. Subliminal sentences are not read syntactically, or are read so only under special circumstances. However, there seems to be a highly emotional unconscious appraisal of the individual words presented, and the outcome of this may result in complex psychodynamic activation effects on the dependent variables. However, the simple messages presented in this study should not be problematical. Each of the two provoking subliminal words, "fd," individually or in any combination, should result in a steering of the interpretation of the tachistoscopic stimuli in the intended direction.

The problem of subliminal reception was recently discussed at length (Holender, 1986). Ideas on the topic vary widely, but there seems to be some agreement on an operational definition of subliminality: the subject's inability to discriminate the experimental from a control stimulus at the time of the experiment. The usual method of assessing this is a forced-choice guessing task. This is of course the strategy that, following the lead of Silverman (1966), has been implemented in this experiment. Yet, as was clear from discussion by Holender, such an empirical approach is not accepted by certain savants on philosophical grounds, and in the bargain raises some theoretical issues. An interesting one was pointed out by Robles, Smith, Carver, and Wellens (1987), following Collins and Loftus (1975). Subliminal stimuli may produce partial memory activation, and this activation can increase the possibility of subsequent discrimination of these same stimuli (even if the original processing was totally outside awareness). Furthermore, such stimuli may produce affective reactions (indeed, that is the starting point of the present study). Discrimination of such stimuli in terms of endogenous affective signals, while the information content of the stimuli is outside awareness, is not impossible. These ideas indicate that the guessing task may be overly conservative. Yet, it seems to fulfil its function and be a reasonable procedure.

In attempts to experimentally provoke intrapsychic conflict—such as in the present study—not all predictions have the same theoretical status. A simple diagram of the hypothetical process would involve the following components: experimental provocation–(activated impulse)–threat/danger–anxiety signal–defense–eventual outcome, possibly iterated in a number of loops before a conscious representation is achieved and reported in the dependent measure. This is a statement within the directional topographic model of psychoanalysis, a type of model I with Reyher (Moses & Reyher, 1985) hold to be indispensable in the conceptual understanding of the type of process studied here. Its consequences are that while, ceteris paribus, valid experimental and control conditions give rise to different reported spectra of defense, it is probable but not necessary that they will produce differences in reports of danger, fear, and anxiety, and of the "defensive struggle," what has here been called general indications of psychological conflict. A specific danger may be countered by an efficient defense, inhibiting conscious unpleasure and different in form from defensive reports in the baseline condition, but not in, for example, number or place in the series of reports. A number of content and intensity factors will determine the outcome. This is seen in, for example, a series of studies on experimentally manipulated superego functioning in men and women (Westerlundh & Terjestam, 1987). In these, the general indications sometimes show, sometimes fail to show condition differences.

What then are the results of the present study? The design is not invalidated by sequence effects. The only significant differences of this type are found for incorrect sex attributions, which are reported by fewer subjects in the second series. This type of result has been reported for the DMT (Sjöbäck, 1972; Westerlundh, 1976). In the DMT context, this finding has generally been attributed to stimulus differences. Here, an explanation in terms of set, induced by the perception of the first series, is nearer at hand. All three types of general indication show significant results in predicted directions. One-third of the comparisons give such results.

Of the fd/tw predictions, the important one concerning a defense mechanism, reaction formation dominance in Woman fd, is verified. The one concerning fear and anxiety does not receive support. This type of prediction was discussed above. The reports studied as signs of female aggression give interesting results—they seem to be related to girl-woman rather than girl-man interactions, and thus to be topical to the area of interest. On the other hand, they do not differentiate between Woman fd and Woman tw. Possibly, even without subliminal steering the oedipal interpretation of the Girl-Woman stimuli is so close at hand that a number of subjects have given the reports in the control condition.

The predictions for the Man/Woman comparisons concerning the use of repression and isolation by and large receive support. The same is true for the other predictions (aggression, introaggression, fear) with regard to these comparisons. For instance, reports of aggression are much more frequent in both Man fd and Man tw as compared to the Woman conditions. Reactions to percept-genetic stimuli with a pp who really is aggressive and threatening (as in the DMT) are of interest in this context. Interindividual differences do not come to an end when the aggressive content is perceived. Male subjects who see boy–aggressive man stimuli often give reports of the type "Man beats boy." Female subjects who see girl–aggressive woman stimuli hardly ever report "Woman beats girl." Instead, if physical violence is reported by women in this situation, it is with the pp transformed to a man, even though exposure times are quite long. Direct violence belongs to a sphere of male activity. There is a middle ground where the sexes meet: "Man gives boy a rating" and "Woman gives girl a rating" are rather common reports for respective sex. Finally, there is a typically female form of report to this type of stimulus: "She (pp) is so angry and sorry because the girl will not eat what she has served her," etc. Male subjects may report pp as angry and completely mad, or as angry and physically hurt, but the angry-and-sad combination is a distinct female mode of aggression.

Some results were not predicted. Denials of aggression show the same pattern as reports of aggression. This is generally found, but so few subjects use denial that predictions for the category as a rule are not given. Faulty sex ascriptions and reports of a young pp are fairly common in the Woman group, and especially in the neutral condition, Woman tw, they tend to be associated. The subjects report neutral but pleasant scenes with a girl and a boy together. To quote Kragh (1985), "this is not a genuine defense mechanism but rather a sign of object relations."

Thus, this study gives experimental support to aspects of the psychoanalytic theory of the female Oedipus complex and its precipitates in later mental functioning. Of especial importance is the verification of predictions concerning differential use of defense mechanisms (repression, isolation, reaction formation) in contrasting conditions. Of course, what has been studied here relates to the dynamic propositions of psychoanalysis—those concerning unconscious anxieties, wishes, defenses, and fantasies motivating behavior in the "here-and now" (Silverman, 1983). General propositions concerning the nature of mental conflict and specific propositions about types of content frequently involved in such conflict receive support. On the other hand, genetic propositions—those that link present functioning to earlier experiences and events—cannot, in the nature of things, be directly investigated by laboratory techniques. Such propositions serve as connecting frameworks, pointing to probable regularities in the present (in this case with success).

Much can be said about psychoanalytic theory. Its highly colorful and mythographic appearance may make it hard for it to gain adherents among those used to the machine analogies of academic psychology. But—in contrast to the latter—its predictions are not trivial. They concern central aspects of human functioning and development. (For a full and spirited statement of this position, see Kline, 1988.) Many of these predictions are empirically testable if the proper methods—for instance, percept-genetic ones—are used.

References

Bonaparte, M. (1953) *Female sexuality*. London: Imago.

Collins, A.M. & Loftus, E.F. (1975) A spreading-activation theory of semantic processing. *Psychological Review, 82*, 407–428.

Fenichel, O. (1946) *The psychoanalytic theory of neurosis*. London: Routledge and Kegan Paul.

Freud, S. (1961) Some psychical consequences of the anatomical distinction between the sexes. In *The standard edition of the complete psychological works of Sigmund Freud: Vol. 19*. London: Hogarth Press (Original work published 1925)

Holender, D. (1986) Semantic activation without conscious identification in dichotic listening, parafoveal vision, and visual masking: A survey and appraisal. With peer commentary. *Behavioral and Brain Sciences, 9*, 1–66.

Horney, K. (1973) *Feminine psychology*. New York: Norton.

Kline, P. (1988) *Psychology exposed: Or, the emperor's new clothes*. London: Routledge.

Kragh, U. (1969) *Manual till DMT. Defense Mechanism Test*. [Manual of the DMT]. Stockholm: Skandinaviska Testförlaget.

Kragh, U. (1985) *DMT manual*. Stockholm: Persona.

Moses, I. & Reyher, J. (1985) Spontaneous and directed visual imagery: Image failure and image substitution. *Journal of Personality and Social Psychology, 48*, 233–242.

Nagera, H. (1975) *Female sexuality and the Oedipus complex*. New York: Jason Aronson.

Robles, R., Smith, R., Carver, C.S., & Wellens, A.R. (1987) Influence of subliminal visual images on the experience of anxiety. *Personality and Social Psychology Bulletin, 13*, 399–410.

Silverman, L.H. (1966) A technique for the study of psychodynamic relationships: The effects of subliminally presented aggressive stimuli on the production of pathological thinking in a schizophrenic population. *Journal of Consulting Psychology, 30*, 103–111.

Silverman, L.H. (1983) The subliminal psychodynamic activation method: Overview and comprehensive listing of studies. In J. Masling (Ed.), *Empirical studies of psychoanalytic theory: Vol. 1* (pp. 69–100). Hillsdale, N.J.: Erlbaum.

Silverman, L.H. & Geisler, C.J. (1986) The subliminal psychodynamic activation method: Comprehensive listing update, individual differences, and other considerations. In U. Hentschel, G.J.W. Smith, & J. Draguns (Eds.), *The roots of perception* (pp. 49–74). Amsterdam: North-Holland.

Sjöbäck, H. (1972) *Apparatkonstruktion, bildkonstruktion och grundläggande bildprovningsförsök med defense mechanism test.* [The construction of the apparatus, the layout and basic testing of the pictures for the Defense Mechanism Test]. Mimeographed, Department of Psychology, Lund University.

Spence, D.P., Klein, L., & Fernandez, R.J. (1986) Size and shape of the subliminal window. In U. Hentschel, G.J.W. Smith, & J. Draguns, *The roots of perception* (pp. 103–142). Amsterdam: North-Holland.

Westerlundh, B. (1976) *Aggression, anxiety, and defense.* Lund: Gleerup.

Westerlundh, B. (1986) On reading subliminal sentences: A psychodynamic activation study. *Psychological Research Bulletin, Lund University, 26*, 10.

Westerlundh, B. & Sjöbäck, H. (1986) Activation of intrapsychic conflict and defense: The amauroscopic technique. In U. Hentschel, G.J.W. Smith, & J. Draguns (Eds.), *The roots of perception* (pp. 161–216). Amsterdam: North-Holland.

Westerlundh, B. & Terjestam, Y. (1987) Psychodynamic effects of subliminal verbal messages on tachistoscopically presented interpersonal stimuli. *Psychological Research Bulletin, Lund University, 27*, 3.

15
Aspects of the Construct Validity of the Defense Mechanism Test

BARBARA E. SAITNER

There has been an upsurge of interest in the Defense Mechanism Test (DMT) following the publication of reports of its success in predicting personally characteristic patterns of coping with stress (e.g., Kragh & Smith, 1970). However, questions concerning the construct validity of the DMT remain unresolved, and there is continued disagreement about how perceptual distortions observed on the DMT are to be interpreted (Draguns, 1986; Meier-Civelli, 1989; Nilsson, 1982). So far Cooper and Kline (1986) are the only researchers who have chosen to investigate the construct validity of the DMT by comparing it with other established psychological tests. They were able to confirm some of the relationships they had predicted, even though the pattern of their results was far from clear-cut.

This chapter pursues the investigation of the construct validity of the DMT by comparing responses to it with the data from a battery of established psychological tests. This research is different from Cooper and Kline's study in that the sample is made up of problem individuals (who were apprehended for driving under the influence of alcohol). The predictive validity of the DMT for this purpose was established in an earlier study (Saitner, 1991). Hypotheses were derived from the DMT literature (e.g., Kragh, 1985), studies of drunken driving (Kunkel, 1977; Müller, 1976; Richman, 1985), and psychoanalytic theory (e.g., Fenichel, 1945; Hartmann, 1958). The following relationships between the DMT data and the variables assessed by means of the several measures within the test battery were predicted.

Repression will be associated with lowered self-consciousness, lower excitability, and higher composure on the Freiburg Personality Inventory (FPI).

Isolation is expected to be correlated with carefulness and accuracy on the concentration test d2 by Brickenkamp and on the Vienna Determination Apparatus (Wiener Determinationsgerät [WDG]).

Denial will be positively associated with the choices of "gray" (scored for denial on the Color Pyramid Test [CPT]) and "purple" (scored for tension on the same test); a negative relationship is expected between denial and openness and emotional stability (both measured by means of FPI) as well as aggressiveness (as assessed by means of the FPI and the Swedish Personality Questionnaire [SPQ]).

Reaction formation is expected to yield a negative relationship with aggressiveness, as assessed by means of both the FPI and the SPQ.

Introagression is expected to be associated with depression on the FPI.

Identification with the female role is expected to be associated with high scores for "purple" on the CPT, emotional instability on the FPI, and low scores for masculinity on the FPI.

Polymorphous identification is predicted to be associated with depression on the FPI.

Projection is expected to be related to high sensitivity scores on the SPQ.

Regression will be associated with the choice of "orange," scored for regression on the CPT, and emotional instability, as scored on the FPI and marked by the choice of "purple" on the CPT. No hypotheses were formulated for identification with the aggressor because of the low rate of occurrence of the manifestations of this mechanism.

Method

For a detailed description of the procedure, the interested reader is referred to Saitner (1990, 1991). Briefly, members of a random sample of male individuals with several severe traffic offenses, mostly drunken driving, were assessed by means of a test battery for the purpose of determining the probability of future transgressions. The DMT was administered in accordance with its original manual (Kragh, 1969). The DMT scores were weighed: scores for the middle and late phases were multiplied by 2 and 3, respectively. The total scores were then computed by adding the weighted scores for all phases and series.

In addition, the following tests were administered.

1. The d2 measure (Brickenkamp, 1966), a derivative of the concentration test developed by Lauer (1955): it measures "attention to detail."

2. A choice reaction test of sensorimotor and perceptual tasks, the Vienna Determination Apparatus (Wiener Determinationsgerät [WDG]): it was derived from the Driving Apparatus Test developed by Häkkinen (1958). Subjects are required to respond to visual and auditory stimuli of different kinds with specified hand and foot movements. Constancy, speed, and accuracy of performance are measured.

3. The German version of the Wechsler–Bellevue Adult Intelligence Scale (HAWIE: Wechsler, 1964): this test comprises 11 subtests, grouped into Verbal (Information, Digit Span, Vocabulary, Arithmetic, Comprehension, Similarities) and Performance (Picture Completion, Picture

Arrangement, Block Design, Object Assembly, Digit Symbol). With respect to scales, factor analytic techniques have sorted out three factors: Verbal Comprehension with large weights in Vocabulary, Information, Comprehension, and Similarities; Perceptual Organization with large weights in Block Design and Object Assembly, and a Freedom from Distractibility, with loadings in Digit Span, Arithmetic, and Digit Symbol.

4. The Freiburg Personality Inventory (FPI: Fahrenberg & Selg, 1970): it is scored for the following 12 dimensions: nervousness, aggressiveness, depression, excitability, sociability, composure, dominance, self-consciousness, openness, extraversion, emotional instability, and masculinity.

5. The German version of the Swedish Personality Questionnaire: it comprises introversion, sensitivity, and aggressiveness scales.

6. The Color Pyramid Test (Schaie & Heiss, 1964), a color preference measure: subjects arc asked to pick out colored papers (out of 14 different colors) and place them within a pyramid design. They are asked to construct three "pretty" pyramids and then are instructed to build three more pyramids and make them "as ugly as possible." Response to color is thought to relate to the sphere of affect and emotion, which are construed as basic aspects of personality. The "pretty" series is associated with the more overt part of personality while the "ugly" series is designed to tap its more hidden and subconscious emotional sphere.

Research Design

Two extreme groups were formed, based on the frequency of defensive reactions on nine of the ten DMT scales; scale 5 (identification with the aggressor) was excluded because incidence of this sign was low in the sample. On each of these nine scales, the sample was divided, with subjects who had no scores on the scale in question and those whose scores were very low forming one group. The other group included subjects whose scores on that scale were high. Comparisons were then carried out with the scores of these two contrasting groups of subjects on the several tests described above (the d2 measure, the WDG, the HAWIE, the FPI, the SPQ, and the CPT). The percentage of the subjects varied because of the distribution of frequencies on the several DMT scales (see tables). t-Tests were used for all group comparisons.

Results and Discussion

Similarly to the results by Cooper and Kline, the number of significant correlations found was low. Of the several hypotheses pertaining to

TABLE 15.1. Difference in personality measures as a function of occurrence of repression as defense style.

	Repression = 0 (N = 34)		Repression ≥ 7 (N = 34)		
	X	sd	X	sd	p
d2 total of details	376.91	80.24	420.41	86.96	<.05
FPI					
Sociability	6.88	3.49	9.04	2.67	<.05
Self-consciousness	3.73	2.07	2.45	1.88	<.05
CPT/difference	42.08	10.64	36.76	8.98	<.05

repression, only the prediction concerning low self-consciousness (FPI) was confirmed. Additionally, high scores on the repression scale were found to be associated with self-representation characterized by sociability (FPI), stability in the sphere of affects and emotions (CPT), and high capacity to withstand stress (d2). These results appear to indicate that the repressors possess stable and "normal," well-adapted personalities. However, this finding is contradicted by the comparatively high record of traffic offenses of drivers who tend toward repression (Saitner, 1990). On the other hand, Bell and Byrne (1977) found the repressive style of defense to be correlated with emotional stability in self-representation, and also with greater aggressiveness and lower sensitivity in social contacts. Table 15.1 provides a summary of quantitative findings pertaining to repression.

No support for the hypotheses concerning isolation was found (Table 15.2). On the other hand, a significant correlation between carefulness on the WDG and isolation emerged for the entire sample, as reported elsewhere (Saitner, 1990).

A surprising finding was the lower achievement of subjects with a distinct isolating and intellectualizing defense style on the Wechsler Performance Scale and the subtests of Picture Arrangement, Picture Completion, and Block Design. These subjects seem to have a cognitive

TABLE 15.2. Difference in personality measures as a function of occurrence of isolation as defense style.

	Isolation ≤ 2 (N = 21)		Isolation ≥ 10 (N = 29)		
	X	sd	X	sd	p
Wechsler					
Performance scale	106.47	9.91	100.05	9.92	<.01
Picture arrangement	10.28	2.63	9.00	2.01	<.05
Picture completion	11.28	1.70	9.77	2.61	<.05
Block design	10.47	2.48	8.88	1.99	<.05
FPI/dominance	2.08	0.90	3.03	1.71	<.05
CPT/pretty series, purple	3.04	3.78	1.02	1.92	<.05

TABLE 15.3. Difference in personality measures as a function of occurrence of denial as defense style.

	Denial = 0 (N = 78)		Denial $\geq$ 1 (N = 30)		
	X	sd	X	sd	p
d2/vacillating of attention	12.06	4.12	15.00	8.03	<.05
FPI					
Aggression	2.29	2.08	1.34	1.22	<.05
Openness	8.11	2.95	6.60	1.97	<.05

style that makes it difficult for them to form complete "gestalten" and to perform effectively in practical contexts. Moreover, subjects with a high isolation score tend to be dominant and rigid, as measured on the FPI, which may shield them from emotional excitability, as assessed on the CPT. These results support the psychoanalytic view of the link between isolation as a defense style and compulsive personality traits. (See Table 15.2 for the details of these results.)

In keeping with the hypothesis, denial was associated with low scores in openness and aggressiveness on the FPI. There was, however, no emotional instability found, as indexed on the FPI, for subjects characterized by reliance on denial, nor did the high-denial groups make significantly more choices of the color gray on the CPT. The Pearson correlation coefficient between the choice of gray and denial was significant, as reported by Saitner (1990). The relationship of denial to vacillating attention on the d2 measure may be indicative of distractibility and, by implication, emotional instability. Table 15.3 presents these findings in greater detail.

No support was received for the hypothesis pertaining to reaction formation. Specifically, subjects with high scores for this defense mechanism did not produce lower scores in aggression either on the FPI or the SPQ. They tend, however, toward passive adaptation and are inclined to deny their conflicts, as expressed in their choice of gray on CPT, regard-

TABLE 15.4. Difference in personality measures as a function of occurrence of reaction formation as defense style.

	Reaction formation = 0 (N = 32)		Reaction formation $\geq$ 8 (N = 37)		
	X	sd	X	sd	p
CPT					
Gray/pretty series	0.40	1.13	2.18	4.12	<.05
Gray/ugly series	7.90	9.40	3.24	3.42	<.05
FPI					
Excitability	3.04	2.21	1.92	1.57	<.05
Openness	9.00	2.96	7.23	2.94	<.05

TABLE 15.5. Difference in personality measures as a function of occurrence of introaggression as defense style.

	Introaggression = 0 (N = 73)		Introaggression ≥ 1 (N = 29)		
	X	sd	X	sd	p
Wechsler					
Digit span	10.55	2.76	12.75	2.38	<.01
Comprehension	10.47	3.08	12.25	1.94	<.01
CPT/ugly series, black	10.64	7.43	7.50	7.15	<.05

less of situational aspects. In contrast to subjects whose scores in reaction formation are zero, this pattern remains stable and is resistant to change, which may be indicative of the rigidity that is frequently imputed to people who tend toward reaction formation (e.g., Fenichel, 1974). On the basis of their self-description, subjects in the reaction formation group experience themselves as less open and less excitable. Thus reaction formation helps these subjects to control their affects to such an extent that they perceive themselves as basically calm and "unaffected." The findings are presented in Table 15.4.

There was no correlation between the FPI manifestations of depression and an introaggressive defense style, as shown in Table 15.5. Subjects with introaggressive defense style tended, however, toward less intense and less abrupt attenuation of affects, as exemplified by the use of black on the CPT. Thus the better performance of these subjects on some of the Wechsler subtests might be connected with the less inhibited use of their energy. It must be concluded that this pattern of results provides no support for the construct validity of introaggression as measured on the DMT.

The hypothesis concerning the relationship between the masculinity scale on the FPI and the DMT scale for the identification with a female role received no support. However, as hypothesized, subjects who score high on this scale experience excitability and emotional instability, as indicated by the choice of "purple" on CPT, and are sensitive, in light

TABLE 15.6. Difference in personality measures as a function of occurrence of identification with a female role as defense style.

	Identification with a female role = 0 (N = 63)		Identification with a female role ≥ 1 (N = 45)		
	X	sd	X	sd	p
SPQ: Sensitivity	10.74	5.50	13.37	6.15	<.05
CPT/pretty series, purple	0.98	1.83	2.08	3.35	<.05

TABLE 15.7. Difference in personality measures as a function of occurrence of polymorphous identification as defense style.

	Polymorphous identification = 0 (N = 73)		Polymorphous identification ≥ 14 (N = 38)		
	X	sd	X	sd	p
Wechsler: Information	11.47	2.22	9.68	2.62	<.05
CPT/ugly series, white	1.44	2.94	3.42	4.69	<.05

of their SPQ scores. Thus their personality can be described as soft and pliable. In this respect they tend toward a "typical" female self-attribution. (See Table 15.6 for the particulars of these results.)

In reference to the hypothesized relationship between polymorphous identification and depression on the FPI, the results are negative. High scores on this scale are associated with lower intellectual performance (Information and Similarity on the HAWIE), which could be interpreted as depressive inhibition of intellectual functions and lack of flexibility. Low scores on Information suggest retreat from the environment. There is also a relationship between polymorphous identification as defense style and the tendency toward latent aggressions as shown by the use of "white" on the CPT. These findings lend support to the relationship between suppressed anger and depression. All these results are contained in Table 15.7.

Analyses pertaining to projection were entirely inconclusive and shed no light on the characteristic personality variables of individuals who rely on this defense. Regression was not associated with emotional instability in light of either FPI or CPT indicators, nor with the regressive sign of "orange" on the CPT. However, there was a significant relationship between the choice of "orange" and on the DMT regression scale in previous analyses (Saitner, 1990). In this sample subjects with a regressive defense style tend less toward introversion on the SPQ and are not very excitable, as shown by the choice of "red" CPT. They rely less on denial, as marked by the use of "gray" on the CPT, are less achievement

TABLE 15.8. Difference in personality measures as a function of occurrence of regression as defense style.

	Regression = 0 (N = 84)		Regression ≥ 1 (N = 24)		
	X	sd	X	sd	p
SPQ: Introversion	11.83	4.78	9.28	4.88	<.05
CPT/pretty series, red1	2.21	2.92	1.13	1.91	<.05
CPT/pretty series, gray	1.51	3.08	0.47	1.08	<.05
CPT/ugly series, yellow	2.01	2.78	1.04	1.18	<.05
CPT/ugly series, blue4	3.28	5.36	1.69	2.24	<.05

oriented, as indicated by the choice of "yellow" on the CPT, and possess less control over the expression of affect, as expressed by the use of "blue" on the CPT. Their defense mechanisms are incompletely developed, and their selection of environmental stimuli tends to be poorly differentiated. Thus they are easily disoriented when stress occurs and are then not able to control their reactions adequately. These results are summarized in Table 15.8.

Conclusion

The number of significant findings obtained is small. Some defenses have not been clarified at all by the analyses performed. Projection is a case in point. For some scales, such as denial, however, support for construct validity was found. As in earlier studies, the overlap between the personality variables and the DMT scales was slight. However, there was sufficient confirmation of several of the hypotheses to support the conclusion that the defense style is intertwined with structural personality traits. Moreover, the connection between defense and cognitive style, as revealed, for example, for the scales of isolation and polymorphous identification, indicates that the personality as a whole is expressed through the manner in which defensive reactions are structured.

To make the DMT an effective diagnostic tool, further research on this topic is needed. An examination of correlations between the DMT data and the variables from other tests should be carried out with a large-scale heterogeneous sample, and the significance of correlations should be tested by means of Dunn's multiple comparison procedure.

References

Bell, P.A. & Byrne, D. (1977) Repression-sensitization. In H. London & J.E. Exner (Eds.), *Dimensions of personality* (pp. 449–485). New York: Wiley.

Brickenkamp, R. (1966) *Aufmerksamkeits-Belastungs-Test (d2)*. [The Attention Stress Test [d2]] (2nd ed.). Göttingen: Hogrefe.

Cooper, C. & Kline, P. (1986) An evaluation of the Defence Mechanism Test. *British Journal of Psychology*, 77, 19–31.

Draguns, J.G. (1986) Subliminal perception as the first stage of the perceptual process: Can personality be revealed so early in the sequence? In U. Hentschel, G.J.W. Smith, & J.G. Draguns (Eds.), *The roots of perception* (pp. 331–352). Amsterdam: Elsevier.

Fahrenberg, J. & Selg, H. (1970) *Freiburger Persönlichkeitsinventar (FPI)*. Göttingen: Hogrefe.

Fenichel, O. (1946) *The Psychoanalytic theory of neurosis*. London: Routledged Kegan Paul.

Häkkinen, S. (1958) *Traffic accidents and driver characteristics*. A statistical and psychological study. Helsinki: Suomalaisen Kirjalisuuden Kirjapaino.

Hartmann, H. (1958) *Ego psychology and the problem of adaptation*. Madison, CT: International Universities Press.

Kragh, U. (1969) *Manual till DMT. Defense Mechanism Test* [DMT manual]. Stockholm: Scandinaviska Testförlaget.

Kragh, U. (1985) *Defense Mechanism Test. DMT Manual*. Stockholm: Persona.

Kragh, U. & Smith, G.J.W. (1970) *Percept-genetic analysis*. Lund: Gleerup.

Kunkel, E. (1977) *Biographische Daten und Rückfallprognose bei Trunkenheits-tätern im Strassenverkehr*. [Biographic data and prognosis for relapse for drunk offenders in vehicular traffic]. Cologne: TÜV Rheinland.

Lauer, A.R. (1955) Comparison of group paper-and-pencil tests for measuring driving aptitude of army personnel. *Journal of Applied Psychology*, *39*, 318.

Meier-Civelli, U. (1989) Der Defense Mechanism Test (DMT). Eine Evaluations-studie aufgrund publizierter Untersuchungen. [The DMT. An evaluative study based on published investigations]. *Bericht der Abteilung für angewandte Psychologie, Universität Zürich.*, No. 26.

Müller, A. (1976) *Der Trunkenheitstäter im Strassenverkehr der BRD*. [The drunk offender on the roads of the Federal Republic of Germany]. Frankfurt: Lang.

Nilsson, A. (1982) *The mechanism of defence within a developmental frame of reference*. Lund: Gleerup.

Richman, A. (1985) Human risk factors in alcohol-related crashes. North American Conference on Alcohol and Highway Safety. *Journal of Studies on Alcohol, 10*, 21–23.

Saitner, B. (1990) *Die Leistungsfähigkeit des Defense Mechanism Tests (DMT) für die Vorhersage der Verkehrsbewährung von Kraftfahrern*. [The efficiency of the DMT for the prediction of performance of car drivers in traffic]. Unpublished doctoral dissertation, University of Cologne, Germany.

Saitner, B. (1991) Application of the DMT for assessing serious drinking and driving offenders. In M. Olff, G. Godaert, & H. Ursin (Eds.), *Quantification of human defense* (pp. 238–251). Berlin: Springer.

Schaie, K.W. & Heiss, R. (1964) *Color and personality*. Bern: Huber.

Wechsler, D. (1964) *Die Messung der Intelligenz Erwachsener* [Measurement of adult intelligence]. Bern: Huber.

16
Adaptation to Boredom and Stress: The Effects of Defense Mechanisms and Concept Formation on Attentional Performance in Situations with Inadequate Stimulation

UWE HENTSCHEL, MANFRED KIEßLING, and ARN HOSEMANN

The present study stems from a project that was aimed at providing information about what personality characteristics are best suited to predict attentional deficits under boredom and stress. It can be placed in the broader context of man–machine interaction and was planned as a computer simulation task for the attention-related activity of driving a car. Man–machine interactions usually do not attract much interest as long as everything runs smoothly. In the case of obvious problems or disturbances of the system, an analysis is required from which in the best case something can be learned about the optimal functioning of the system. These analyses usually have either a stronger technical impact, directed at the functioning of the machine, or a stronger psychological impact, directed at the user and his or her interaction with the existing technical solutions. The relevance of man–machine interactions for differential or personality psychology is to be found in those examples where personality characteristics have or may have an influence on the reaction to the machine.

A rather famous example is provided by the driver of the tank truck who in spite of a slightly defective transmission decided to drive down a steep hill in Herborn, a small town in Germany. He could not change into a lower gear, the brakes did not hold the extra load put on them, and the truck crashed into an ice-cream parlor and exploded. Five people were killed and a number of neighboring houses completely destroyed. In this case different technical prevention measures would have been possible, ranging from better technical control of trucks in general to forbidding heavy trucks to use that specific road (later pronounced by the local government). But it is also legitimate to ask whether another driver would not have come to a decision better adapted to this situation, which generally would suggest the attempt at better selection and/or training of drivers, to which another question has to follow: selection (and training) on the basis of which criteria?

The contribution of psychology to traffic studies was for a long time dominated by the search for the accident-prone type of driver. On the whole this attempt was not very successful. The majority of accidents are caused by normal drivers, not belonging to this special group (see, e.g., Forbes, 1972). For the study of accident risks it seems generally better (a) to favor a probabilistic approach and (b) try to find a possible link between accident proneness in certain types of situation. The second part of this assumption is based on the idea that the probability for making a mistake changes with different situations, which in turn are related to personal characteristics (cf. McGuire, 1976) and such inner states as, for example, vigilance, which is, as far as external preconditions are concerned, among the variables influenced by noise and vibration (Floru, Damongeot, & di Renzo, 1988). Being tired or being bored has direct consequences for the task of driving. It increases the chance of reacting inadequately, especially in case of an unexpected new situation. There are also interindividual differences in getting bored while, for example, driving on a straight highway with almost no traffic. The driver's activity, basically comparable with many other man–machine interactions, can be summarized as a complex input–output process with a continuous feedback loop (cf. Rockwell, 1972). The input is the attention-related registration and evaluation of changing scenes. The outputs are motor reactions (reactions fitted to fulfill the intentions of accelerating, braking, changing the direction of the car, etc.). With experience, the motor reactions become highly automatized, so that the psychologically more interesting questions seem to be connected with the input side: the observation and evaluation of constantly changing stimulus patterns.

Whether both observation and evaluation of the incoming stimuli can be subsumed under attention control depends on which definition of attention is used. More complex definitions recognize its multidimensional features (e.g., Fröhlich, 1978), consider a potentially unconscious part of it (Dixon, 1981; Dixon, Hentschel, & Smith, 1986), regard attention as an organized set of procedures (Glass, Holyoak, & Santa, 1979), or focus on its contribution to resources of ability (Cooper and Regan, 1982; Hunt, 1980). Seen from a broader perspective, including observation and evaluation, attention is part of a reaction to a complex social environment (Chance, 1976), an aspect of attention that is certainly relevant for the activity of driving a car as well as for many other types of man–machine interaction. Within the aims of the project, we intended to study the effect of three basic situations: understimulation, overstimulation, and a normal input level, with two variants for each of the inadequate stimulation conditions: monotony and satiation for the condition of understimulation and two levels of information overload (stress1 and stress2) for the overstimulation condition. With that characterization, we have clearly abandoned a merely physical description of the stimuli.

Monotony, satiation, and stress are terms related to subjective experience, but through their operationalization there is, of course, a relation with physical characteristics too. It should be noted, however, that no complete congruence is possible. The experience of monotony or stress is ultimately a subjective one, but a possible goal that we also tried to reach in the present study is to create situations that at least for most of the subjects, if not all, are boring, stressful, etc. (i.e., the attempt to create situations prototypical in that respect). Our general research question can be formulated in everyday language as follows: What kind of people lose their composure in conditions of inadequate stimulations and what kind of people can manage these situations better? We wanted to control the differential effect in being able to cope with these different conditions with the basic hypothesis of an interaction of defense mechanisms and cognition; thus we had to select the set of variables to be used from the whole test battery with these prerequisites in mind. From the cognitive tests we wanted to include a test requiring logical thinking. The most difficult in the battery was a concept formation test, called Symbol Maze Test (SMT: Hentschel & Kießling, 1983). We knew from analyses of the project data (Hentschel & Kießling, in press; Hentschel, Kießling, & Hosemann, 1989, 1991) that the perceptual defense mechanisms of the Defense Mechanism Test (DMT: see Chapter 7) interact with anxiety but not with concept formation on attentional performance. From earlier research and from the project data, we knew also that since the defense mechanisms registered by the FKBS (Fragenbogen zu Konfliktbewältigungsstratigien: Inventory for Conflict-Solving Strategies—see Chapter 5) and the DMT reveal no substantial correlations, the cognition defense interaction hypothesis could get another chance by using the FKBS defenses. The computer simulation task for the measurement of attentional performance is described in greater detail in the method section. A schematic overview of the design of the study is given in Fig. 16.1. Based on studies using the FKBS (e.g., Hentschel & Schneider, 1986) and in contrast to the DMT defenses, we did not expect that all the FKBS defense mechanisms would hamper the attention performance. A higher score of Turning Against Object (TAO, see Chapter 5) seems to be a rather positive sign in many situations. For the other clusters of defense, the general hypothesis was that higher defense scores in interaction with a poor concept formation ability are related to more errors in the understimulation and overstimulation conditions of the attention task.

Method

The Construction of the Experimental Conditions and the Attentional Performance Measure

The main dimension in the construction of the dependent variable in the experiment taken from the analogy of driving a car is the variation of

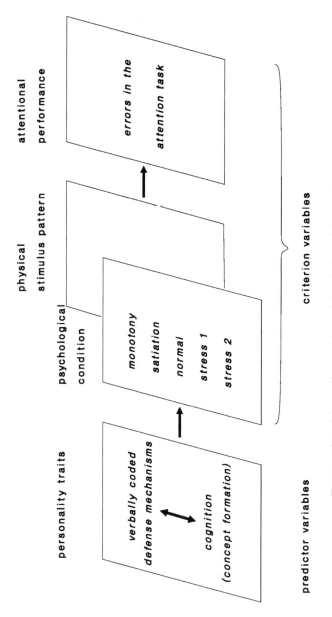

FIGURE 16.1. Schematic overview of the design of the study.

information load. This dimension was to be introduced into the psychological conditions of monotony, satiation, normal, stress1, and stress2, which should give a higher level of stress in comparison to stress1. Monotony, provoking a state of lower vigilance with the feeling of being bored, usually comes about by a lack of variation in the surrounding. A possible way to introduce it into an attention control task is to use a low frequency of the events to be controlled. Kurt Lewin (1935) and his coworkers made the first experiment on the effects of satiation. Karsten (1928) asked her subjects to make strokes in a certain rhythm until they did not want to continue any longer even upon slight pressure from the experimenter. She described in detail how subjects became bored, tired, and inattentive and tried to introduce minor variations until finally they could not be persuaded to go on. The main characterization for satiation is repetition. It is less easy to trace it in the activity of driving a car, although a longer stop-and-go condition might provoke it, especially in cars that do not have automatic transmissions. In our experiment we tried to operationalize it through the requirement of repetitive motor reactions (pressing the keys of the keyboard in a certain ordered sequence in reaction to visual stimuli). From the deviations of a normal information load hitherto mentioned, normal conditions can be delineated: a higher frequency of the events to be controlled, nonrepetitive, and at a manageable speed.

Stress1 and stress2 were both conditions featuring an overload of information, and it was impossible to react to the stimulus without making

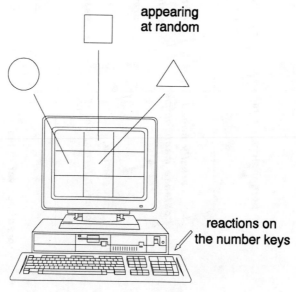

FIGURE 16.2. The task of the subjects: to react at the "relevant" symbol on a computer monitor.

TABLE 16.1. Parameters of the experimental conditions.

	Monotony	Satiation	Normal	Stress1	Stress2
Relevant symbol	Square	Circle	Triangle	Circle	Circle
Presented in color	Green	Yellow	Green	Changing	Changing
Background color	Black	Black	Blue	Black	Changing
Number of symbols	1	1	Max. 3	Max. 3	Max. 3
Number of trials	25	594	200	250	300
Error feedback	No	No	Yes	Yes	Yes
Minimum time between two trials (0.1 s)	300	10	10	5	3
Acceleration factor	1	1	15	50	50
Exposure time (0.1 s)	7	5	8	4	4

errors, although there was enough space for interindividual differences. The stress situations were planned to provoke feelings of being ill at ease, of nervous tension, and of hyperactivity. The order of the different conditions was monotony, stress1, normal, satiation, and stress2. The subjects were seated in front of a computer monitor and had to give their reactions on the keyboard. The basic setting is graphically presented in Fig. 16.2. In each of the conditions, reactions were required to a specific relevant symbol. A more detailed description of the different conditions is given in Table 16.1. For the condition of satiation, the appearance of the symbols was restricted to the four upper left fields corresponding to the key numbers 7, 8, 4, and 5, which for correct reactions had to be pressed as a repeated series of the following order, 7, 8, 4, 5, 7, 5. Errors in reaction times were registered automatically; errors were scored when subjects pressed the wrong key, missed the reaction, or did not respond within the given time limit, which varied for the different conditions. An adequate measure for interindividual comparison of the performance is the error rate (i.e., the percentage of the maximally possible errors in each of the conditions). This measure is used in all group comparisons to follow.

The Predictor Variables

Defense Mechanisms Registered by Questionnaire: FKBS

The FKBS is described in greater detail in Chapter 5, which also considers how far the psychodynamic idea can be kept alive by measuring defenses by means of questionnaires. The basic scores of the FKBS corresponding to the Defense Mechanism Inventory (Gleser & Ihilevich, 1969) are Turning Against Object (TAO), Projection (PRO), Principalization (PRN), Turning Against Self (TAS), and Reversal (REV) (cf. Chapter 5). In the present study the overall scores (combining the answers for the feeling and behavior level) were used.

Concept Formation

To measure concept formation, we developed a new test, the Symbol Maze Test (SMT: Hentschel & Kießling, 1983; Hentschel & Kießling, in preparation), the validity of which has been studied in different experiments (cf., e.g., Hentschel & Kießling, 1986; Hentschel, Kießling, & Ternes, 1984). The SMT is a computer-controlled experimental task. It is presented to the subject in form of a mental maze in which the "right way" has to be found. Getting at the right way implies the need to find a symbol (i.e., a correct combination of signs indicating this way). There are no real blind alleys as in other mental mazes, but when the subject enters a forbidden way (i.e., a way with a combination of signs other than the correct one), he or she receives an error feedback in form of a low tone. On the way through the maze there are 25 decision points, which allow the subject to learn the concept asked for in that specific maze. When the solution is found, the further way through the maze can be made without any errors. From earlier studies, the characteristics that make a maze more or less difficult are known. The difficulty depends on the redundancy of symbols in a specific maze and the kind of combination rule: that is, how often the subject encounters the same combination of signs in a maze and what the required rule of combination is ("and," "or," "and plus or": e.g., a red square and a blue triangle, a red square or a blue square, a red square and a blue triangle, or a blue square and a red triangle). Subjects are confronted with a series of eight mazes (two with houses, three with abstract figures, and three with faces). The score is the weighted sum of errors in a particular maze, which can be summed up to the whole series or separately for subseries of difficult and easy mazes. The task is process oriented and within the tradition of microgenesis (cf. Hentschel, 1984) has been labeled "schematogenetic" (Hentschel & Kießling, 1983). According to our experience, concept formation has an intermediate position between intelligence tests and more complex problem-solving tasks (Hentschel & Kießling, 1986).

TABLE 16.2. Analysis of variance: TAS by concept formation by understimulation.

Source of variation	df	F	p
TAS	1	3.93	.05
Concept formation	1	15.93	<.001
TAS by concept formation	1	2.11	.15
Within cells	72		
Understimulation	2	17.60	<.001
TAS by understimulation	2	2.31	.10
Concept formation by understimulation	2	4.89	.009
TAS by concept formation by understimulation	2	3.04	.05
Within cells	144		

Sample

One hundred subjects (48 males, 52 females, mean age 34 years) voluntarily took part in the experiment; they were tested individually and received renumeration. Each one had to have a driving license. It was necessary to exclude from the sample 24 subjects in the condition of understimulation and 23 subjects in the condition of overstimulation because of data missing from either the SMT and/or the attention task.

Results

On the Differentiation of the Situations of Inadequate Stimulation

The results of a pilot study ($N = 5$) gave a first indication that the construction of the different psychological conditions was successful. With the main sample ($N = 77$ resp. 76), for the 10 nonredundant possibilities of comparison between the five different conditions, t-tests were calculated which were all significant ($p < 0.005$). The stress2 condition following the stress1 situation resulted, however, in a lower number of errors. Moreover, the two stress conditions were highly correlated ($r = .83$).

The Effect of Defense Mechanisms and Concept Formation on Attention Control Under the Conditions of Inadequate Stimulation

To compare the differences within the conditions of understimulation and overstimulation, the different situations were grouped in threes (monotony, normal, satiation and stress1, normal, stress2), using the normal stimulation for both conditions as a control. The effects of the defense mechanisms in concept formation were controlled by using separate median splittings for all five defense scores and the error score in the concept formation task. The significant results for the condition of understimulation are presented in Table 16.2, which shows a very significant main effect for concept formation, already known from analyses of the project data (cf. Hentschel & Kießling, in press), and also a main effect for TAS and an interaction effect between TAS, concept formation, and the sequence. The results are graphically presented in Figs. 16.3 and 16.4. Figure 16.3 gives the attention task results for the groups with good versus bad concept formation. Figure 16.4 shows the interaction between TAS and concept formation. A higher score of TAS combined with a higher score in the concept formation task results in higher error scores in

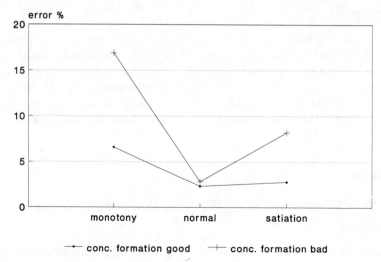

FIGURE 16.3. Performance in the concept formation task and errors in the attention task under the condition of understimulation.

the attentional task in both understimulation situations, with the worst result in the monotony situation.

Tables 16.3 give the significant results for the overstimulation condition. Two out of the five defenses show a main effect. In three cases there are

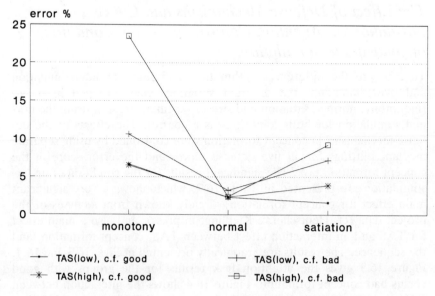

FIGURE 16.4. Performance in the concept formation task, high versus low TAS scores, and errors in the attention task under the condition of understimulation.

TABLE 16.3. Analysis of variance.

REV by concept formation by overstimulation

Source of variation	df	F	p
REV	1	3.12	.08
Concept formation	1	4.88	.03
REV by concept formation	1	.56	.46
Within cells	72		
Overstimulation	2	485.13	<.001
REV by overstimulation	2	3.31	.04
Concept formation by overstimulation	2	3.13	.05
REV by concept formation by overstimulation	2	.43	.65
Within cells	144		

TAS by concept formation by overstimulation

Source of variation	df	F	p
TAS	1	5.56	.02
Concept formation	1	8.20	.005
TAS by concept formation	1	.82	.37
Within cells	72		
Overstimulation	2	531.40	<.001
TAS by overstimulation	2	4.67	.01
Concept formation by overstimulation	2	5.70	.004
TAS by concept formation by overstimulation	2	1.19	.31
Within cells	144		

TAO by concept formation by overstimulation

Source of variation	df	F	p
TAO	1	7.01	.01
Concept formation	1	5.10	.03
TAO by concept formation	1	.14	.71
Within cells	72		
Overstimulation	2	517.34	<.001
TAO by overstimulation	2	5.30	.006
Concept formation by overstimulation	2	3.48	.03
TAO by concept formation by overstimulation	2	.24	.78
Within cells	144		

interaction effects with the sequence too. There is no interaction of the defense groups with concept formation. Concept formation shows, however, a main effect and an interaction effect with sequence, which are both also known from other analyses (cf. Hentschel & Kießling, in press).

The results are graphically presented in Figs. 16.5 and 16.6. In both stress situations the group with higher TAO scores makes fewer errors in

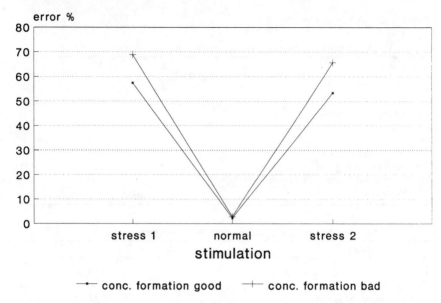

FIGURE 16.5. Performance in the concept formation task and errors in the attention task under the condition of overstimulation.

the attention task, although there seems to be a learning effect also for the group with lower TAO scores from stress1 to stress2. The group with higher TAS scores makes more errors in both stress situations, and for REV there is a significant difference for the stress2 situation, indicating fewer errors for the group with lower REV scores. This group shows also a significant learning effect from stress1 to stress2.

Discussion

The results show some support for the general hypothesis that defense mechanisms, concept formation, and attentional performance are related. As far as concept formation, exclusively in relation to attention control, is concerned, we have only summarized the results of another study (Hentschel & Kießling, in press) in this chapter. Moreover, the relation of the SMT to the attention task might to a certain degree be influenced by an overlap of the predictor with the criterion. Attention is also important for the microgenetic concept formation task. Nevertheless, the results would be interesting if it were possible to show a close relation between the computer simulation task of attention control and real car driving. Then the SMT could be regarded as a really valuable predictor. In this stage of our research we do not know if this is the case.

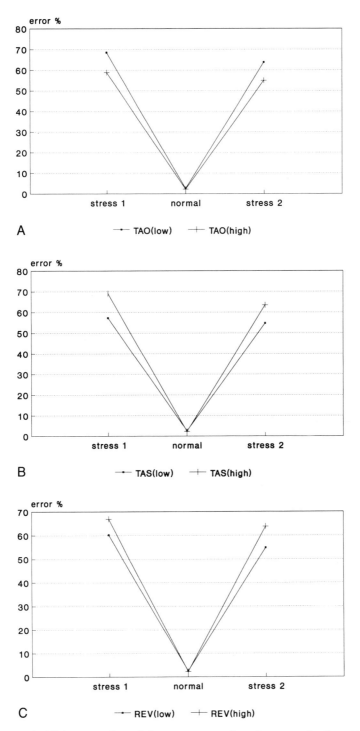

FIGURE 16.6. High versus low defense scores and performance in the attention task under the condition of overstimulation: (A) TAO, (B) TAS, and (C) REV.

In formulating our hypothesis for this study we were more interested in the potential effects of the FKBS defense mechanisms and, especially, in the interaction between defense mechanisms and concept formation with regard to the criterion. In the latter respect, one result appeared for the condition of understimulation, namely for the combination of TAS and concept formation, especially in the monotony situation. A lower concept formation ability combined with a tendency to ascribe the faults to oneself hampers attentional performance under monotony. Formulated as a probabilistic statement, this would mean that given the condition of understimulation, the risk of making a mistake is greater for people showing this combination of personality characteristics (25% of the sample). Concept formation also shows a main effect for the condition of overstimulation, but no interaction with defense mechanisms is found here. Among the defense mechanisms, TAS, REV, and (with an opposite direction) TAO give the significant effects as presented in Fig. 16.6. To summarize the FKBS results in both conditions of inadequate stimulation, one could say that attributing faults to oneself (TAS) results in a decrease of performance in both conditions. REV hampers learning, and a higher TAO score seems to have a favorable influence on managing the attention task under stress.

From earlier research with the FKBS it can be concluded that these results are partly in line with the results of other studies. TAO, for example, has shown a positive influence on creativity under very different experimental conditions (Hentschel & Schneider, 1986), TAS a negative effect on cognitive performance (Hentschel & Kießling, 1990), and REV significantly lower learning effects in a complex sorting task (Udenhout & Bekker, 1990). Although we did include PRO in the analyses of variance, we did not expect an effect to come from it under the given conditions. Our basic hypothesis did however cover PRN, which actually showed no effects. When we try to come to a conclusion based on the results available thus far from our research project on attention control, which was focused on the predictor side on defense mechanisms, anxiety, and concept formation, a clear method effect regarding the measurement of defenses appears, leading to predictive validities that are method specific for different defense mechanisms and different interactions. It seems very difficult to use one theoretical umbrella for these results. The problem of method specificity has been discussed to a greater extent in a theoretical context in two of the introductory chapters of this book (cf. Chapters 5 and 7), but it remains a concrete obstacle in empirical research. We do not share the opinion of Lazarus and Folkman (1984) that persisting with one method and ignoring others is a good way out of the dilemma. An intermediate solution could be to look for an optimalization of the predictors to this end—in our case, the possibility of cross-validating the set of predictor variables would be a necessary step; specifically, more information about the relation of the computer task to real driving is needed also. This goal could not be achieved with the available data.

The state of affairs is thus unsatisfying mainly from a theoretical point of view and provides better perspectives in regard to practical applications. Drivers of tank trucks as well as pilots, flight controllers, railway operators, or captains of ships should have a certain tolerance for inadequate stimulation (some unexpected stress seems to be as unavoidable in these jobs as well as certain forms of understimulation). Understimulation is a somewhat neglected topic in traffic research, but it constitutes a real safety problem (cf. Coblentz, Mollard, & Cabon, 1989; McDonald, 1984). Personnel selection on the basis of defense mechanisms could reduce the probability of errors under these circumstances of inadequate stimulation. The validity of the DMT regarding the prediction of performance under stress in real-life situations has been shown. For the FKBS, the generalizability of the results reported here remains to be proved. The application of the FKBS in combination with the microgenetic SMT seems to be promising, however. Some of the FKBS scales seem to exert a filter function with respect to attention control: TAS and REV in a negative, TAO in a positive direction.

The requirements in attention control are rather complex, and it could be that perceptually and verbally coded defense mechanisms predict different aspects of this complex task. Reducing the attentional complexity to its hypothetical elements is of doubtful value. One could think, for example, of the basic cognitive dimensions of focusing and scanning (Gardner, Holzman, Klein, Linton, & Spence, 1959; Hentschel, 1980), which Wachtel (1967) has compared to a torch directed at a dark object, where you can distinguish between the size of the circle of the light and its movements over the object. But in our task there is a double matching of the symbols shown on the screen with the relevant one, and its location on the screen with the number keyboard in a disjunctive reaction sequence.

Validity estimates for the elements, if they could be achieved, would not necessarily end up in the prediction of the complex task. A criterion-related optimization of the predictors seems to be more promising. Especially interesting in this respect are interactions of defenses with emotional and cognitive variables. One major aim to which the present study also is devoted to would be to enlarge the mere correlational proof of the interrelatedness of defenses with these variables by experimental evidence. Another important aspect for our project would be to submit the results found here to a reality test of actual driving. Possible conclusions to be expected from this research are not only in regard to person-related decisions but also to other variables in the system that can be used for the prevention of inadequate stimulation.

Acknowledgment. The study has been supported by a grant from Daimler-Benz, Stuttgart, Germany.

References

Chance, R.M.A. (1976) Social attention: Society and mentality. In M.R.A. Chance & R.A. Larsen (Eds.), *The social structure of attention* (pp. 315–333). London: Wiley.

Coblentz, A., Mollard, R., & Cabon, P. (1989) Vigilance and performance of human operators in transport operations. Applications to railway and air transport. *Proceedings of the ESTEC-Workshop: A task-oriented approach to human factors engineering*. November 21–23. Noordwijk: ESA.

Cooper, L.A. & Regan, D.T. (1982) Attention, perception and intelligence. In R.J. Sternberg (Ed.), *Handbook of human intelligence* (pp. 123–169). Cambridge: Cambridge University Press.

Dixon, N.F. (1981) *Preconscious processing*. Chichester, England: Wiley.

Dixon, N.F., Hentschel, U., & Smith, G.J.W. (1986) Subliminal perception and microgenesis in the context of personality research. In A. Angleitner, A. Furnham, & G. van Heck (Eds.), *Personality psychology in Europe: Vol. 2. Current trends and controversies* (pp. 239–255). Lisse, The Netherlands: Swets & Zeitlinger.

Floru, R., Damongeot, A., & Di Renzo, N. (1988) Vigilance et nuisances physiques. 2. Effets de l'association du bruit et des vibrations sur la vigilance du conducteur. Etude expérimentale [Combined effects of noise and vibrations on vigilance during driving. Experimental investigation]. *INRS, Cahiers de notes documentaires*, *130*, ND 1661.

Forbes, T.W. (1972) Introduction. In T.W. Forbes (Ed.), *Human factors in highway traffic safety research* (pp. 1–22). New York: Wiley.

Fröhlich, W.D. (1978) Stress, anxiety and the control of attention. In C.D. Spielberger & I.G. Sarason (Eds.), *Stress and anxiety: Vol. 5* (pp. 99–130). Washington, DC: Hemisphere.

Gardner, R.W., Holzman, P.S., Klein, G.S., Linton, H., & Spence, D.P. (1959) Cognitive control: A study of individual consistencies in cognitive behavior. *Psychological Issues*, *1*, No. 4.

Glass, A.L., Holyoak, K.J., & Santa, J.L. (1979) *Cognition*. Reading, MA: Addison-Wesley.

Gleser, G.C. & Ihilevich, D. (1969) An objective instrument for measuring defense mechanisms. *Journal of Consulting and Clinical Psychology*, *33*, 51–60.

Hentschel, U. (1984) Microgenesis and process description. In W.D. Fröhlich, G. Smith, J.G. Draguns, & U. Hentschel (Eds.), *Psychological Processes in cognition and personality* (pp. 59–70). Washington, DC: Hemisphere.

Hentschel, U. (1980) Kognitive Kontrollprinzipien und Neuroseformen [Cognitive styles and forms of neuroses]. In U. Hentschel & G. Smith (Eds.), *Experimentelle Persönlichkeitspsychologie* [Experimental personality psychology] (pp. 227–321). Wiesbaden: Akademische Verlagsgesellschaft.

Hentschel, U. & Kießling, M. (1983) On the predictability of performance in a serial problem-solving task: First results with the Symbol Maze Test. *Archives of Psychology*, *135*, 85–101.

Hentschel, U. & Kießling, M. (1986) Über die Beziehung von Intelligenz-Konzeptbildungs- und Problemlöseleistung: Eine theoretische Skizze und einige empirische Ergebnisse [On the relation of intelligence, concept formation and problem-solving performance: A short theoretical outline and some empirical results]. *Archives of Psychology*, *138*, 287–294.

Hentschel, U. & Kießling, M. (1990) Are defense mechanisms valid predictors of performance on cognitive tasks? In G. van Heck, S. Hampson, J. Reykowsky, & J. Zakrzewski (Eds.), *Personality psychology in Europe: Vol. 3. Foundations, models, and inquiries* (pp. 203–223). Lisse: Swets & Zeitlinger.

Hentschel, U. & Kießling, M. (in press) *Möglichkeiten der differentiellen Vorhersage von Reaktionen in Fehlbelastungssituationen* [On the differential predictability of reactions in situations with inadequate stimulation].

Hentschel, U. & Kießling, M. (in preparation) *Manual for the Symbol Maze Test (SMT)*.

Hentschel, U., Kießling, M., & Hosemann, A. (1989) The effect of cognitive and affective personality variables on attention control. *Proceedings of the ESTEC-Workshop: A task-oriented approach to human factors engineering*. November 21–23. Noordwijk: ESA.

Hentschel, U., Kießling, M., & Hosemann, A. (1991) Anxiety, defense and attention control. In R.E. Hanlon (Ed.), *Cognitive microgenesis: A neuropsychological perspective* (pp. 262–285). New York: Springer.

Hentschel, U., Kießling, M., & Ternes, G. (1984) *Kognitive Aspekte des Problemlösens bei Konzeptbildungsaufgaben* [Cognitive aspects of problem-solving in concept formation tasks]. Mainz: Arbeitsbericht aus dem DFG-Forschungssprojekt "Symbol-Labyrinthe" [Working report from the DFG research project "Symbol Mazes"].

Hentschel, U. & Schneider, U. (1986) Psychodynamic personality correlates of creativity. In U. Hentschel, G.W.J. Smith, & J.G. Draguns (Eds.), *The roots of perception* (pp. 249–275). Amsterdam: North-Holland.

Hunt, E. (1980) Intelligence as an information processing concept. *Journal of British Psychology*, *71*, 449–474.

Karsten, A. (1928) Psychische Sättigung [Psychic satiation]. *Psychologische Forschung*, *10*, 142–254.

Lazarus, R.S. & Folkman, S. (1984) *Stress, appraisal, and coping*. New York: Springer.

Lewin, K. (1935) *A dynamic theory of personality. Selected papers*. New York: McGraw-Hill.

McDonald, N. (1984) *Fatigue, safety and the truck driver*. London: Taylor & Francis.

McGuire, F.L. (1976) Personality factors in highway accidents. *Human Factors*, *18*, 433–442.

Rockwell, T. (1972) Skills, judgment and information acquisition in driving. In T.W. Forbes (Ed.), *Human factors in highway traffic safety research* (pp. 133–164). New York: Wiley.

Udenhout, M.Y. & Bekker, F.J.B. (1990) *Defensiemechanismen, een barrière voor het feedbackproces?* [Are defense mechanisms hampering the feedback process?]. Leiden University (mimeographed).

Wachtel, P. (1967) Conceptions of broad and narrow attention. *Psychological Bulletin*, *68*, 417–429.

Part IV
Clinical Assessment and Psychotherapeutic Interventions

17

The Structure and Process of Defense in Diagnosis of Personality and in Psychoanalytic Treatment

Wolfram Ehlers

Freud (1917) considered the psyche to be a hierarchy of super- and subordinated instances, corresponding to the multitude of the individual's drives and relations with the external world. Very often there are opposite and incompatible relations among those instances. He attributed the defense process and the object of it, "the defended," to separate systems according to the contradictory nature of their function and their conceptual meaning. The defense process is activated in the "ego" (A. Freud, 1936), whereas the defended is generated in the "id" and "superego." For the conscious observation of a defense mechanism, the ego is the medium through which an image of the two other instances can be grasped. The ego senses oncoming urges, as well as increased tension with its concomitant feelings of displeasure, and finally the resolution of the tension in the satisfying experience of pleasure.

In contemporary psychoanalysis this structural theory of the psyche has been discussed with respect to its misleading metapsychological consequences for clinical thinking. One of the prominent representatives of American ego psychology has concluded that "It is anything but agreeable to have to realize that one has dedicated most of one's career to a worthless theory as which metapsychology has proven itself" (Holt, 1989). On the other hand, Arlow and Brenner (1988) strive to promote ego psychology. Many psychoanalysts see research as the only way out of the crisis (Edelson, 1988). The research presented here is based on three empirical clinical studies of the application of defense mechanisms in the diagnostic phase of inpatient psychoanalytic treatment of severely disturbed patients as well as in single case studies of two outpatient treatments with analytical psychotherapy.

The aim of the studies is to determine which structures of defense mechanisms can be described by quantitative methods. These empirical data were gathered by psychoanalysts in the course of psychoanalytic treatment and in the diagnostic phase.

Clinical Definitions of Defense Mechanisms

The classical psychoanalytical defense doctrine worked out by Anna Freud (1936) describes the defense process as an activity of the ego. This ego is conceptualized as Sigmund Freud (1923) described it in his structural theory. Whenever a conflict arises between ego, id, and superego, the function of defense mechanisms enables the ego to reject unconscious desires and affects from consciousness.

The release of defense is activated by the anxiety signal. The ego must have access to the unconscious processes emanating from the other structures. Thus the goal of defense is to prevent the reactivation of traumatic situations (Moser, 1965), so that these are reactivated in less severe forms. If repression fails as the main defense mechanism, other defense mechanisms assume the duty of making the "repressed" acceptable to the consciousness. Symptoms and character traits can be interpreted as a result of this defense process (Freud, 1908).

Earlier dynamic conceptions of defense focused on the functional aspects. The psychodynamic conception of defense is based on repression. If some new situation is similar to former events where repression occurred, repressed and unconscious powers may have a permanent and pathogenic influence. Thus, suppressed impulses develop bonds to other traces of reminiscence and attempt to gain access to consciousness in a less offensive manner. This dynamic concept is a model for the regulation of impulses and affects as we can find in modern cognitive interpretation of defense mechanism by Moser, von Zeppelin, and Schneider (1968). The conflict model of defense is supplemented by Moser, von Zeppelin, and Schneider (1981) with the aspect of limitations of the information processing capacity of the ego. The dosage of incoming information is controlled by selecting the level and stages of processing. This is an important extension of the structural conception of defenses. A defense is not limited to solving unconscious conflicts; it can also modulate images the subject has developed in himself during the course of life (Sandler & Rosenblatt, 1962). It is therefore possible today to envisage defense mechanisms as modifiers of self- and object representations (Kernberg, 1984), thus contributing to the regulation of the self-image. Models of these steering processes clearly show that defense mechanisms cannot be defined as fixed structures as postulated by psychoanalytic structure theory and personality theory (Ehlers and Czogalik, 1984b). Nevertheless we can identify stable defense patterns in the psychoanalytic diagnosis of personality. But in the psychoanalytic process of treatment one can observe the change in these structures. Therefore the modification of classical structure theory with respect to a regulation model is necessary. The logical structure of the controlling devices of the defense models can define the clinical description of defense mechanism in their logical structure.

I therefore followed the suggestion of Suppes and Warren (1975) to define a defense mechanism as the logical relation between the behaving subject and the object to which the action of the subject is directed. In a generalized form such a sentence can be defined as follows: a subject (s) only partly activates, modifies, or erases a drive-impulse (d) or an affect (a) with respect to an object (o) in/to his consciousness or behavior. By replacing subject (s), drive-impulse (d), affect (a), or object (o) with concrete meanings, and by inserting the correct verb of the defense action, this very abstract sentence permits the definition of a great number of defense mechanisms. The abstract definitions show the psychoanalytic evaluator the logical structure of the algorithm, allowing him to solve the more complex problems of identifying the drive and affect in the behaving subject and object in communication with the patient. The material can be a transcript of a first interview or a clinical assessment after a treatment session. In discussions about interview transcripts I experienced little difficulty in achieving interrater agreement on the logical structure of defense, but it is much more difficult to come to agreement about the identification of the single components of the algorithm. The discussion can be shortened by this specific identification of disagreement because the logical structure of the defense definition affords a common basis for the assessment.

Dahl (1991) prefers the concept of affect to the concept of drive in the definition of defense mechanisms. Thus the theory of defense is allowed to free itself from instinct psychology. For the more general definition of a defense mechanism in our algorithm, we need only exclude the instinct model (d), and we can work on the surface of the linguistic material with the expression of affect in the transcript. These mechanisms are the major regulation tools of self- and object relations (Steffens & Kächele, 1988) in libidinally and aggressively determined representations.

Different project groups worked with this algorithm and found their own specification of the single defense mechanisms depending on their material. A study of interrater agreement (Ehlers, & Czogalik, 1984a) on 20 definitions of defense mechanisms found a mean of .51 for the interrater reliability according to Ebel (1951). Other research studies done by Aeschelmann (see Chapter 24) found an interrater agreement of $\kappa = .42$ ($p < 0.001$).

The Structure of Diagnostic Evaluations of Defense Mechanisms

Structure designates the wholeness of elements among which there are relations. For the mathematical aspects, the relations of the structural elements are computed by correlations among variables on representating the elements. The concentration of research on single elements often neglects this relation, which may be very important in clinical research.

Anna Freud (1936) worked out the isolated evaluation of defense mechanisms. This resulted in a relatively differentiated description of ego functions. French (1938) argued that the isolated description produces a distorted and fragmentary image of the synthetic ego activity. Therefore he proposed a combination of isolated defense mechanisms in a defense pattern. This idea was taken up by Suppes and Warren (1975) when they formulated a macrodefinition of defense mechanism. Ehlers and Czogalik (1984a) showed empirically that there is a structure of defense based on the interaction or combination of isolated defense mechanisms as assessed by psychoanalysts. With the statistical method of correlation analysis and principal component analysis of these correlations, independent dimensions (factors) of defense could be constructed, to which the different isolated defense mechanisms show a higher or a lower contribution. We found five factors that correspond particularly to the systematic classification of defense by Anna Freud (1936), who made the distinction between drive rejection, affect rejection, symptom formation, permanent defense phenomena in character traits, and resistance. Here we extend the empirical study of the defense structure to the aspects of defense in object relation and narcissistic development. This extension of the conceptualization of defense is based on Kernberg's (1977, 1984) differentiation between the neurotic and the borderline levels of defensive organization. The neurotic level is centered around more mature defenses like repression and reaction formation. The more primitive defensive operations on the borderline level are centered around the mechanisms of splitting and devaluation.

Method, Sample, and Instrument

In one research project (Ehlers & Czogalik, 1984a), 11 analytic psychotherapists made a diagnostic classification using a list of 16 defense mechanisms and 4 symptoms for their 147 patients before beginning inpatient treatment (CADM, Clinical Assessment of Defense Mechanisms; German: KBAM). The nosological classification of the patients showed the following distribution: hysterical neurosis, ($N = 16$, median age = 31 years) neurotic depression ($N = 70$, median age = 40 years), borderline personality disturbance ($N = 22$, median age = 31 years), and compulsion neurosis ($N = 9$, median age = 33 years). Thirty cases were unclassified. A five-point scale ranging from very probable to very improbable was created to permit a clinical assessment on each defense mechanism.

The correlation matrix of these quantitative evaluations was factorized to get a quantitative description of the similarity of the defense mechanisms. We used factor analysis to construct dimensions for these similarities of subgroups. With this principal component analysis (SPSS program) we found five dimensions that explained 41.1% of the variance in the data. These five dimensions of defense were named after the main loading of each defense mechanism on these dimensions. For the similarity of the main defense mechanism on each dimension we found the following expressions: superego defense (turning against self, introjection, identification, regression, projection), impulse defense (undoing, reaction formation, reversal), affect defense, (isolation, inhibited affect expression), consequences of affect defense (equivalents of affect, conversion), and displacement of libido (displacement of libido or aggression, denial).

Four symptoms corresponded to the following dimensions: self-pity and resignation (superego defense), compulsion (impulse defense), avoiding social contacts (affect defense), and affect equivalent (consequences of affect defense). In the present study we expanded the list of defense mechanisms to the aspect of object relation and narcissistic development. On the basis of Kernberg's descriptions (1977), we formulated abstract definitions of primitive idealization, the mechanism of splitting, projective identification, devaluation of external object, fantasies of omnipotence, and primitive denial (see Table 17.1).

We analyzed 284 evaluations of patients from 11 analytic psychotherapists. The nosological and age distributions of the patients were quite similar to the published examination of defense mechanisms. Data analysis was done with the same procedure as in the study described previously. Our intention was to study the application of the factorial structure of the classic defense mechanisms in a new data set.

Results and Discussion

The factor analysis of the defense items (CADM) was carried out by means of the calculation of an R-similarity matrix of the correlations of the 20 scales from 284 patients. On the criteria of the Scree test we found five dimensions for the structure of the defense system. All the five dimensions of the first publication (Ehlers & Czogalik, 1984a) could be replicated for this larger sample. Only the order of the extracted factors changed in this replication and the factor loadings of some defense mechanisms. This can be seen by the amount of the extracted variance. The first dimension showed an extracted total variance of 9.7%. Turning against self and introjection characterize this dimension of superego defense.

The second dimension (extracted total variance 6.1%) can be called the "defense of impulse information" because the main loadings on isolation, rationalization, denial, and reversal characterize the defense style of the compulsive neurosis, which is accompanied by so much trouble with the control of conflictual drive and affect information.

The third dimension (extracted total variance 17.9%) can be called "defense of affect" because the inhibition of affect is the denominator of

TABLE 17.1. Dimensions of defense: Abstract definitions of defense mechanisms (S = subject, D = drive/impulse, O = object).

Superego defense/Affect defense	Defense of impulse	Consequences of defense of affect	Libido displacement	Narcissistic defense
Turning against self S turns aggression (D) against himself (O).	*Rationalization* S disguises existence of impulses (D) toward object (O) through logical and morally accepted explanations.	*Dominance of affect equivalence* S is not aware of the affective significance of physical reaction usually accompanying the affect.	*Regression* S condemns oedipal impulse (D_1) and retreats to pregenital impulse (D_2).	*Primitive idealization* S idealizes an object (O), which is to protect him from own aggressive impulses (D^-) and from negative external objects (O^-)
Introjection S unites himself with the whole object (O), which represents the repressed impulse (D).	*Denial* S denies existence of threatening perception or action concerning impulse (D) with regard to self or to external object (O).	*Identification* S unites himself with parts of the object (O) that represents impulse (D).	*Displacement of aggression* S cathexes an image toward a neutral object (O) with destruction (D).	*Mechanisms of splitting* S feels negative (D^-) and positive (D^+) impulses or expresses negative (O^-) and positive (O^+) object images concerning the same object (O), which have a character of exclusiveness, and he acts accordingly. S is not affected by contrast of his emotions and imaginations.
Delayed affect expression S delays affect expression to avoid connection between impulse (D) and object (O).	*Repression* S excludes images, memories, and thoughts of threatening impulse (D).	*Conversion* S shows expression of impulse (D) through bodily reaction.	*Displacement of libido* S cathexes a less threatening thought or behavior toward an object (O) with libido (D).	*Projective identification* S displaces own defended impulse (D) onto object (O) and at the same time feels linked empathically with object (anxious empathy).

Undoing (compulsive rituals)
S takes back a prohibited impulse (D) in regard to an object (O).

Reaction formation
S shows toward object (O) controversial attitude and behaviors, other than what would be expected from the repressed impulse (D).

Reversal into the opposite
S shows controversial impulse toward the object (O), other than what would be expected from the stimulated situation.

Primitive denial
S is aware of emotional significance of denied impulse (D). Yet S denies existence of threatening perception of thought or emotion toward self or object (O).

Isolation
S divides related associations or actions as well as images and affects to avoid contact between repressed impulse (D) and self (O).

Projection
S displaces the repressed impulse (D) onto the object (O).

Devaluation of external object
S devalues (dropping, shifting, denigrating of) external object (O) because of feelings of revenge for being frustrated and feeling defenseless.

Fantasies of omnipotence
S clings to "magically" overrated object or develops overrated self, claiming special privileges or the devotion of objects (O) in regard to the subject (S).

such high loading defenses as delayed affect explosion, isolation, rationalization, undoing, and denial.

The fourth dimension (extracted total variance 7.4%) can be called "consequences of affect-defense" because the main loading of the items conversion and equivalence of affect refers to the forbidding of consciousness of bodily information as part of a rejected affect, which the patient tries to avoid.

The fifth dimension (extracted total variance 8.8%) can be called "displacement of impulse information" because the displacement of aggression and libido belongs to the main loading items. In a factor solution with five dimensions, the results from a second factor analysis with 26 scales, which included narcissistic defense variables like splitting and devaluation, showed that the first dimension concurred with the third dimension, so that the items of superego defense and defense of affect loaded on the same dimension (see Table 17.1).

The new dimension in this factor solution is characterized by the highest loadings on such defense mechanisms from object relation and narcissistic development as primitive idealization, the mechanism of splitting, projective identification, fantasies of omnipotence, devaluation of external object, and primitive denial. Therefore one can call this dimension the "narcissistic defense."

In conclusion one can say that the structure of the first study could be replicated very well in this new study. Second, we must postulate a further defense dimension if we expand our concept of defense in the domain of narcissistic development and object relation.

This quantitative description of the structure in defense evaluation demonstrates that clinicians have defense styles in mind that generate a profile of defense mechanisms, resembling the contemporary development of psychoanalytic theory (Gedo & Goldberg, 1973). The structural concept of Anna Freud (1936) on impulse defense, affect defense, and formation of symptoms can be reconstructed empirically. One can assume that the 11 analytical psychotherapists were not aware of these correlations of the isolated defense mechanism. On the other hand, the new defense concept of object relation theory and narcissism can be identified by clinicians in the diagnostic classification of their patients.

Personality Diagnosis as a Determinant of Defense Structure

The diagnosis of personality structure depends on two determinants. On the one hand the psychoanalyst diagnoses the fixation of the subject at a specific level of development (e.g., "oral fixation combined with depressive personality structure"). On the other hand he diagnoses a defense pattern, as I described earlier. The last diagnosis suggests both adaptive and psychopathological modifications of personality. The clinical personality theory of psychoanalysis postulates high correlations between developmental fixations and defense (Ehlers & Czogalik, 1984b). For the depressive personality structure, a distortion of superego development is postulated, which results in a dominance of a defense pattern with high values on introjection, projection, and turning against self. The compulsive personality structure, on the contrary, develops more mature defense mechanisms (e.g., reaction formation and isolation) because libido fixation taken place later in psychosexual development. These defense mechanisms work on behalf of the drive defense, where the drive impulse, contrary to the mechanism of repression, can be detected in compulsive behavior. Hysterical illness shows a symptomatology that is determined by the mechanism of conversion and displacement, as we can see in phobic patients and repression. This clinical hypothesis should be tested with an objective personality diagnosis which can be reconstructed from self-evaluation questionnaires. For the clinical evaluation of defense by means of CADM (Ehlers & Czogalik, 1984a), the differences between the hysterical, the compulsive, and the depressive character structure should be tested empirically.

Method, Sample, and Instrument

The method of objective personality diagnosis is based on the semantic arrangement of various questionnaire scales for three dominant personality conceptions: depressive, compulsive, and hysterical personality structure. With a factorial analysis of the test scales, we found three characteristic profiles for depressive, compulsive, and hysterical subgroups. The stability of this classification was calculated by means of a replication of the taxonomy in a new clinical sample with discriminant analysis (Ehlers & Czogalik, 1984a). For the new sample, an average hit rate of 75% could be calculated with the classification function of the discriminant analysis (SPSS program). This classification function is the basis for the selection of three subgroups, which were evaluated on the clinical rating scales for the defense mechanism (CADM) version with 20 items. The factor scores of the five dimensions from the 20-item version of defense mechanisms were computed for the three subgroups of depressive, compulsive, and hysterical personality structure. With an analysis of variance for the mean values of each dimension between these subgroups, I tested the postulated differences for the personality structure.

Results and Discussion

The automatic classification of patients with a discriminant function guarantees a maximum of objectivity for testing the psychoanalytic hy-

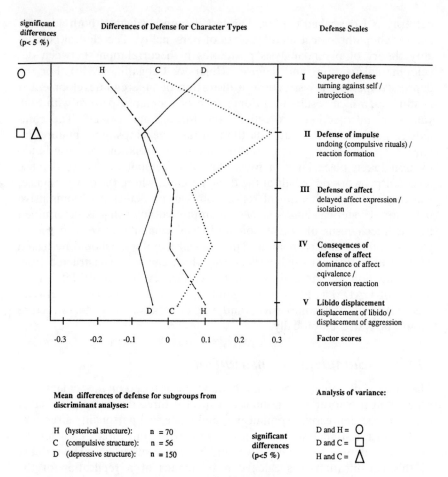

significant differences (p< 5 %)

Differences of Defense for Character Types

Defense Scales

O

□ Δ

I   Superego defense
    turning against self /
    introjection

II Defense of impulse
    undoing (compulsive rituals) /
    reaction formation

III Defense of affect
    delayed affect expression /
    isolation

IV Conseqences of
    defense of affect
    dominance of affect
    eqivalence /
    conversion reaction

V   Libido displacement
    displacement of libido /
    displacement of aggression

-0.3   -0.2   -0.1   0   0.1   0.2   0.3   Factor scores

Mean differences of defense for subgroups from discriminant analyses:

			Analysis of variance:	
H	(hysterical structure):	n = 70	D and H =	O
C	(compulsive structure):	n = 56	D and C =	□
D	(depressive structure):	n = 150	H and C =	Δ

significant differences (p<5 %)

FIGURE 17.1. Three character types with differences on five CADM scales.

pothesis of the correlation between personality structure and defense. The significant differences between means for the depressive, compulsive, and hysterical personality diagnoses show the following results (see Fig. 17.1). The depressive subgroup is characterized by significantly higher superego defense than the hysterical subgroup. This higher extension of superego defense is caused by the interaction of turning against object, introjection, and inhibited affect expression. The compulsive subgroup is significantly higher in the dimension of impulse defense compared to the depressive and hysterical subgroups. This means dominance of the defense mechanisms isolation, rationalization, denial, reaction formation, and repression for the compulsive patients. For the hysterical subgroup we cannot find any significant differences. Therefore we conclude that for the depressive and compulsive subgroups we can demonstrate the postulated clinical hypothesis for the combination of personality structure and defense for the depressive and the compulsive structures—but not for the hysterical personality. This means that the dimensions of defense mechanisms in the differentiation of the personality structure have a differential validity.

Defense Variables of the Process in Psychoanalytic Treatment

Introduction

The justification for discussing the connectedness of structure and process in psychoanalysis is established by the genetic perspective of psychoanalysis. During early development, parts of the contents of the id are absorbed by the ego and elevated into the subconscious. Others remain in the id as the unconscious. During the development of the ego, however, through the defense process against conflict-related psychological impressions and events, these parts come to be excluded from the subconscious. These contents are described as being repressed. The analytical work on repression is developed by the exploitation of the normal regression of the ego functions in that the analyst enters into an alliance with the ego, thus extending self-awareness and so making lost contents accessible to the consciousness once more. This takes place through interpretation of what the patient remembers and numerous nonverbal interactions, which, with the interpretation, decisively codetermine transference and can lead to deepening regression. With increased depth of regression, less mature defense mechanisms are employed, which offers the verbal interaction of emotional control an increasingly greater scope. By increasing regression, therefore, the ego resorts to earlier methods of defense. For the examination of this thesis, we compare the development of the defense process in a female patient with a hysterical personality structure and in a female patient with a borderline level depressive personality structure. It is expected that the patient with the hysterical personality structure will show fewer immature defense mechanisms. Thus, during the analytical process a less intense ego regression will be observed, which will express itself contentwise in the dominance of oedipal themes.

Method

Assessment of the development of the defense process was enabled by the psychoanalyst's assessment (after each session) of the dominant defense mechanisms in the respective sitting. The assessment was carried out on a scale for the Clinical Assessment of Defense Mechanisms (CADM) for 26 single items.

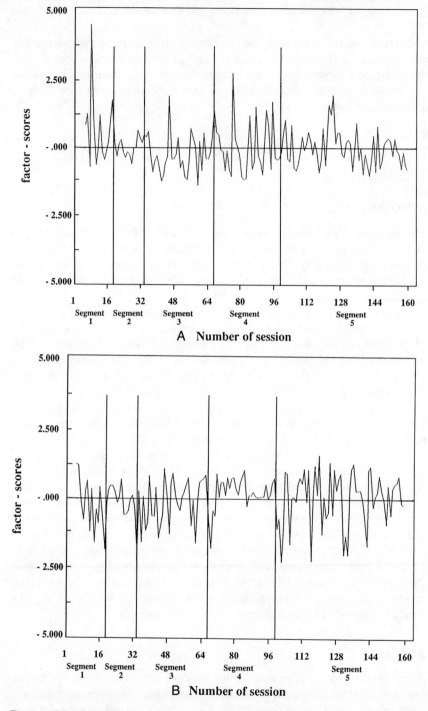

FIGURE 17.2. CADM factor scores (P-technique) for 160 theapy sessions of patient G. A. Factor 1: Turning against self/introjection/regession/dominance of affect equivalence. B. Factor 2: Rationalization/isolation/repression.

The data were then presented statistically with reference to the process development. A factor analysis for each patient was established from the correlation of the item assessment throughout the whole process of psychoanalysis. After the extraction of these course factors (P-analysis), the factor values of the extracted dimensions were presented graphically (see Figs. 17.2 and 17.3) for the determination of therapy segments, which were then described with regard to content quality. The presentation of the process development with regard to quality was produced by a structured content analysis. Using the protocol of the session as a base, a paraphrase of the central conflict, or transference and/or resistance, was written according to the dominance of each aspect. These were then summarized in an account of the therapy segments. The limits of the therapy segments were determined by the graphical results of the quantitative process analysis.

Patient G was diagnosed as a hysterical depressive personality structure with a high structure level. Symptomatically she belonged to the large patient group in which recurrent headaches with a background of conversion neurosis appear. The somewhat vague description "tension headache" (Beyme, 1966) abstains from making a psychological neurosis classification. Such a headache can be attributed to muscular contractions in connection with tension, depression, and fear. Specific "trigger" situations in life, mostly connected with ambition, jealousy, and envy, could be explored. Psychoanalytical therapy, in the prone position, was carried out three times weekly and lasted for 160 sessions over a period of two years.

Patient S was diagnosed as a depressive personality structure at borderline level. Symptomatically she had a major depression. The patient was apathetic, without drive, and her psychomotoric functions had slowed down. Mood changes were not fixed to certain times of day. Feelings of guilt and the need for punishment were strongly marked. She had extreme fear of failure and of being unable to master her professional responsibilities. In her household she was incapable of satisfactory work performance. There were sleep disturbances like waking up to early in the morning. Moods of depression, fear of failure, and feelings of inferiority had existed since puberty. There were recurrent depressive episodes to explore. Analytical psychotherapy, in the sitting position, was carried out two or three times a week and lasted for 370 sessions over a period of 5.5 years, with a break of one year. Data collection ended with session 305, because of a change in the contract with the patient. The health insurance stopped its contribution.

Results

The Quantitative and Qualitative Process Analysis of a High Structure Level (Patient G)

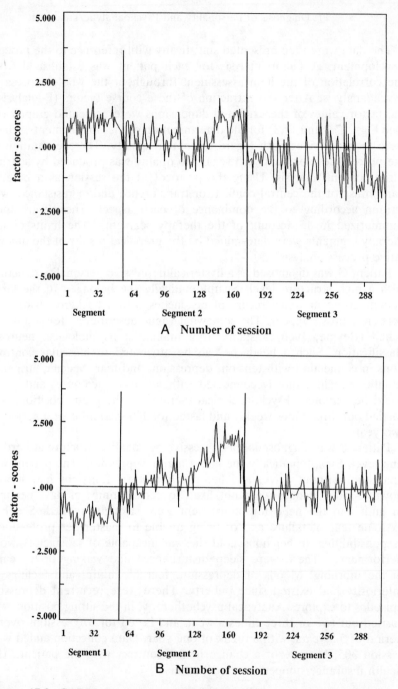

FIGURE 17.3. CADM factor scores (P-technique) for 305 therapy sessions of patient S. A. Factor 1: Self-pity/turning against self/introjection. B. Factor 2: Primitive denial/devaluation of external objects/mechanism of splitting. C. Factor 3: Primitive idealization/fantasies of omnipotence. D. Factor 4: Reversal into opposite/undoing.

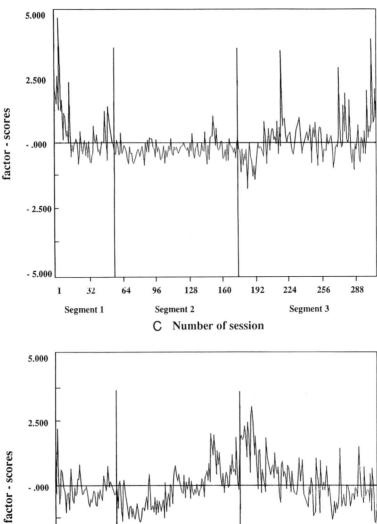

C Number of session

D Number of session

Process Development and Segment Determination

In factor 1 there is no significant segmentation of the process. The structure analysis of the development (P-factor analysis) of the 26 defense mechanisms of the CADM produced two factors that account for 9.8 and 9.1% of the total variance. Factor 1 contains immature defense mechanisms such as turning against self (factor loading .53), introjection (.49), regression (.47), and the domination of affect equivalents (.59). Factor 2, in comparison, is determined by such mature defense mechanisms as rationalization (.65), isolation (.61), and repression (.58).

Only in the portrayal of the development of factor 2, which is the mature defense dimension in this therapy, is it possible to distinguish individual therapy segments from one another (see Fig. 17.2). After a decrease in mature defense from session 1 to 20 (segment 1), it moves from session 21 to 34 to a relatively stable high defense level (segment 2), which from session 35 to 68 is replaced by a segment (3) of great defense fluctuation. From session 69 to 99 a relatively stable high defense level is again shown (segment 4). Segment 5 is determined by a great fluctuation in defense, while the first factor independent of these segments fluctuates over the process. With the maximum D of this rather immature factor, an inverse relationship to factor 2 emerges. Whereas the immature defense shows the highest values, the mature defense in these areas shows lowest values and vice versa. In process development, apparently, the maturity of defenses can, factorially, vary independently of each other and can exclude each other if extremely pronounced (see Fig. 17.2).

Qualitative Process Analysis

Therapy Segment 1. The first therapy segment enables the development of the oedipal incestuous conflict situation with reference to the relationship with a married lover. Mrs. G. seeks his presence so that he can free her from the slur of being a silly little girl. She is torn between the wish for a proper marriage and the romance with an already married lover. If it became known that she is in love with a married man, then she would be open to strong moral persecution. Because of cramplike pains in the back and lower abdomen, she has to take analgesic tablets all day. She again lives together with her lover for several days although she has already parted from him. In a dream full of the desire to destroy, she breaks into the house of a couple, who are her friends, and wrecks the living room. She remembers how her lover deceived her with another woman. She must keep it secret from her parents that she is still keeping up this relationship.

Therapy Segment 2. The guilt-ridden aspect of the rivalry to the lover's wife and her parents swings into the foreground. In transference an ever-increasing resistance to open herself in the therapy process develops, because she fears personal contempt as experienced earlier from her maternal grandfather. At the same time, outside the therapy, she builds a new unstressed relationship, from which nothing may infiltrate into the therapy process. Especially, even in dreams, this extratherapeutic trust relationship is veiled and only implied.

Therapy Segment 3. Ambivalence to the desires for the old and new lovers develops. A leading theme of the sessions is a fight against the pressing demands of her old lover and against being treated as a child by her mother or her boss. The necessary moving out from the parent's home to detach herself from her parents causes much pain. When Mrs. G. informs her old lover of her new relationship, she experiences increasingly strong courting from his side. The incestuous relationship to her father is so strongly activated that in dreams it is experienced as sexually oppressive. The consuming feelings change into a playful state of being in love as between children. In this form the feelings can be realized with the new lover. The identification with the strengths and the powers of a woman lets her experience the powers of a mature woman in regard to the old lover and, in regard to the new lover, allows the wish for children to awake. Because the analyst now has the role of protecting her from seduction by her old lover, the state of being in love in the new relationship can develop uninhibited so that she receives a proposal of marriage. Finally, she renounces flight to the United States with her old lover—deciding to continue with therapy.

Therapy Segment 4. The treatment of intrapsychic conflicts is in the foreground. Mrs. G. tries now to involve herself more in the analysis of her personal development and does not just see herself as pushed here and there between men. Rivalry to other women and mistrust make her conceal her marriage plans. She fights against an analysis of the new relationship; instead, she brings up the themes of her rivalry to her mother, her childish affection for her father, and the alliance with her father, which was directed against her mother and brother. The acute illness of her mother makes it clear to her that she will personally have to take over the preparations for her wedding. In the therapy process the work on repression resistance in the detailed examination of mature defense mechanisms is of significance, whereby a thorough study of the incestuous bond is possible.

Therapy Segment 5. The wedding takes place after the bridegroom has passed the test of not deceiving her with other women, as repeatedly experienced with the old lover and with the father. The patient experiences the honeymoon as a sensual mountain climb in a dream, in the course of which she is always accompanied by her envious mother. She has increasing discussions and arguments with her archaic mother, who wants to prevent her from having children. She must conceal from her husband her jealousy of his earlier companion, although she is at every turn confronted with traces of this woman in the apartment. In the marriage bed she has to take the responsibility for contraception, since neither spouse has finished schooling. She fears being unable to have children. After she has finally made up her mind to finish the analysis, she sets up house with her husband, from which she happily reports in the last therapy session. In a catamnestic talk 18 months later, she proudly reports her motherhood and her new role as a doctor's wife since her husband's qualification as a specialist for internal medicine.

To summarize the process of defense for patient G: in the second therapy segment a stronger resistance to transference establishes itself, which apparently leads to a stabilization of mature defense mechanisms (factor 2). In the fourth segment the intensive work on the intrapsychic conflicts leads to an increase of repression resistance, which stabilizes over a period of 31 sessions. In the other three therapy segments the fluctuation in mature defense is so strong that no uniform defense level results.

The Quantitative and Qualitative Process Analysis for a Low Structure Level (Patient S)

Patient S was diagnosed as having undergone a major depression, with depressive personality structure at borderline level. The structural analysis of the development of the defense mechanisms produces four P-factors, which by way of their main loaded defense mechanisms were characterized as follows. Factor 1 is characterized by self-pity, turning against self, and introjection. Factor 2 is marked by such typical immature defense mechanisms in the coping with archaic aggression as primitive denial, devaluation of external objects, and a mechanism of splitting. Factor 3 is also to be seen as an immature defense mechanism, which relates to narcissistic defenses (e.g., primitive idealization and fantasies of omnipotence). Factor 4 can be seen as a more mature defense form, which is characterized by mechanisms such as reversal into opposite and undoing what has been done (see Fig. 17.3).

Segmentation and Qualitative Development Description

For the segmentation of the development of the factors just described, the interaction of the first two appears to be very suitable for the presentation of the segments. In this process the qualitative description must summarize larger units, because the process lasts twice as long. It appeared meaningful because of the greater complexity of the interplay of the factors that the qualitative description follows immediately after each formal segment description.

Therapy Segment 1. The first segment reaches from session 1 to session 60 and is distinguished by a contrary development of factors 1 (turning against self) and 2 (primitive denial and splitting), while the mature factor 4 (reversal into opposite) lessens increasingly up to session 23 and then levels off. The simultaneous lessening of mature defense (factor 4) and archaic defense (denial, splitting, and devaluation) as well as the increase of typical depressive defense (self-pity, turning against self, and introjection) corresponds contentwise to the inner struggle for an oral provision by simultaneous refusal of erotic activity, which is expressed in a strong interest for the fairy tale "Sleeping Beauty." The devaluation of her own marriage stands opposite her high expectations of the analyst, who should free her from the poisoned relationship. The analyst's neutrality, however, leads to massive disappointment, which expresses itself in increasing paralysis. She wants to stop teaching school; she wants to give up and wants to be awkward. She observes arguments between other couples intently. She avoids clearing arguments in her own relationship. She cannot explain her dissatisfaction in her relationship to her husband and wishes for deliverance by the analyst. When the principal at the school where she works tries to win her back into teaching, from which she is on sick leave, she refuses. When sleeping with her husband, she acts dead. She is active only in transference, especially in dreams. The absence of the analyst during the Easter break causes everything to collapse again. Then the school superintendent presses for a transfer after the summer holiday, and great fear of the future arises. First experiences in the new school after the summer holiday give rise to strong disappointment in the school superintendent who, supposedly, made her false promises.

Therapy Segment 2. The second segment describes the development between sessions 61 and 175. While the immature defense of factor 2 (splitting) increases more and more, this trend is first found by factor 1 in session 117. With factor 3 this increasing trend begins in session 103, whereby it is interspersed with phases of steep increase and decrease. The increase of archaic defense in factor 2 corresponds contentwise to the increasing experience of slights, which are answered with regressive withdrawal into passivity, inactivity, and resistance by refusal. Her husband's waning interest in her leads to an intensification in the experience of slights in the analysis. She wants to prove to me that she can cope with the children in school. But she can only report again and again her failure and must more and more come to terms with the shame she feels before me. Her fear of the school superintendent, who observes her twice in lessons and advises her, increases immeasurably. She is appalled at her supposed failure and increasingly devalues herself and sinks into greater and greater regression, which is expressed as silences of more than 20 minutes during analysis. The analyst can maintain contact with her only through the utmost sensitivity for her unspoken thoughts and feelings. After ideas of suicide arise, antidepressive medication therapy in teamwork with a psychiatrist is begun, which takes effect.

After the husband clearly states his plans for separation, she wants to break off the outpatient therapy and, as a psychotherapy inpatient, be cared for passively like a baby. By the refusal of food she forces her husband to feed her, just as the analyst, after long periods of silence, administered her emotional nourishment by speaking to her about her possible feelings. Session 159 results in the first stay in a clinic, during which time the therapy is continued. After the husband has left here resistance to therapy becomes so strong that only a separation from the psychoanalyst can be fantasized as the solution. She arranges admission into an out-of-town clinic for psychotherapeutic treatment and finally fantasizes that she accompanies the analyst, symbolizing an idealized object, on holiday sitting on the back seat of his car, as she did as a child when she went away alone with her father. The separation cannot be spoken of. The decrease in archaic defense from session 174 on is explained by the inner decision to break off the therapy and so terminate the negative therapeutic transference.

Therapy Segment 3. The last segment, from sessions 176 to 305, is marked by a comparatively low level of defense in factors 1 and 2. After continuation of therapy after one year (from session 184), the narcissistic defense in factor 3 (primitive idealization and fantasies of omnipotence) reaches its maximum. In the meantime the fourth, rather mature defense factor shows a greater frequency of sessions with high defense. Toward the end of the process this defense form (from session 282) increases continually. Contentwise this therapy segment is marked by a more realistic working alliance, by which, in spite of the decrease in the idealization of the analyst, therapeutic work can be continued. One year after discontinuing therapeutic contact, she wants to resume outpatient psychotherapy. Analysis in sitting is continued with a weekly frequency of two sessions. After the idealization of the analyst could be made an object of analysis, work on the present relationship to the analyst was possible. Through this her own tendencies toward regressive retreat in critical situations of narcissistic vulnerability in the relationship could be verbalized. When neither the principal nor the school superintendent was pleased by her decision about taking up teaching again, suicidal ideas were activated, which could be worked on. After the husband's move out of their house, she experiences her need for dependence on the support of a family, which is now given only by the analysis relationship. Here she tests the possibilities of defining her own powers without loss of domestic security. Work on the pitfalls of her very critical and self-destructive self-ideals arises while coping with examination fears and work inhibitions during finals of the second state examination. Work on sadomasochistic relationship patterns in the therapeutic relationship becomes increasingly possible. In the struggle between the wish for passive care and aggressive self-fulfillment in the transference relationship, she faces up to the realities in her professional life after completing the finals of the examination. Only after this development is an identification with her wishes for feminine bodily potence possible. In a central dream she creeps out of her narrow cave, baring her breasts, and seduces a shy man sitting in front of the cave. She tests her bodily expression in an upright gait.

Summary

Psychoanalytical treatment leads to a revival of childish consciousness contents, which are represented in the relationship to the analyst. Resistance toward this transference relationship presents itself as defense structures whose relation to each other can be established empirically. In the treatment development of patients with oedipal and pre-oedipal neurotic disturbances, these defense structures differ at symptomatological levels and with regard to the organizational level of the personality.

A patient with hysterical symptomatology and a phallic hysterical personality structure develops a mature defense structure in a process development that can be described as mature within the frame of repression resistance.

In contrast, a patient with depressive symptomatology and a personality structure at a lower structural level develops an immature defense structure in process development. This is so decisively marked by archaic defense mechanisms or primitive denial or splitting that transference resistance from the point of negative therapeutic reaction leads to a temporary breaking off of therapy. The activation of narcissistic defense (primitive idealization and omnipotence fantasies) and the successful, thorough study of this defense after the resumption of therapy represents an important side condition for the overcoming of an immature defense structure in the transference relationship. The segmental process description is based on the composition of defense mechanisms with the corresponding mature and immature defense patterns.

References

Arlow, J.A. & Brenner, C. (1988) The future of psychoanalysis. *Psychoanalytic Quarterly, 57*, 1–14.

Beyme, F. (1966) Der Verlauf der Migräne mit und ohne Psychotherapie [The course of migraine with and without psychotherapy]. *Psychotherapy and Psychosomatics, 14*, 90.

Dahl, H. (1991) The key to understanding change: Emotions as appetitive wishes and beliefs about their fulfillment. In J.G. Safran (Ed.), *Emotion, Psychotherapy and Change* (pp. 130–165). New York: Guilford Press.

Ebel, R.L. (1951) Estimation of the reliability of ratings. *Psychometrica, 16*, 4.

Edelson, M. (1988) *A theory in crisis.* Chicago: University of Chicago Press.

Ehlers, W. & Czogalik, C. (1984a) Dimensionen der klinischen Beurteilung von Abwehrmechanismen [Dimensions of clinical assessment of defense mechanisms]. *Praxis der Psychotherapie und Psychosomatik, 29,* 129–138.

Ehlers, W. & Czogalik, D. (1984b) Taxonomic aspects of clinical character typology in psychotherapy. *Psychotherapy and Psychosomatics, 42,* 156–163.

French, T.M. (1938) Defense and synthesis in the function of the ego. *Psychoanalytic Quarterly, 7,* 537–553.

Freud, A. (1936) *The ego and the mechanisms of defence.* Vienna: Internationaler Psychoanalytischer Verlag.

Freud, S. (1908) Charakter und Analerotik [Character and anal eroticism]. In *The standard edition of the complete psychological works of Sigmund Freud: Vol. 9* (pp. 169–175). London: Hogarth Press.

Freud, S. (1917) Metapsychologische Ergänzungen zur Traumlehre [A metapsychological supplement to the theory of dreams]. In *The standard edition of the complete psychological works of Sigmund Freud: Vol. 14* (pp. 222–235). London: Hogarth Press.

Freud, S. (1923) Das Ich und das Es [The ego and the id]. In *The standard edition of the complete psychological works of Sigmund Freud: Vol. 19* (pp. 19–27). London: Hogarth Press.

Gedo, J.E. & Goldberg, A. (1973) *Models of the mind.* Chicago: University of Chicago Press.

Holt, R.R. (1989) *Freud reappraised: A fresh look at psychoanalytic theory.* New York: Guildford Press.

Kernberg, O.F. (1977) The structural diagnosis of borderline personality organization. In P. Hartocollis (Ed.), *Borderline personality disorders* (pp. 87–121). Madison, CT: International Universities Press.

Kernberg, O.F. (1984) *Severe personality disorders. Psychotherapeutic strategies.* New Haven, CT: Yale University Press.

Moser, U. (1965) Zur Abwehrlehre. *Jahrbuch der Psychoanalyse, 4,* 56–85.

Moser, U. Zeppelin, I. v, & Schneider, W. (1968) Computersimulation eines Modells neurotischer Abwehrmechanismen. Ein Versuch zur Formalisierung der psychoanalytischen Theorie (Bulletin 2) [Computer simulation of a model of neurotic defense mechanisms. An attempt at formalizing psychoanalytic theory]. Department of Psychology, University of Zürich.

Moser, U. Zeppelin, I. v, & Schneider, H. (1981) Wunsch, Selbst, Objektbeziehung. Entwurf eines Regulierunsmodells kognitiv-affektiver Prozesse [Wish, self, object-relation. Concept of a model for the regulation of cognitive and affective processes]. (*Berichte aus der interdisziplinären Konfliktforschungsstelle no. 9*) unpublished report. Department of Psychology University of Zürich.

Sandler, J. & Rosenblatt, B. (1962) The concept of the representational world. *Psychoanalytic Study of the Child, 17,* 128–145.

Steffens, W. & Kächele, H. (1988) Abwehr und Bewältigung—Vorschläge zu einer integrativen Sichtweise [Defense and coping. Proposal for an integrative perspective]. *Psychotherapie Psychosomatik Medizinische Psychologie, 38,* 3–7.

Suppes, P. & Warren, H. (1975) On the generation and classification of defense mechanisms. *Journal of Psychoanalysis, 56,* 405–414.

18
The Measurement of Ego Defenses in Clinical Research

HOPE R. CONTE and ROBERT PLUTCHIK

Among the more important contributions of psychoanalysis to personality theory and to the theory of psychological adaptation is the concept of ego defenses. The term "defense mechanism" first appeared in Anna Freud's *The Ego and the Mechanisms of Defense* (1936). This work described 10 methods of functioning used by the ego to ward off dangerous drives or wishes that would lead to painful feelings of anxiety, depression, or shame. Since that time, there has been general agreement that the defenses may be triggered by both internal and external stressors: that is, by both internalized prohibitions on the one hand and external reality on the other. There has also been substantial agreement on a number of aspects or facets of defense mechanisms: (a) they are the major means that the ego uses to manage instinct and affect and forestall potential conflict; (b) they are unconscious; (c) although a patient may be characterized by his or her most dominant defense, each patient uses several defenses; (d) the defenses are dynamic and reversible; and (e) they may be adaptive as well as pathological (Freud, 1936; Perry & Vaillant, 1990).

Variations in the Concept of Ego Defenses

However, there is considerably less agreement among psychoanalysts and other clinicians on just how many defenses there are and over what should or should not be considered a defense mechanism (Brenner, 1973; Moore & Fine, 1990; Plutchik, Kellerman, & Conte, 1979; Vaillant, 1977; Wong, 1989). While Anna Freud (1936) originally described 10 defenses, Vaillant's (1971) glossary defines 8 and Brenner's (1973) textbook lists 11. In DSM-III-R the American Psychiatric Association (1987) identifies 18 ego defenses, and the most recent edition of the *Comprehensive Textbook of Psychiatry* defines 32 (Wong, 1989).

These schemata identifying differing numbers of defenses exist partly as a result of the differing theories on which they are based. They are, however, also a function of the extensive overlap of meanings. There are, for example, no distinct boundaries differentiating one defense from another. Noyes and Kolb (1963) point out that projection is, in many respects, a form of identification, while Arieti (1974) notes that isolation and splitting are merely two names for the same concept.

Regarding what should be included as an ego defense, Brenner (1973), for example, does not include "suppression" as a defense mechanism, considering it rather to be a conscious activity (i.e., the familiar decision to forget about something and think no more about it). It is also not included by Plutchik et al. (1979) in their Life Style Index or by Perry and Cooper (1989) in the Defense Mechanism Rating Scales. In contrast, Andrews, Pollock, and Stewart (1989), Bond (1983), Meissner, Mack, and Semrad (1975), and Vaillant (1985) do include suppression as a defense mechanism. They also include "humor." It appears that the decision to include suppression, humor, and other mechanisms such as altruism and anticipation depends to a great extent on an investigator's willingness to admit the more conscious mechanisms as defenses.

This issue leads directly to that of the classification of the ego defenses. Here, too, there is disagreement. They can be classified developmentally, whereby they are categorized according to the libidinal phase in which they are presumed to arise. Denial and projection would thus be assigned to the oral stage. But some defenses, such as regression, cannot be classified in this manner. They may also be divided hierarchically into narcissistic, immature, neurotic, and mature categories (see Wong, 1989, pp. 375–376).

The point to be made is that an investigator's choice of classification depends largely on that investigator's theoretical model. For example, some investigators include in their models, in addition to the more unconscious regressive aspects of defenses, the more conscious, adaptive aspects of an individual's functioning. For these authors, empathy, substitution, suppression, humor, altruism, and asceticism are all part of defensive functioning (Bond, Gardner, Christian, & Sigal, 1983; Haan, Stroud, & Holstein, 1973; Meissner et al., 1975; Semrad, Grinspoon, & Feinberg, 1973; Vaillant, Bond, & Vaillant, 1986). Others, like the present authors, remain closer to the original Freudian notion of defenses as unconscious mechanisms, preferring rather to label the more conscious, adaptive processes as a separate category, that is, as coping styles (Plutchik & Conte, 1989). The present chapter is not concerned with processes in the latter category.

One final area in which there exists little agreement concerns the issue of how to measure, reliably and validly, the presence and extent of defensive functioning in an individual. Over the past 20 years or so a modest literature has evolved that is concerned with this problem. Some techniques of measurement—for example, Kragh's (1969) Defense Mechanism Test, which utilizes subliminal perception—derive from projective testing. However, the validity of this type of assessment has been questioned (Cooper & Kline, 1986; Kline, 1987). Other techniques require the judgments of an interviewer (e.g., Ablon, Carson, & Goodwin, 1974; Hackett & Cassem, 1974), while still others depend on self-reports (e.g., Gleser & Ihilevich, 1969; Kreitler & Kreitler, 1972; Marshall, 1982; Sarason, Ganzer, & Singer, 1972). However, most of these exhibit a narrow preoccupation with only one or two defenses. More important, none of these defense mechanism tests provide a theoretical framework for explicating the relations among the defenses and related constructs.

In 1979, Plutchik, Kellerman, and Conte described a new self-report instrument, the Life Style Index for the measurement of ego defenses, that does provide such a theoretical framework. This framework is based on Plutchik's general theory of affect, which has been fully described elsewhere (Plutchik, 1962, 1980). Basically, this model provides a rationale for the choice of defenses to be measured, and at the same time, it helps to define the relations among those defenses. The model assumes that a circumplex or circular structure is most appropriate for the relations among the ego defenses. The circumplex indicates the relative similarity of the different defenses and ensures that an adequate sample of this hypothetical domain is obtained by making certain that every sector of the circle is sampled. The rationale for the proposed relations among the ego defenses and between the ego defenses and diagnostic constructs is presented more fully elsewhere (Plutchik et al., 1979).

In the following sections, we present a description of the Life Style Index, examples of its use in clinical research, and suggestions for its use in future research projects.

The Life Style Index

Originally, the Life Style Index (LSI) consisted of 224 items designed to represent 16 defense mechanisms. These 16 were selected on the basis of a review of a large number of psychoanalytic, psychiatric, and psychological sources. A series of studies designed to determine the psychometric properties of the test was then conducted. During the course of these studies, the number of items was systematically reduced to 97, and some of the items were reworded. In addition, as the result of an analysis of an intercorrelation matrix that indicated considerable overlap among the defenses and a factor analysis of the matrix, it was concluded that 16 defenses were too many. Thus, on the basis of these empirical data as well as psychoanalytic theory, which holds that anxiety is at the core of the development of any defense, the items were regrouped into eight scales: compensation (including identification and fantasy), denial, displacement, intellectualization (including sublimation, undoing, and rationalization), projection, reaction formation, regression (including

TABLE 18.1. Synthesized definitions of eight ego defense scales.

Compensation, identification, fantasy	Intense attempt to correct or find a suitable substitute for a real or imagined physical or psychological inadequacy; unconscious modeling of attitudes and behaviors after another person as a way of increasing feelings of self-worth or coping with possible separation or loss; retreat into imagination to escape realistic problems or to avoid conflicts.
Denial	Lack of awareness of certain events, experiences, or feelings that would be painful to acknowledge.
Displacement	Discharge of pent-up emotions, usually of anger, on objects, animals, or people perceived as less dangerous than those that originally aroused the emotions.
Intellectualization, sublimation, undoing, rationalization	Unconscious control of emotions and impulses by excessive dependence on rational interpretations of situations; gratification of a repressed instinct or unacceptable feeling, particularly sexual or aggressive, by socially acceptable alternatives; behavior or thoughts designed to cancel out an act or thought that has much anxiety or guilt attached to it; use of plausible reasons to justify actions caused by repressed, unacceptable feelings.
Projection	Unconscious rejection of one's emotionally unacceptable thoughts, traits, or wishes, and the attribution of them to other people.
Reaction formation	Prevention of the expression of unacceptable desires, particularly sexual or aggressive, by developing or exaggerating opposite attitudes and behaviors.
Regression, acting Out	Retreat under stress to earlier or more immature patterns of behavior and gratification; reduction of the anxiety aroused by forbidden impulses by permitting their direct or indirect expression, without the development of guilt.
Repression, isolation, introjection	Exclusion from consciousness of an idea and its associated emotions, or an experience and its associated emotions; recollection of emotionally traumatic experiences or situations, without the anxiety originally associated with them; incorporation of values, standards, or traits of other people in order to prevent conflicts with, or threats from, these people.

acting out), and repression (including isolation and introjection). These defenses are listed in Table 18.1, along with their definitions.

Each scale contains between 10 and 14 items. Coefficient alphas were computed on two samples of subjects, 60 inpatients on the psychiatric wards of a municipal hospital and 75 Midwestern college students. Table 18.2 presents these coefficients, along with the items ranking highest on relevance for each of the eight ego defense scales as rated by 17 experienced clinicians with an average of 13 years of experience (Plutchik et al., 1979). As is evident from the table, these coefficients show considerable variation, both within a sample of subjects and between the two samples, but in all instances internal consistency is higher for the patients. The median alpha for the patients is .62, with a range from .54 to .86. For the students, the median is .54, with coefficients ranging from .30 to .75.

It is likely that the alphas for the patient sample are higher than those for the students because for each of the scales, the patients' scale variance was higher, and greater variability influences the magnitude of the correlation. It is a more difficult task to explain the considerable variation in internal consistency among the scales themselves. Defense mechanisms are difficult, abstract concepts about which there is much difference of opinion, even among the experts. Some defenses, however, appear to be clearer than others. Projection, for example, may be one of the concepts whose components are more readily agreed upon and one that is, therefore, more easily operationalized in statements about behavior. Inspection of Table 18.2 suggests that when one combines several abstract concepts into a single, relatively short scale, even when there are both empirical and theoretical reasons for doing so, one is bound to sacrifice a certain amount of internal consistency for that scale. The scale combining intellectualization, sublimation, undoing, and rationalization is a case in point.

A study comparing the use of ego defenses by 29 schizophrenic patients in a state hospital and 70 college students provides some evidence of the discriminant validity of the LSI. The schizophrenic patients scored significantly higher than the students on seven of the eight defenses (Plutchik et

TABLE 18.2. Coefficient alphas and items ranking highest on relevance for the eight ego defense scales.

	Scale coefficient alpha	
	Inpatients (N = 60)	Students (N = 75)
Compensation, identification, fantasy		
In my daydreams I'm always the center of attention.	.59	.43
Denial		
I am free of prejudice.	.54	.52
Displacement		
If someone bothers me, I don't tell it to him, but I tend to complain to someone else.	.69	.62
Intellectualization, sublimation, undoing, rationalization		
I am more comfortable discussing my thoughts than my feelings.	.58	.30
Projection		
I believe people will take advantage of you if you are not careful.	.86	.75
Reaction formation		
Pornography is disgusting.	.73	.63
Regression		
I get irritable when I don't get attention.	.65	.56
Repression, isolation, introjection		
I rarely remember my dreams.	.55	.38

al., 1979). These findings are consistent with a comparison of the mean scale scores for the 60 inpatients and 75 students whose test data served as the basis for the computation of the LSI's internal consistency. For all scales, the patients' means were greater than the students. In general, it could be said that increasing psychiatric symptomatology leads to increasing anxiety, which in turn leads to a greater use of ego defenses.

A degree of construct validity for the scales of the LSI was obtained when it was found that all but one of the scales correlated positively with the Taylor Manifest Anxiety Scale (Bendig, 1956) and that there were negative correlations between five of the eight defenses and total score on a test of self-esteem based on the Tennessee Self-Concept Scale (Fitts, 1965).

The Life Style Index and Clinical Research

Since the publication of the original description of the LSI (Plutchik et al., 1979), normative data, derived from test data of 147 normal adults (no history of psychiatric difficulties), have been constructed. They are available both as percentiles and as *T*-scores. In addition, the LSI has been used in a number of studies relating the use of ego defenses to outcome data and to the clinical variables of risk of suicide and risk of violence.

Ego Defenses and Outcome for Hospitalized Schizophrenics

As part of an attempt to examine the possible relations between psychodynamic variables assessed at admission to the hospital and outcome after discharge, 30 schizophrenics, 15 male and 15 female, on an inpatient ward of a large municipal hospital were asked to complete the LSI (Conte, Plutchik, Schwartz, & Wild, 1983). The profile presented in Fig. 18.1 represents their percentile scores based on the normative group of 147 adults. The outcome measure consisted of readmission to the hospital.

Patients were followed for 2 years after their index admission. It was found that 16 of the 30 were not rehospitalized during either the first or second year subsequent to their discharge. Point-biserial correlations were computed that related scores on each of the eight ego defenses obtained at the time of admission to whether the patients had been readmitted to the hospital during the 2-year follow-up.

In general, variables reflecting patients' psychodynamics proved to be less predictive of whether a schizophrenic patient would be rehospitalized than did more traditionally used predictors such as reduction of overall symptomatology. However, significant positive correlations were found

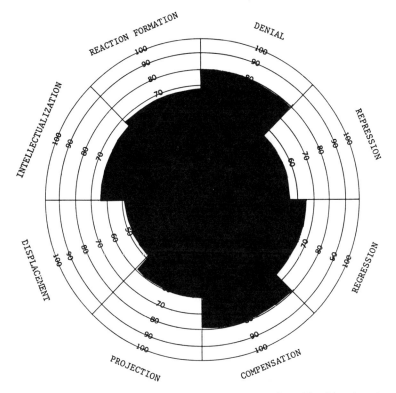

FIGURE 18.1. Life Style Index: Ego defense profile based on 30 schizophrenics.

between the use of the ego defenses of repression ($r = .40$, $p < .03$), displacement ($r = .36$, $p < .05$), and denial ($r = .35$, $p < .05$) and the likelihood of readmission. It is interesting to note that repression and denial have been considered to be primative or immature defenses (Bond et al., 1983; Plutchik et al., 1979; Wong, 1989), and displacement has at best been termed "intermediate" or "neurotic" (Vaillant, 1985; Wong, 1989). Thus, while there are undoubtedly multiple causal factors that determine rehospitalization, it appears that patients high in the use of these relatively immature defense mechanisms are more likely candidates than those who report lower levels of their usage.

Ego Defenses and Outcome of Long-Term Psychotherapy

More recently, the Life Style Index has been used in a study of variables that might predict the outcome of psychotherapy (Buckley, Conte,

Plutchik, Wild, & Karasu, 1984). In this study, 21 medical students were seen in psychotherapy, averaging 42 sessions. At intake, each student completed a battery of self-report tests that included the LSI. Outcome was evaluated by psychiatrists' ratings on a termination form that consisted of 13 items, each rated on a four-point scale ranging from "got worse" to "markedly improved." The items included such symptoms as depression and suicidal impulses, paranoid ideation, sexual problems, and difficulties with academic work.

Of the statistically significant pretreatment predictors of outcome, two, reaction formation and projection, were self-report assessments of ego defenses as measured by the LSI. The first of these, reaction formation, characterizes a person who substitutes socially acceptable behavior, thoughts, or feelings for his or her diametrically opposed unacceptable ones. This implies at least an openness to change that would enable the individual to benefit from psychotherapy.

The use of projection as a predictor of good outcome is somewhat surprising, since projection is regarded as a low level defense, more typical of serious pathology. However, a comparison of the percentile scores obtained for the patients who were rated most improved by the psychiatrists with those rated least improved sheds some light on this finding. Those rated most improved ($N = 11$) were at the 31st percentile on the norms based on normal adults, the majority of whom fall at approximately the 50th percentile, whereas those rated least improved ($N = 10$) fell at the 4th percentile. This suggests that projection may reflect a capacity for emotional engagement, albeit distorted, a certain amount of which is necessary for therapeutic change. This raises the possibility that the use of either too little or too much of any defense may be maladaptive.

Defense Mechanisms in Relation to Risk of Suicide and Risk of Violence

Psychodynamic theorists have addressed the role of defense mechanisms in relation to suicide. Freud (1957), for example, assumed that suicidal behavior may result as an individual turns toward him- or herself the originally repressed anger felt against another person who has been lost. Yet there have been few attempts to use empirical methods in the study of the defense mechanisms of suicidal or outwardly violent patients.

Apter and his colleagues, using the LSI to assess defenses, did conduct such a study (Apter, Plutchik, Sevy, Korn, Brown, & van Praag, 1989). Shortly after admission, 60 patients on the psychiatric inpatient wards of a municipal hospital center were administered a Suicide Risk scale (SR), a Past Feelings and Acts of Violence scale (PFAV), and the LSI as part of a battery of tests designed to identify correlates of suicide and violence risk in psychiatric patients. It should be mentioned that the SR and PFAV scales are not meant to predict future suicides or acts of violence, but, rather, the probability that an individual will make a suicide attempt or perform a violent act. No attempt was made to select any particular diagnostic category of patients, but 30 were selected because they had been admitted subsequent to a suicide attempt. These were matched according to sex, age, and diagnosis with nonsuicidal control patients. Of the group of 30 suicidal patients, 20 had to be secluded or restrained for assaulting a staff member or fellow patient. These constituted the violent group and were compared with the other 40 patients.

Risk of suicide and risk of violence were highly correlated ($r = .62$) with one another. For this reason, partial correlations were computed between each of the defenses and risk of suicide or violence. Application of the Bonferroni correction indicated that correlations greater than .32 were significant. It was found that repression, denial, and displacement were significantly correlated with risk of suicide after risk of violence was partialed out ($r = .47, -.51; p < .001$; and $r = .34, p < .01$, respectively). When the risk of suicide was partialed out, risk of violence correlated .46 ($p < .001$) with projection and .32 ($p < .01$) with denial. The remaining correlations were not significant. Thus, patients who scored high on repression had a relatively high probability of making a future suicide attempt, whereas the risk for suicidal behavior of those scoring high on denial was relatively low. However, their risk for violent behavior was high.

Interpretation of why an individual who scored high on displacement would be considered to be at risk for suicide is somewhat less obvious. It is, however, possible that these individuals turn the anger that low scorers on displacement would normally express toward those who rejected or frustrated them back on themselves. In so doing, they would increase their risk for self-destructive behavior. High scorers on the use of projection as a defense also were at significant risk for violence, but were at little risk of suicidal behavior. These findings are in accord with what one would predict from psychoanalytic theory and provide a degree of validity to the scales.

Suicidal patients were also compared with nonsuicidal patients and violent patients with nonviolent ones. Suicidal patients scored significantly higher on regression ($t = 2.61$, df $= 58$, $p < .01$) than did the nonsuicidal patients. Comparing the violent with the nonviolent patients, two significant differences were found. The violent group scored significantly higher on displacement ($t = 2.96$, df $= 58$, $p < .01$) and lower on reaction formation ($t = 2.64$, df $= 58$, $p < .01$).

That use of regression was significantly greater in the suicidal patients than in the nonsuicidal ones is consistent with the clinical observation that suicidal patients have greater potential for severe infantile, impulsive acting out behavior in the face of intolerable life stress than do nonsuicidal patients. The finding that displacement was more marked in the violent than in the nonviolent patients also provides support for clinical impressions and expectations from psychodynamic theory. Many acts of violence appear to represent displacement of aggression from primary objects onto symbolic representations of or substitutes for those objects. That the violent patients should score lower on the use of reaction formation is also consistent with both theory and what is noted in clinical practice. Individuals prone to violence have little tendency to adopt attitudes or behavior opposite to their feelings. Their aggressiveness is more often expressed directly.

The extent to which an individual uses the different ego defenses is thus seen to play an integral role in determining the probability that he or she will engage in suicidal or violent behavior. The ability to actually quantify the role of the defenses in this regard may have important implications for the management and treatment of patients.

Clinicians' Conceptions of Ego Defenses in Relation to Psychotherapy Outcome

Clinicians have implicit beliefs about characteristics that make some patients more likely to benefit from psychotherapy than others. As one way of looking at this issue, 20 clinicians, 15 psychiatrists, 4 social workers, and a psychologist with an average of 12 years post-training, were asked to respond to the 97 items of the Life Style Index in the following way. They were to assume that a patient had answered "yes" to each item, indicating that the item described him or her. They were then asked to indicate whether a "yes" response to each of the items was indicative of a probable "good" or "poor" prognosis in psychodynamic psychotherapy, or whether they believed that this description was "irrelevant" to outcome. Table 18.3 presents a brief summary of the data obtained.

Included under the heading of "Good prognosis" are items to which 70% or more of the clinicians responded that an individual who fit these descriptions would do well in psychotherapy. Top candidates for a good prognosis would be those who use the defenses of intellectualization and compensation. There was almost total agreement that an individual who is willing to listen to all sides of an argument would do well. Slightly less predictive of good outcome, but still endorsed by 70% of the clinicians, was the item describing an individual who describes him or herself as being logical in arguments. Two items from the compensation scale were endorsed by 80% of the clinicians as predicting good prognosis. The first, "There has always been a person whom I wished I were like" suggests that a patient who responds "yes" would readily develop a positive transference. The second, descriptive of someone who is willing

TABLE 18.3. Defense mechanisms as prognostic indicators of psychotherapy outcome as rated by clinicians ($N = 20$).

	Clinicians' response (%)
Good Prognosis	
Intellectualization	
I am always willing to listen to all sides of an argument.	95
In arguments, I'm usually more logical than the other person.	70
Compensation	
There has always been a person whom I wished I were like.	80
I work harder than most people to be good at what I like.	80
Poor Prognosis	
Regression	
I lie a lot.	90
I "fly off the handle" easily.	80
When I'm upset, I often get drunk.	75
I can't seem to finish anything I start.	70
Projection	
Most people are obnoxious.	80
I am irritated because people can't be trusted.	70
Most people annoy me because they are too selfish.	70
Displacement	
When I've been rejected, I've sometimes felt suicidal.	85
Sometimes I wish an atom bomb would destroy the world.	70
Repression	
When I read or hear about a tragedy, it never seems to affect me.	70

to work hard to realize a gain, suggests that the person is persistent and not easily discouraged, characteristics that are an asset in making progress in therapy.

The clinicians rated considerably more items of the LSI as reflective of poor prognosis. Consistent with the notion that patients who utilize relatively immature defenses are not likely to have a good outcome is the finding that these poor prognosis items represent the ego defenses of regression, projection, displacement, and repression. As illustrated in Table 18.3, a large percentage of the rating clinicians (70–90%) indicated their belief that patients who regress under stress to immature patterns of behavior or gratification would have a poor prognosis for psychotherapy. In addition, 70–80% responded that patients who attribute their own unacceptable characteristics to others would not do well. Similarly, 70–85% of the clinicians considered the prognosis to be poor of patients who do not deal directly with their pent-up emotions or whose emotional responses have become blunted.

Further research is necessary to determine the accuracy of these clinicians' predictions about who would and who would not do well in therapy. It would be interesting, for example, to administer the Life Style Index to a sample of patients before they enter treatment and to follow them over the course of therapy to determine which patients, in fact, had a good or a poor outcome. Nevertheless, it is unlikely that the raters were merely responding to stereotypes. They were asked to make predictions about specific items, not to the use of a given defense per se. What is likely is that the items they endorsed as good prognosticators described individuals with whom they believed they could work well. That in itself might make for a good prognosis.

Conclusions and Directions for Future Research

We believe that we have constructed a reasonable test for measuring some important ego defenses. Among its salient characteristics, the LSI has a self-report format and is thus easy to administer and to score. It is of special significance that the selection of defenses to be measured was based on a general theory of affect (Plutchik, 1980, 1990). This theory assumes that ego defenses are basic adaptive mechanisms that function to deal with specific emotional conflicts. Displacement, for example, functions to handle conflicts involving anger or aggression. Projection handles conflicts over issues of acceptance of self or others, while repression deals with conflicts produced by intolerable anxiety.

While the connections between emotions, ego defenses, and diagnoses is at this stage hypothetical, the theory also assumes that individuals with particular personality disorders such as borderline, schizoid, or antisocial, are likely to emphasize the use of specific ego defenses. In the case of these three disorders, they might be regression, fantasy, and projection, respectively. In addition, the theory postulates a systematic structuring of the ego defenses that closely approximates a circumplicial, or circular, order that reflects the degree of similarity among the defenses. The Life Style Index is thus based on a theory that permits systematic inferences to be made about the relations among the ego defenses themselves and about their relation to other clinical domains.

The relation between defense mechanisms and psychiatric diagnoses is an area that is in need of clarification. One reason for this is that while DSM-III-R has provided a relatively well-accepted standardized classification of diagnoses, no comparable standardized classification system exists for the ego defenses. This is not really surprising. Vaillant and Drake put it well when they state: "Defenses are, after all, metaphors; they are a shorthand way of describing different cognitive styles and modes of rearranging inner and outer realities" (1985, p. 601). As such, they reflect integrated processes that are both difficult to identify and to define.

It is our belief that the Life Style Index represents a comprehensive and relatively well agreed upon selection of defense mechanisms when they are defined as unconscious mental processes. It might prove productive, therefore, to test the notion of Laplanche and Pontalis (1973) that the type of illness a patient has in large measure determines which defense mechanisms will predominate. Vaillant and Drake (1985) related Axis II of the DSM-III to patients' dominant choice of ego defenses and found that two-thirds of the men with personality disorders used primarily immature defense mechanisms. Bond and Vaillant (1986) compared patients' defense styles with their diagnoses on Axes I, II, and IV of DSM-III and found that a significant relationship existed between defense style and only one diagnosis, major affective disorder.

Further investigations of this sort would help to provide a clearer picture of the extent to which defense mechanisms relate to an aspect of human functioning that is distinct from that encompassed in diagnoses or whether the use of particular defenses is an integral part of a given diagnostic status. In addition to investigating the relations between defense mechanisms and diagnoses, future research should address the relationship between ego defenses and general level of adjustment in varying psychiatric populations.

Research in the area of psychotherapy has been concerned with such issues as predictors of outcome, factors influencing process, matching of therapist and patient, and identification and training of good psychotherapists. We believe that the use of measures of ego defenses are important parameters for investigations in these areas. Furthermore, their use should enrich the findings in these investigations by adding psychodynamic insights to the more traditional demographic, symptom, and personality-oriented variables.

References

Ablon, S.L., Carlson, G.A., & Goodwin, F.K. (1974) Ego defense patterns in manic-depressive illness. *American Journal of Psychiatry*, *131*, 803–807.

American Psychiatric Association Committee on Nomenclature and Statistics (1987) *Diagnostic and Statistical Manual of Mental Disorders* (3rd ed., rev.). Washington, DC: American Psychiatric Association.

Andrews, G., Pollock, C., & Stewart, G. (1989) The determination of defense style by questionnaire. *Archives of General Psychiatry*, *46*, 455–460.

Apter, A., Plutchik, R., Sevy, S., Korn, M., Brown S., & van Praag, H. (1989) Defense mechanisms in risk of suicide and risk of violence. *American Journal of Psychiatry*, *146*, 1027–1031.

Arieti, S. (Ed.) (1974) *American handbook of psychiatry*. New York: Basic Books.

Bendig, A.W. (1956) The development of a short form of the Manifest Anxiety Scale. *Journal of Consulting Psychology*, *20*, 384–387.

Bond, M. (1986) Defense Style Questionnaire. In G.E. Vaillant (Ed.), *Empirical studies of ego mechanisms of defense* (pp. 146–152). Washington, DC: American Psychiatric Press.

Bond, M., Gardner, S.T., Christian, J., & Sigal, J.J. (1983) Empirical study of self-rated defense styles. *Archives of General Psychiatry, 40*, 333–338.

Bond, M.P. & Vaillant, J.S. (1986) An empirical study of the relationship between diagnosis and defense style. *Archives of General Psychiatry, 43*, 285–288.

Brenner, C. (1973) *An elementary textbook of psychoanalysis*. Madison, CT: International Universities Press.

Buckley, P., Conte, H.R., Plutchik, R., Wild, K.V., & Karasu, T.B. (1984) Psychodynamic variables as predictors of psychotherapy outcome. *American Journal of Psychiatry, 141*, 742–748.

Conte, H.R., Plutchik, R., Schwartz, B., & Wild, K. (1983) *Psychodynamic variables related to outcome in hospitalized schizophrenics*. Paper presented at the Convention of the American Psychological Association, Anaheim, CA.

Cooper, C. & Kline, P. (1986) An evaluation of the Defense Mechanism Test. *British Journal of Psychology, 77*, 19–31.

Fitts, W.H. (1965) *The Tennessee Self-Concept Scale*. Nashville: Counselor Recordings & Tests.

Freud, A. (1936) *The ego and the mechanisms of defense*. Madison, CT: International Universities Press.

Freud, S. (1957) Mourning and melancholia. In *The standard edition of the complete psychological works of Sigmund Freud: Vol. 14*. London: Hogarth Press.

Gleser, G.C. & Ihilevich, D. (1969) An objective instrument for measuring defense mechanisms. *Journal of Consulting and Clinical Psychology, 33*, 51–60.

Haan, N.A., Stroud, J., & Holstein, C. (1973) Moral and ego stages in relationship to ego processes: A study of "hippies." *Journal of Personality, 41*, 596–612.

Hackett, T.P. & Cassem, N.H. (1974) Development of a quantitative rating scale to assess denial. *Journal of Psychosomatic Research, 18*, 93–100.

Kline, P. (1987) The scientific status of the DMT. *British Journal of Medical Psychology, 60*, 53–59.

Kragh, U. (1969) *The Defense Mechanism Test*. Stockholm: Testfoerlaget.

Kreitler, H. & Kreitler, S. (1972) The cognitive determinants of defensive behavior. *British Journal of Social and Clinical Psychology, 11*, 359–373.

Laplanche, J. & Pontalis, J.B. (1973) *The language of psychoanalysis*. London: Hogarth Press.

Marshall, J.B. (1982) *Psychometric and validational studies of an objective test of Freudian defense mechanisms*. Unpublished doctoral dissertation, University of North Carolina at Chapel Hill, NC.

Meissner, W.W., Mack, J.E., & Semrad, E.V. (1975) Theories of personality and psychopathology: Classical psychoanalysis. In A.M. Freedman & H.I. Kaplan (Eds.), *Comprehensive textbook of psychiatry: Vol. 11* (pp. 535–536). Baltimore: Williams & Wilkins.

Moore, B. & Fine, B.D. (Eds.) (1990) *Psychoanalytic terms and concepts*. New York and New Haven, CT: American Psychoanalytic Association and Yale University Press.

Noyes, A.P. & Kolb, L.C. (1963) *Modern clinical psychiatry*. Philadelphia: Saunders.

Perry, J.C. & Copper, S.H. (1989) An empirical study of defense mechanisms. I. Clinical interview and life vignette ratings. *Archives of General Psychiatry, 46*, 444–452.

Perry, J.C. & Vaillant, G.E. (1990) Personality disorders. In H.I. Kaplan & B.J. Sadock (Eds.), *Comprehensive textbook of psychiatry: Vol. 2* (5th ed.) (pp. 1352–1395). New York: Plenum.

Plutchik, R. (1962) *The emotions: Facts, theories, and a new model.* New York: Random House.

Plutchik, R. (1980) *Emotion: A psychoevolutionary synthesis.* New York: Harper & Row.

Plutchik, R. (1990) Emotions and psychotherapy: A psychoevolutionary perspective. In R. Plutchik & H. Kellerman (Eds.), *Emotion: Theory, research, and experience: Vol. 5* (pp. 3–41). New York: Academic Press.

Plutchik, R. & Conte, H.R. (1989) Measuring emotions and their derivatives: Personality traits, ego defenses, and coping styles. In S. Wetzler & M.M. Katz (Eds.), *Contemporary approaches to psychological assessment* (pp. 239–269). New York: Bruner/Mazel.

Plutchik, R., Kellerman, H., & Conte, H.R. (1979) A structural theory of ego defenses and emotions. In C.E. Izard (Ed.), *Emotions in personality and psychopathology* (pp. 229–257). New York: Plenum.

Sarason, I.G., Ganzer, N.J., & Singer, M. (1972) Effects of modeled self-disclosure on the verbal behavior of persons differing in defensiveness. *Journal of Consulting and Clinical Psychology, 39,* 483–490.

Semrad, E.V., Grinspoon, L., & Feinberg, S.E. (1973) Development of an ego profile scale. *Archives of General Psychiatry, 28,* 70–77.

Vaillant G.E. (1971) Theoretical hierarchy of adaptive ego mechanisms: A 30-year follow-up of 30 men selected for psychological health. *Archives of General Psychiatry, 24,* 107–118.

Vaillant, G.E. (1977) *Adaptation to life.* Boston: Little, Brown.

Vaillant, G.E. (1985) An empirically derived hierarchy of adaptive mechanisms and its usefulness as a potential diagnostic axis. *Acta Psychiatrica Scandinavica, 71,* (Suppl. 319), 171–180.

Vaillant, G.E., Bond, M., & Vaillant, G.O. (1986) An empirically validated hierarchy of defense mechanisms. *Archives of General Psychiatry, 43,* 786–794.

Vaillant, G.E. & Drake, R.E. (1985) Maturity of ego defenses in relation to DSM-III, Axis II personality disorder. *Archives of General Psychiatry, 42,* 597–601.

Wong, N. (1989) Theories of personality and psychopathology. In H.I. Kaplan & B.J. Sadock (Eds.), *Comprehensive textbook of psychiatry: Vol. 1* (5th ed.) (pp. 356–410). Baltimore: Williams & Wilkins.

19
Validation of the German Version of Bond's Questionnaire of Defensive Styles

GERHARD REISTER, ROLF MANZ, ROLAND FELLHAUER, and WOLFGANG TRESS

Bond, Gardner, Christian, and Sigal (1983) introduced a questionnaire designed to study defense mechanisms that did not rely on the rater's subjective judgment. Because of the immense problems of measuring intrapsychic phenomena that are for the most part unconscious, the results of this effort were rather modest. Bond et al. argued, that their questionnaire "taps possible derivative of defense mechanisms" (p. 333). They conceded, however, that no direct avenue for measuring specific defense mechanisms existed; what could be measured instead were the characteristic defense styles. Bond et al. construed defense as a mode of mastering conflicts and stress, involved in reconciling internal and external demands. In this sense, defense mechanisms are not only pathological patterns, but resources of adjustment in general. Taking as a base the concepts of Vaillant (1971, 1976), Haan (1977), and Semrad, Grinspoon, and Fienberg (1973), Bond et al. classified 24 defense mechanisms on the basis of developmental states. In other words, they proposed a sequence of defensive styles from immaturity to maturity.

The questionnaire is intended to supplement clinical experts' ratings and aims to avoid their specific shortcomings, such as dependence of judgment on individual clinical experiences and poor interrater reliability.

Bond et al. asserted that unconscious defense processes can be measured by self-rating. As for defensive styles, they developed the following arguments:

1. Unconscious defense mechanisms become apparent in behavior, which is close to consciousness.
2. Other persons often comment on or criticize the person's behavior; these remarks can be absorbed through reflection.
3. Persons can accurately comment on their behavior at a distance.
4. Defenses fail temporarily and at those times subjects may become aware of their unacceptable impulses and their usual styles of defending against them.

The questionnaire consists of 88 items. Each item refers to one of the 24 defense mechanisms. Of the 209 volunteers who participated in the validation study, 98 were patients from psychiatric wards or psychiatric outpatient departments. Their ages ranged from 15 to 69 years. Principal component factor analyses were carried out. The results indicated that a four-factor solution provided an adequate representation of the data:

1. Defense style 1 consisted of immature defense mechanisms (such as withdrawal, regression, and acting out), which generally imply a person's inability to deal with impulses by means of constructive action. This style has been described in terms of "maladaptive action patterns."
2. Defense style 2 was called "image distortion." It includes mechanisms such as splitting, primitive idealization, omnipotence, and devaluation. All these mechanisms are image oriented rather than action oriented.
3. Defense style 3 was labeled "self-sacrificing." Its component defenses were reaction formation and pseudoaltruism. The items designed to test these defenses reflect a need to perceive one's self as being kind, helpful to others, and never angry.
4. Defense style 4, "adaptive defense style," seems to be clearly associated with good coping. Defense mechanisms such as humor, repression, and sublimation establish a constructive type of mastery of the conflict.

In addition to these four styles, a control scale to measure frankness of self-report was included in the measure. It was found that 60% of the patients used defense style 1 in conjunction with other styles and 16% used it exclusively. By contrast, 90% of the nonpatients used defense style 4 in conjunction with other styles and 42% used it exclusively.

Correlations with indicators of ego strength also provided empirical support for the defense styles listed above. Correlations with ego strength increased from maladaptive through image-distorting to self-sacrificing and, finally, to adaptive defense styles.

The German Version of the Questionnaire

Bond's questionnaire was translated into German. We then asked 12 psychoanalysts with extensive clinical experience of the Psychosomatic Department of the Central Institute of Mental Health in Mannheim to provide their precise assessment of every single item. Specifically, these raters were asked whether the item represented a defense mechanism and, if so, which one. Multiple assessments (i.e., ratings of more than one mechanism per item) were possible. The modifications we introduced into the procedure were minimal; in this manner cross-cultural equivalence

TABLE 19.1. Several items of the questionnaire.

Defense[a]	Strongly disagree							Strongly agree
4. I'm always treated unfairly.	1 2 3 4 5 6 7 8 9
9. I act like a child when I'm frustrated.	1 2 3 4 5 6 7 8 9
63. I often find myself being very nice to people who by all rights I should be angry at.	1 2 3 4 5 6 7 8 9
16. People say I'm like an ostrich with my head buried in the sand. In other words, I tend to ignore unpleasant facts as if they didn't exist.	1 2 3 4 5 6 7 8 9
53. As far as I'm concerned, people are either good or bad	1 2 3 4 5 6 7 8 9
35. I withdraw when I'm angry.	1 2 3 4 5 6 7 8 9

[a] Key: 4, projection; 9, regression; 63, reaction formation; 16, denial; 53, splitting; 35, withdrawal.

was maintained as much as possible. At the same time, the procedure we adopted was designed to maximize the clinical relevance of the items.

Some of the items used can be seen in Table 19.1. The German questionnaire with 88 items was presented to 310 probands drawn from the general population; 301 persons sent back the questionnaire, a return rate of 97%. Ages ranged from 16 to 76 years (mean 36 years, standard deviation 13.9 years). Fifty-one percent of the subjects were women, 49% men. There was a very high proportion of university students and graduates (43.5%). Fifty four percent of the probands were practicing a profession, and 48.5% were salaried employees or wage earners.

The 88 statements were factor analyzed (principal axis factoring, SPSS-X, PAF). After Varimax rotation and Scree test, five- to seven-factor solutions could be accepted. Factor 6 consists of only four items with low factor loadings. We therefore accepted the five-factor solution, which has the same composition as that reported by Bond et al. (1983) (see Table 19.2).

There were some minor differences in detail from the factorial structure of Bond et al. Only 22% of the variance was captured by the five factors. This finding is rather disappointing.

TABLE 19.2. Comparison of the factors of the original and the German version of the questionnaire (88 items).

Defense styles by Bond	Defense styles of the German version
Factor 1: Maladaptive action patterns	Factor 1: Immature defense
Factor 2: Image-distorting mechanisms	Factor 3: Narcissistic defense
Factor 4: Adaptive defense style	Factor 4: Mature defense
Factor 3: Self-sacrificing defense style	Factor 5: Control of impulse and affects
Factor 5: [control scale]	Factor 2: Frankness, social desirability

TABLE 19.3. Factors of the revised German version of the questionnaire (35 items).

Factor 1: Immature defense (paranoid projection, projection, regression)
Factor 2: Neurotic symptoms (withdrawal, inhibition, . . .)
Factor 3: Omnipotence (omnipotence, devaluation, . . .)
Factor 4: Frankness [control scale]
Factor 5: Mature defense (altruism, identification, repression)

For statistical and test construction reasons, we attempted to optimize the items. The selection of items was done according to their commonality (>.40) and the Fürntratt criterion ($a^2/h^2 > .50$; Fürntratt, 1969). There remained 28 items. We added 7 items using the face validity criterion (10 of 12 experts had agreed in labeling the defense mechanisms); thus little information of any clinical relevance was discarded.

We expanded the sample by adding 96 inpatients from the wards of the departments for Psychosomatic Medicine and Psychotherapy at the universities of Mannheim and Düsseldorf. Another factor analysis of the data based on the total of 397 subjects produced a five-factor solution, with the explained variance amounting to 41%. The labels for the factors extracted from the short form of the questionnaire, comprising 35 items, are presented in Table 19.3.

The defense mechanisms included in factor 2 (withdrawal, inhibition) apparently represent neurotic symptoms. The internal consistencies ranged from .48 to .82.

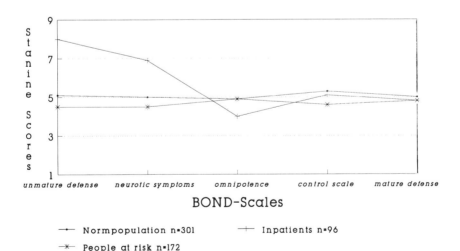

FIGURE 19.1. Differences among three groups on the Bond scales: graph represents data corrected for control scale scores.

TABLE 19.4. Sex differences of the stanine scales for inpatients and general population in parentheses.

Scales	Men ($N = 184$)	Women ($N = 205$)	Significance level (%)
Immature defense	5.6 (2.4)	5.9 (2.6)	n.s.
Neurotic symptoms	5.2 (2.2)	5.7 (2.1)	2
Omnipotence	5.3 (2.0)	4.3 (1.9)	0.1
Frankness	5.4 (1.8)	4.7 (2.1)	0.1
Mature defense	4.7 (2.0)	5.2 (2.1)	1

There was another sample of 172 subjects, so-called people at risk (i.e., individuals exhibiting a certain risk to fall ill with psychosomatic, neurotic, or personality disorders). They were interviewed in the context of an epidemiological research project, the Mannheim Cohort Study (Schepank, 1987, 1990). They had the highest scores on the immature defense and neurotic symptoms factors (see Fig. 19.1, p. 293). The scores corrected with the control scale show also that the inpatient sample had the lowest value on the "omnipotence" factor. It is possible that this factor could represent a behavior pattern connected with health; subjects with high values on this scale seem to have better self-esteem. This result, however, must be cross-validated with larger samples.

Gender differences emerged (see Table 19.4). In their defense styles, women seem to use more neurotic mechanisms and mature defenses than men; at the same time, they rely less on omnipotence mechanisms. Women's control scale scores are also lower.

Discussion

The questionnaire of Bond et al. as adapted and modified for this study is principally a trait-oriented instrument, because its focus is on habitual defense styles. Moreover, the wording of the items is rather general and does not apply to specific situations that generate stress or embarrassment. Yet we think that in emotionally stressful situations that demand mechanisms of adaption and coping, not only aspects of the situation, but also aspects of the personality with a relative low rate of change are of importance. In this respect our questionnaire can tap defensive behavior only partially and incompletely. The advantage of this questionnaire is that it lends itself well to individual ratings by going beyond binary (yes–no) categorization and providing for individual ratings of the subject's complex defense behavior. Cluster analyses for different diagnoses in the field of psychogenic diseases would be important to undertake.

In any case, our questionnaire has demonstrated its practical utility. It can be completed by the patient within 15 minutes. Because of the similarity of its basic structure with the pattern of expert ratings, we have reasonable assurance of being able to measure defense styles, not neurotic symptoms.

We were unable to show a complete hierarchy of defenses as described by Vaillant (1971), although we did identify clearly immature and mature factors, indicative of the two poles of the theoretical continuum. On the other hand, the use of factor analysis is problematic for the description of hierarchies, because a continuum should be reflected as a bipolar factor. Thus, at the moment we cannot conclusively say whether the ranking of defense mechanisms according to maturity is realistic throughout the entire range of defenses.

We hope to obtain some more information about the validity and reliability of the questionnaire by comparing it with other self-administered instruments such as the inventory for conflict-solving strategies (FKBS: Fragenbogen zu Konfliktbewältigungsstrategien) used in the study by Hentschel, Kießling, and Hoscmann (cf. Chapter 16).

References

Bond, M., Gardner, S.T., Christian, J., & Sigal, J.J. (1983) Empirical study of self-rated defense styles. *Archives of General Psychiatry, 40*, 333–338.

Fürntratt, E. (1969) Zur Bestimmung der Anzahl gemeinsamer Faktoren in Faktoranalysen psychologischer Daten [Definition of the number of common factors in factor analyses of psychological data]. *Diagnostica, 15*, 62–75.

Haan, H. (1977) *Coping and defending. Processes of self environment organization.* New York: Academic Press.

Schepank, H. (1987) *Epidemiology of psychogenic disorders.* Berlin: Springer.

Schepank, H. (Ed.) (1990) *Verläufe Seelische Gesundheit und psychogene Erkrankungen heute.* Berlin: Springer.

Semrad, E.V., Grinspoon, L., & Fienberg, S.E. (1973) Development of an ego profile scale. *Archives of General Psychiatry, 28*, 70–77.

Vaillant, G.E. (1971) Theoretical hierarchy of adaptive ego mechanisms. *Archives of General Psychiatry, 24*, 107–118.

Vaillant, G.E. (1976) Natural history of male psychological health: The relation of choice of ego mechanisms of adult adjustment. *Archives of General Psychiatry, 33*, 535–545.

20
Regulative Styles and Defenses: Some Relationships Between the Serial Color-Word Test and the Defense Mechanism Test

I. Alex Rubino and Nicola Ciani

The frame of the present study stems from a certain number of theoretical statements that were advanced about 40 years ago (Smith & Klein, 1953): (a) the concept of defense expresses "a stabilized coping mechanism concerned with mediation of conflict"; (b) personality rests on some preferred styles of cognitive organization, which are reflected in the course of adaptation to various types of conflicting situation; and (c) these regulative styles are "especially evident in serials (i.e., in the manner in which response unfolds in a situation)", thus paying attention to temporal patterning and not to average achievement level scores.

The instrument chosen by Klein and Smith to assess regulative styles was a serial version of the Color-Word Test (Stroop, 1935), currently known as Serial Color-Word Test (S-CWT; Smith, Nyman, & Hentschel, 1986). The task involves two conflicting response tendencies, reading the printing hue or reading the name of a number of color-words printed in incongruent colors: the subject is asked to read the color, resisting the interference effect. The only published systematic attempt to correlate S-CWT patterns with defenses (Almgren, 1980) employed the Meta-Contrast Technique (MCT: Smith, Johnson, & Almgren, 1982), a well-validated tachistoscopic method, which provides information on anxiety and defenses. The subjects with high nonlinear change of reading times on the three first S-CWT subtest (viz., dissociative style) had more signs of repression and fewer signs of isolation, compared to nondissociative subjects; furthermore, more isolations and fewer repressions were found among probands characterized by high initial times, followed by a series of stabile and much lower times (viz., initial types, IT). The latter finding confirmed the high positive correlation between IT and isolation that had been reported earlier, in a paper devoted more to the different clinical significance of S-CWT and MCT than to their interrelationships (Smith, Nilsson, & Johnson, 1964).

Subsequently, Westerlundh (1983) studied the relationships of the S-CWT with the defenses reported by subjects who were administered the stimuli of the other major percept-genetic method designed to assess defensive organization, the Defense Mechanism Test (DMT; Kragh, 1985); however, the DMT's anxiety-arousing pictures were administered not tachistoscopically, but limiting perception to peripheral vision (Sander's ambient focal technique). In agreement with Almgren's data, the dissociative style was significantly linked with a group of repression variants (but with a rather low probability level). A number of clinical investigations employed both the S-CWT and the MCT, frequently contrasting combinations of adaptive patterns and codings of defense against symptom constellations and outcome criteria (see, e.g., Kragh & Smith, 1970, pp. 286–318), but they seem only marginally relevant in this context.

A different line of research compared the DMT codings of defense with patterns of adaptation on the Spiral Aftereffect Technique (SAT: Andersson, Nilsson, Ruuth, & Smith, 1972). The main significant results opposed repression to introaggression; repression (but not the repetition of a repression variant) correlated with diminishing durations of the aftereffect in the course of the 10 massed trials of the SAT, while introaggression on the central figure (but not on the object with which the latter is concerned) corresponded to linearly increasing durations (Andersson & Weikert, 1974; Andersson & Bengtsson, 1985). In line with his interpretation of the SAT variables, Andersson argued that repression and introaggression reflect respectively an orientation toward nonself and toward self factors. Furthermore, the strongest variant of isolation (viz., barrier isolation) was linked to an extraceptive orientation, like introaggression on the hero. It may be added that no simple relationship exists between SAT and S-CWT patterns, because, for instance, rising curves of aftereffect durations do not significantly correspond to rising curves of reading times (Andersson, 1967). The present investigation into the relationships between regulative styles and types of defense was originally thought of as a four-instrument endeavor (MCT, DMT, CWT, and SAT). Unfortunately, technical problems allowed the administration of the MCT and SAT to only a minor portion of the sample. Therefore only the hypotheses and findings relative to DMT and S-CWT are reported here.

Assuming a basic relatedness between codings of defense in the MCT and DMT, the following major hypotheses about the DMT/S-CWT interrelationships could be advanced: (a) correspondence between dissociative style and repression (or some repression variants) and (b) positive correlation between IT and the strongest isolation variants. Since further correlational suggestions and data on the other defenses and adaptive patterns were lacking in the available literature, the study had also obvious exploratory aims.

Method

Subjects

The S-CWT and the DMT were administered to 119 clinical and non-clinical subjects in the age range of 18–60 years. Only subjects with a canonical primary S-CWT classification (see below) were included; therefore, the size of the sample was reduced to 58 (38 women and 20 men). Aside from 15 nonclinical volunteers from the university administration staff, the subjects included in the study were psychiatric or psychosomatic patients, belonging to the following broad diagnostic classes: neurosis, bronchial asthma, psoriasis, and eczema. Psychotic or neurologic patients and color-blind subjects were excluded.

Instruments

The Serial Color-Word Test

The subjects were given a page with 10 lines of color-words printed in incongruent hues and were asked to read the printing hue, disregarding the color names. Instructions, administration, and calculations followed strictly the S-CWT manual (Smith et al., 1986). Italian norms, stratified for age and sex, were employed for classification (cf. Rubino, Grasso, & Pezzarossa, 1990). The same color-words plate was read five times (viz. subtests), with one-minute pauses in between. Reading times were taken every couple of lines, for a total of five reading times for each subtest. The two fundamental measures of the S-CWT are linear regression (R) and residual variability (V). A sequence of continuously augmenting reading times (e.g., 11, 13, 14, 16, 17 s) has a high R and no V; if there are sudden drops, (e.g., 15, 12, 16, 11, 15 s), R is low and V is high; eventually, a substantial increment of reading times intermingled with decrements corresponds to a high R and a high V (e.g., 12, 14, 18, 12, 23 s). R and V were calculated for each of the five subtests and were compared with the normative medians. The following four patterns were derived:

Stabilized (S), when both R and V were below the norms.
Cumulative (C), when R was above and V was below the norms.
Dissociative (D), when R was below and V was above the norms.
Cumulative-Dissociative (CD), when both R and V were above the norms.

If one of these patterns was present in at least three subtests (and at least in two of the first three subtests), it was indicated as the primary type of the subjects. Protocols that did not meet these conditions for primary classification were excluded from the present study (although also less strict rules are usually applied.)

TABLE 20.1. Distribution of subjects on S-CWT types ($N = 58$).

Primary types	R-types	V-types	ITa	ITb	Rad
S ($N = 14$)	Sr ($N = 15$)	Sv ($N = 14$)	ITA$^+$ ($N = 26$)	ITb$^+$ ($N = 27$)	Rad$^+$ ($N = 30$)
C ($N = 10$)	Cr ($N = 14$)	Cv ($N = 17$)	ITa$^-$ ($N = 32$)	ITb$^-$ ($N = 31$)	Rad$^-$ ($N = 28$)
D ($N = 17$)	Dr ($N = 10$)	Dv ($N = 14$)			
CD ($N = 17$)	CDr ($N = 19$)	CDv ($N = 13$)			

As a second step, R and V were calculated on the Rs of the five sub-tests (R-secondary classification or R-types) and on their Vs (V-secondary classification or V-types). Confrontation with the norms permitted to classify R- and V-types according to the same four patterns listed above. Thus, for instance, a subject found to be Stabilized on the primary types, Cumulative on the R-types, and Dissociative on the V-types was classified S/Cr/Dv. Furthermore, two initial types (ITa and ITb) were calculated. High initial types indicate a sudden initial drop in reading times, followed by only minor decreases; the ITa applies to the initial reading times of the five subtests, while ITb applies to the reading times within the first subtest. Eventually, an "index of adaptation," called Rad, was obtained from the logarithms of the initial times of the subtests; the value of the Rad is typically high when the initial times of the first two subtests (especially of subtest 1) strongly exceed the initial times of the last two subtests (especially of subtest 5). ITa, ITb, and Rad were marked with a plus sign when values exceeded the norms. Table 20.1 shows the distribution of subjects on S-CWT types.

The Defense Mechanism Test

In the DMT the subject is administered two TAT-like pictures representing a central figure (hero, H) and a threatening peripheral person of the same sex as H (Pp); these stimuli are presented tachistoscopically at gradually longer exposure durations (two series of 22 steps, from 5 ms to 2 s). Verbal and graphic reports are coded for evidence of defensive alterations, according to the classical psychoanalytic list of defense mechanisms. Administration and coding followed the DMT manual (Kragh, 1985). The DMT apparatus employed was the standard one (by Persona, Sweden). A .5 gray filter was used throughout; no distracting stimulus was presented during testing.

The following codings were found to be relevant in the present study:

1. 1:42 (Stimulus-distal repression). Pp is an object. Particular attention was paid to the exclusion of reports of objects not clearly in the position of Pp. Instances of two objects, one on each side of the H, and reports of repression combined with isolation (e.g., "a lighted reflector") were not included into calculations on 1:42.

2. 2:10a (Barrier isolation). H and Pp are isolated by a separating line or area. Only clear reports of 2:10a were coded.
3. 2:10b (Second variant of isolation between H and Pp). H and Pp are placed in different frames of reference (levels of reality or space).
4. 2:10c (Third variant of isolation between H and Pp). The distance between H and Pp increases (typically, Pp turns away from H).
5. 2:32 (Pp discontinuity). Pp disappears after having been reported in the preceding phase.
6. 3: (Denial). Threat is explicitly denied or made light of.
7. 4:10 (First variant of reaction formation). H and Pp have a mutual, positive relationship.
8. 4:12 (Third variant of reaction formation). Pp is positive or tries to establish positive contact with H.
9. 4: (Reaction formation). The two variants above and 4:20 (the total mood is specified as agreeable).
10. 7:31 (A variant of introjection). H's sex is changed from correct to incorrect.
11. 8:71 (A variant of polymorphous identification). H is below 7 years of age.
12. 10:30 (Color regression). Color is seen even though the stimulus picture is black and white. Also weak reports were coded (e.g., "a brown table" or "a pink face").

Three codings that are not included in the manual were introduced: (a) WTP (without T-phase), Pp lacks a threatening character even at the 22nd exposure; (b) Ster (stereotypy), a single defensive variant is repeated in more than five phases directly following each other; and (c) BAPP (belated appearance of Pp), Pp is reported more than eight phases after the first reporting of H as a human figure. Furthermore, all the scores of defense of each DMT protocol were summed together, to give a number of defensive scorings (NDS). A sample of 20 protocols was independently coded by a psychologist with several years of experience in DMT coding. The interrater agreement on the 13 variants listed above was always high, ranging from 100 to 85%.

Results

Variant 1:42 was the only coding of repression for which there were significant differences of distribution among S-CWT types. Table 20.2 shows that it was rare among S and C subjects, while being common in the D and CD primary types; furthermore, 1:42 was more frequently associated with Rad[+] than with Rad[−] types.

As predicted, subjects with evidence of initial types had more frequent codings of isolation variants 2:10a and/or 2:10b; more specifically, Table

TABLE 20.2. Stimulus-distal repression and S-CWT types.

Group	S + C	D + CD	(One-tailed)
Subjects with 1:42	2	15	.002
The rest	22	19	
Group	Rad⁺	Rad⁻	(One-tailed)
Subjects with 1:42	13	4	.024
The rest	17	24	

20.3 shows that 2:10a (barrier isolation) was reported by more ITa^+ than ITa^- subjects. When subvariant 2:10c was added to the list two, the probability level of comparisons was found to be considerably lowered. Therefore 2:10c was treated separately and appeared to be linked with the absence of initial types; the same trend was apparent for sign 3: (denial), and the lowest section of Table 20.3 shows that when 2:10c and 3: were combined, their correspondence with IT^- reached significance.

The disappearance of Pp (isolation variant 2:32) was significantly linked with several S-CWT patterns (see Table 20.4). This kind of percept-genetic defense was far more common among D and CD subjects than among S and C ones. Somewhat surprisingly, 2:32 was more often reported by Sv subjects than by persons with the other V secondary classifications (in particular, the Cv type was rarely associated with 2:32). Eventually, a significant correspondence between Rad^+ and 2:32 was noted.

It may be seen from Table 20.5 that the lack of recognition of the threatening character of Pp (WTP) also was significantly linked with a number of primary and secondary S-CWT classifications. As for 2:32, D and CD types were more often associated with WTP than was the case for S and C primary types. The same held true for Dr and CDr, compared

TABLE 20.3. Isolation variants and initial types.

Group	ITa^+	ITa^-	(One-tailed)
Subjects with 2:10a	9	4	.035
The rest	17	28	
Group	ITa^+	ITa^-	(One-tailed)
Subjects with 2:10a or/and 2:10b	15	9	.016
The rest	11	23	
Group	IT^+	IT^-	(One-tailed)
Subjects with 2:10a or/and 2:10b	21	3	.004
The rest	18	16	
Group	IT^+	IT^-	(Two-tailed)
Subjects with 2:10c or/and 3:	6	8	.048
The rest	33	11	

TABLE 20.4. Disappearance of peripheral person and S-CWT types.

Group	S + C	D + CD	(Two-tailed)
Subjects with 2:32	4	21	.001
The rest	20	13	
Group	Sv	Cv + Dv + CDv	(Two-tailed)
Subjects with 2:32	10	15	.026
The rest	4	29	
Group	Sv	Cv	(Two-tailed)
Subjects with 2:32	10	2	.001
The rest	4	15	
Group	Rad$^+$	Rad$^-$	(Two-tailed)
Subjects with 2:32	17	8	.042
The rest	13	20	

with Sr and Cr. A stronger probability level characterized the correspondence of Dv with WTP, compared with the other three V secondary types. Also in this case, the defense was more often coded in protocols belonging to Rad$^+$ than to Rad$^-$ patterns.

The primary C type was tightly linked with sign 4: (reaction formation); furthermore, Table 20.6 shows that among the R secondary types, the Cr pattern corresponded significantly to the variant 4:10 (H and Pp are doing something together). The most clear-cut evidence of reaction formation (i.e., 4:12: Pp is friendly toward H) was again typical of the primary Cumulative type of adaptation. Furthermore, the most pathological S-CWT pattern (combination of two high secondary Vs) was characterized by the significantly low association with codings of reaction formation.

Among the many variants of introjection and of polymorphous identification listed in the DMT manual, only 7:31 (sex of H changes from correct to incorrect) and 8:71 (age of H below 7) presented significant correspondences with adaptive patterns; they both were clearly more frequently employed by subjects classified as Dissociatives than by subjects with other primary types (see Table 20.7).

TABLE 20.5. Lack of recognition of the threat and S-CWT types.

Group	S + C	D + CD	(Two-tailed)
Subjects with WTP	5	19	.012
The rest	19	15	
Group	Sr + Cr	Dr + CDr	(Two-tailed)
Subjects with WTP	7	17	.012
The rest	22	12	
Group	Dv	Sv + Cv + CDv	(Two-tailed)
Subjects with WTP	11	13	.002
The rest	3	31	
Group	Rad$^+$	Rad$^-$	(Two-tailed)
Subjects with WTP	18	8	.024
The rest	12	20	

TABLE 20.6. Reaction formation and S-CWT types.

Group	C	S + D + CD	(Two-tailed)
Subjects with 4:	9	24	.036
The rest	1	24	
Group	Two high secondary Vs	The rest	(Two-tailed)
Subjects with 4:	4	29	.012
The rest	11	14	
Group	Cr	Sr + Dr + CDr	(Two-tailed)
Subjects with 4:10	6	3	.006
The rest	8	41	
Group	C	S + D + CD	(Two-tailed)
Subjects with 4:12	9	14	.001
The rest	1	34	

Because of the low number of codings of the sensitivity–projection cluster, no information could be obtained about the relationships of these important defenses with S-CWT types. The same was true for the most pathological regression variants; on the other hand, color regression (10:30) was more frequently linked with the CD type than with other primary patterns, and the probability level was strengthened when CD was compared only with S. It may be seen from Table 20.8 that a weak significance signaled a correspondence between CDr and 10:30.

The belated appearance of Pp (BAPP) was more frequently coded in subjects with D or CD, with CDr and with Rad$^+$ types (see Table 20.9). The CDr pattern was found to be clearly linked with the stereotyped repetition of the same defensive variant, especially compared with the Sr type (see Table 20.10).

Last but not least, no one-to-one correspondence between number of defensive scorings and S-CWT types could be ascertained; from Table 20.11 it may be inferred that a very low number of defensive scorings (1 sd below the mean) characterized the DMT protocols of that minority of subjects who were neither Rad$^+$ nor ITa$^+$. Table 20.11 also shows that surprisingly more Ss than CDs had either a very high or a very low number of defensive scores; this was confirmed regarding R-types, for which CDr corresponded to intermediate numbers of scores, whereas Sr was more frequent in the two extreme quartiles. The reverse was true

TABLE 20.7. Introjection variants and Dissociative type.

Group	D	S + C + CD	(Two-tailed)
Subjects with 7:31	10	10	.022
The rest	7	31	
Group	D	S + C + CD	(Two-tailed)
Subjects with 8:71	11	7	.001
The rest	6	34	

TABLE 20.8. Color regression and Cumulative–Dissociative type.

Group	CD	S + C + D	(Two-tailed)
Subjects with 10:30	8	6	.02
The rest	9	35	
Group	CD	S	(Two-tailed)
Subjects with 10:30	8	0	.006
The rest	9	14	
Group	CDr	Sr + Cr + Dr	(Two-tailed)
Subjects with 10:30	8	6	.048
The rest	11	33	

for V-types: here the Cumulative-Dissociatives were significantly more extreme scorers than the Stabilizers.

Discussion

Primary Dissociation (either alone or in conjunction with primary Cumulation) showed the most telling correspondences with types of defense. It was strongly linked with stimulus-distant repression, disappearance of Pp, WTP, and BAPP. The latter three codings share a common formal feature (i.e., the absence of something that ought to be present); this seems to parallel the sudden gaps that characterize the dissociative style. Not all the defense variants with discontinuity features showed this correlation, but probably only for interfering reasons: (a) 2:30 (structure disappears over the whole field) may be due to blinking, is often hardly distinguishable from 2:31 (disappearance of H), and perhaps has no specific meaning when coded in between the very first phases; (b) 2:33a (threat disappears, after having been recognized) is not compatible with WTP, therefore the high ratio of WTP among Ds and CDs automatically lowered the frequency of 233a; and (c) 10:10 (sudden breakdown of stimulus adequacy) was too rare in this nonpsychotic sample.

Although WTP and BAPP are not listed as such in the DMT manual, definitions close to these two codings are included by Kragh among the

TABLE 20.9. Related appearance of peripheral person and S-CWT types.

Group	D + CD	S + C	(Two-tailed)
Subjects with BAPP	19	5	.012
The rest	15	19	
Group	CDr	Sr + Cr + Dr	(Two-tailed)
Subjects with BAPP	12	12	.030
The rest	7	27	
Group	Rad[+]	Rad[−]	(Two-tailed)
Subjects with BAPP	17	7	.022
The rest	13	21	

TABLE 20.10. Stereotyped repetition of the same variant and S-CWT types.

Group	CDr	Sr + Cr + Dr	(Two-tailed)
Subjects with Ster	16	17	.006
The rest	3	22	
Group	CDr	Sr	(Two-tailed)
Subjects with Ster	16	5	.004
The rest	3	10	

variants of isolation (i.e., the typical obsessive–compulsive defense). Present findings suggest a different interpretation of 2:32 and WTP and BAPP (for similar variants, the MCT manual employs the categories of regressive discontinuity and of depressive stereotypy; cf. Smith et al., 1982). Furthermore, the clustering of stimulus-distal repression together with these three codings points toward unexpected conceptual relationships: a common regulative style embraces the transformation of Pp in an inanimate object, the disappearance of Pp, its belated appearance, and its total lack of threatening character. Even more radically, one might wonder what kind of link is the well-known one between primary Dissociation and stimulus-distal (phobic) repression.

The following hypothetical explanation might perhaps be advanced: repression corresponds basically to a disappearance from consciousness of a drive derivative, of a traumatic event, etc., its most typical product being infantile amnesia. In other words, repression is the lack of something that ought to be there. Thus, its affinity to primary Dissociation and

TABLE 20.11. Number of defensive scorings (NDS) and S-CWT types.

Group	ITa$^-$ or/and Rad$^+$	ITa$^-$ and Rad$^-$	(Two-tailed)
Subjects with NDS >35	12	0	.004
Subjects with NDS <10	4	6	
Group	S	CD	(Two-tailed)
Subjects with NDS >35 or <10	9	2	.006
Subjects with intermediate NDS	5	15	
Group	Sr	CDr	(Two-tailed)
Subjects with NDS >35 or <10	8	3	.042
Subjects with intermediate NDS	7	16	
Group	Sv	CDv	(Two-tailed)
Subjects with >35 or <10	2	8	.026
Subjects with intermediate NDS	12	5	

to 2:32, WTP, and BAPP comes under focus; only when displacement is added to repression may a perceptual defense like 1:42 (or for that matter, a phobic symptom) be resorted to. Apart from the concept of deplacement, reports of 1:42, with their distance from the real stimulus, suggest an element of overimagination that reminds one of what Smith and Klein (1953) observed about the Dissociative style: ". . . another property of the D style which was only vaguely implied before, namely, that Ds are more autistically disposed than are Cs and Ss; i.e., at least intermittently they lean less upon objective supports or cues."

When attention is shifted from the correspondences between 2:32, WTP and BAPP, and primary Dissociation to those between these defenses and the secondary Vs, interesting differences appear: (a) disappearance of Pp is typical of the Sv pattern (!) and does not correspond to any R-type; (b) WTP strongly characterizes the Dv pattern and is significantly linked with Dr and CDr and with the concomitance of two high secondary Vs; and (c) BAPP has no correspondence with V-types and is more frequent among subjects of the CDr type. Thus, WTP is a superdissociative defense, while 2:32 is a dissociative defense on a more superficial level, being an antidissociative strategy on the deeper, secondary level, and BAPP lies midway between 2:32 and WTP on a continuum of dissociation. Clearly, from present findings, WTP may be considered to be the most pathological type of defense evidenced in the DMT. Unfortunately, it is unclear to which defense mechanism observable in the psychoanalytic situation the WTP might refer. Perhaps to denial (as distinguished from negation)? The "lack of something that ought to be there" could be thought of as a defensive strategy, with varying degrees of gravity, from the waiving of a wish or emotion, to the waiving of simple or complex memories, up to the waiving of parts of current external reality (see Fenichel, 1945). We hypothesize that this progression from repression to true denial may correspond to the escalation from primary dissociation without accompanying secondary dissociation, toward concomitant primary, R-, and V-dissociation. While the foregoing considerations are equally valid for the primary types D and CD, two variants of introjection/identification characterized type D per se: change of sex of H from correct to incorrect (7:31) and very low age of H (8:71). The instability of identity inherent in these codings is well in accordance with primary Dissociation, but perhaps the surprisingly strong link between D type and 8:71 also deserves closer attention, because 8:71 is a poorly considered variant. The assumption of earlier roles, to escape the dangers connected with more advanced conflicts is perhaps the natural counterpart of the danger of stepping backwards, which lies at the heart of primary Dissociation in its purest form (D type).

As predicted, the CD type was significantly connected with color regression, that is, with the trend toward faulty reality testing; this finding provides a validation for one of the most "psychotic" DMT defenses.

However, the link between 10:30 and CDr barely reached significance, and there was no significant correspondence of 10:30 with Dv, CDv, or two concomitant high secondary Vs; the poor significance of color regression on the level of secondary Dissociation indicates perhaps a circumscribed, temporary meaning of this perceptual sign of ego regression. The cluster of "compulsive" defenses was found to be clearly divided into codings associated with IT^+ (barrier isolation) and codings associated with Cumulation (reaction formation). The very low rate of reports coded for reaction formation among subjects with two high secondary Vs confirms that this defense (and especially its strong variant, 4:12) is the prototype of the C style, to be opposed to the dissociative defenses discussed above. The IT^+, being a type of adaptation "stamped by attempts at a sudden pseudo-objective mastery of reality" (Nyman & Smith, 1961), seems to be well in accord with a defense like barrier isolation, which does not directly alter the disturbing percept but grants a safe distance from the threat. It is less easy to grasp the common grounds between C type and reaction formation, even if the anxious, rigid overcontrol and the highly structured, actively defensive style reflected in cumulative patterns seem to share formal features with the reaction formation strategy. In the clinical S-CWT literature, IT^+ (especially ITa^+) has been most frequently bound to the obsessive–compulsive personality, while the C type has been described as typical of "subjects with symptoms of anxiety coupled with averting defenses against insight" (Nyman & Smith, 1961).

The conceptual and ontogenetic closeness between "turning away of the threat," barrier isolation, intellectualization, and negation (MCT codings roughly corresponding respectively to 2:10c, 2:10a, 2:10b, and 3: in the DMT) was suggested by Smith and Danielsson (1982, p. 44); present findings draw attention to an unpredicted stylistic opposition of turning away of the threat and negation (IT^-) versus barrier isolation and intellectualization (IT^+). The much higher frequency of stereotyped repetitions of the same coding among subjects of the CDr type confirms the usefulness of this R-type as a signal of extreme rigidity and defective functioning (Smith et al., 1982, pp. 48–49) but indicates that Cr and CD rare not wholly overlapping patterns, as they have been frequently considered.

Unexpectedly, the Rad^+ type corresponded to the "dissociative" defenses (1:42, 2:32, WTP, and BAPP); one way to make sense of this convergence between Dissociation and Rad^+ is to realize that the latter represents the opposite of a Cumulation of initial times.

Types derived from initial times were the only ones with significant relationships with the very high number of defensive scorings (ITa^+ or/and Rad^+) and with the very low NDS (ITa^- or/and Rad^-). Lacking any difference on these variables between Stabilizers and other types, it is impossible to decide whether it is more adaptive to have many or few defenses. On the other hand, it could be expected that it is more adaptive to have an intermediate NDS than one of the two extreme NDS forms; but on this issue both primary and R-Stabilizers were strangely more extreme scorers than their CD counterparts—a finding that remains in search of a reasonable explanation and is partially counterbalanced by the higher frequency of extreme scorers among CDv than among Sv.

The complex and sometimes surprising relationships between patterns of adaptation to interference and DMT defenses reported here seem to support the heuristicity of studying defense mechanisms and strategies on the background of the tradition of "cognitive controls." It may be added that only a part of S-CWT information was exploited in this chapter, inasmuch as a more detailed study should have considered the relationships among defense variables and combinations of primary, secondary, and initial S-CWT patterns; very large numbers of subjects are obviously needed for the latter research purpose.

Acknowledgment. The research presented in this chapter has been supported by the Italian National Research Council.

References

Almgren, P.E. (1980) Die Beziehungen zwischen Abwehrformen in der Meta-Contrast-Technik und verschiedenen Anpassungsstilen in zwei serialen Wahrnemungstests [The relationships between forms of defense in the MCT and different styles of adaptation in two serial perceptual tests]. In U. Hentschel & G.J.W. Smith (Eds), *Experimentelle Persönlichkeitspsychologie* [Experimental personality psychology] (pp. 94–106). Wiesbaden: Akademische Verlagsgesellschaft.

Andersson, A.L. (1967) Adaptive visual aftereffect processes as related to patterns of color-word interference serials. *Perceptual and Motor Skills, 25,* 437–453.

Andersson, A.L. & Bengtsson M. (1985) Perceptgenetic defenses against anxiety and a threatened sense of self as seen in terms of the Spiral Aftereffect Technique. *Scandinavian Journal of Psychology, 26,* 123–139.

Andersson, A.L. & Weikert, C. (1974) Adult defensive organization as related to adaptive regulation of spiral aftereffect duration. *Social Behavior and Personality, 2,* 56–75.

Andersson, A.L., Nilsson, A., Ruuth, E., & Smith, G.J.W. (1972) *Visual aftereffects and the individual as an adaptive system.* Lund: Gleerups.

Fenichel, O. (1945) *The psychoanalytical theory of neurosis.* New York: Norton.

Kragh, U. (1985) *DMT Manual.* Stockholm: Persona.

Kragh, U. & Smith, G.J.W. (1970) *Percept-genetic analysis.* Lund: Gleerups.

Nyman, G.E. & Smith, G.J.W. (1961) Experimental differentiation of clinical syndromes within a sample of young neurotics. *Acta Psychiatrica Neurologica Scandinavica, 37,* 14–31.

Rubino, I.A., Grasso, S., & Pezzarossa, B. (1990) Microgenetic patterns of adaptation on the Stroop task by patients with bronchial asthma and duodenal peptic ulcer. *Perceptual and Motor Skills, 71*, 19–31.

Smith, G.J.W. & Danielsson, A. (1982) Anxiety and defensive strategies in childhood and adolescence. *Psychological Issues*, No. 52. Madison, CT: International Universities Press.

Smith, G.J.W. & Klein, G. (1953) Cognitive controls in serial behavior patterns. *Journal of Personality, 22*, 188–213.

Smith, G.J.W., Johnson, G., & Almgren, P.E. (1982) *MCT—Metakontrasttekniken. Manual* [Manual of the Meta-Contrast Technique]. Stockholm: Psykologiförlaget.

Smith, G.J.W., Nilsson, L., & Johnson, G. (1964) Differentiation of character neurosis and symptom neurosis on the basis of differences between two serial experiments. *Scandinavian Journal of Psychology, 5*, 234–238.

Smith, G.J.W., Nyman, G.E., & Hentschel, U. (1986) *Manual till CWT-Serialtfärgordtest* [Manual of the Serial Color-Word Test]. Stockholm: Psykologiförlaget.

Stroop, J.R. (1935) Studies of interference in serial verbal reactions. *Journal of Experimental Psychology, 18*, 643–661.

Westerlundh, B. (1983), Personal organization of the visual field: A study of ambient to focal reports of threatening stimuli. *Archives of Psychology, 135*, 17–35.

21
Change in Defense Mechanisms Following Intensive Treatment, As Related to Personality Organization and Gender

PHEBE CRAMER and SIDNEY J. BLATT

In this chapter we discuss how defense mechanisms change following intensive treatment and show how different defense mechanisms are related to gender and personality organization in psychiatric patients. In a large-scale study of psychological change following intensive treatment, Blatt, Ford, Berman, Cook, and Meyer (1988) found it useful to differentiate between the anaclitic and the introjective personality configurations. According to theory, there are two parallel developmental lines in personality development (Blatt & Shichman, 1983). One of these—the anaclitic—relates to the development of stable, mutually satisfying interpersonal relationships. The other—the introjective—is concerned with the development of a stable, realistic, and positive self-identity. These two lines interact throughout the course of development. Various forms of psychopathology have been conceptualized as an over-emphasis and exaggeration of one of these developmental lines at the expense of the other. Thus, psychiatric patients with an anaclitic personality configuration (e.g., the infantile personality of a hysteric character) show an excessive and distorted preoccupation with establishing satisfying interpersonal relationships and a corresponding neglect of development of self. Patients with an introjective personality configuration (e.g., paranoid, obsessive–compulsive, guilty depression) manifest a peremptory and distorted concern around establishing and maintaining a consolidated definition of self, and a corresponding neglect of establishing meaningful interpersonal relationships. Recent findings (Blatt et al., 1988) indicate that these two groups of patients change in different ways during long-term, individual treatment.

The anaclitic and introjective personality configurations have also been characterized as using different defense mechanisms (Blatt & Shichman, 1983; Cramer, Blatt, & Ford, 1988). Anaclitic defenses are primarily avoidance maneuvers—denial, repression, and displacement. Their aim is to maintain interpersonal relationships, while neglecting the development of self. Introjective defenses, on the other hand, are primarily counteractive, including projection and externalization, aiming to protect and preserve the self, while neglecting the establishment of satisfying interpersonal relationships.

The study of anaclitic and introjective personality configurations also indicates a significant relationship to gender (Blatt et al., 1988). Within a sample of 90 patients, for example, the majority of those clinically rated anaclitic were female, while the majority of the patients rated introjective were male. This result is consistent with gender stereotypes: females are typically described as being more concerned with and oriented toward affiliation, while males are described as being more concerned with personal autonomy and achievement (e.g., Blatt & Shichman, 1983; Gilligan, 1982). It appears, then, that developmental demands, cultural stereotypes, and perhaps biological predispositions contribute to an increased proclivity for females to focus more on the anaclitic developmental line, while males more often focus on the introjective line of development. Defense mechanisms, also, have been found to be gender-related. Consistently, denial has been found to be a "female defense," while projection is characteristically used more often by males (see Cramer, 1991). Thus, in predicting that anaclitic patients will use more avoidant defenses such as denial, it may be important to consider that denial is more typically a female defense. Anaclitic males may not utilize denial as fully. Likewise, in predicting that introjective patients will be higher on counteractive defenses such as projection, it may be important to note that projection is a male defense; introjective females may not use projection as fully as introjective males.

If, in fact, there is a congruence among the anaclitic/introjective configuration, defense use, and gender, it becomes interesting to compare gender-congruent and gender-incongruent individuals. It is important to determine whether male anaclitics' and female introjectives' defense use is determined more by gender, by the anaclitic/introjective personality configuration, or by some interaction of the two. It is equally important to determine whether these gender-incongruent patients experience more conflict and thus manifest greater defensiveness than their gender-consistent counterparts (female anaclitics and male introjectives).

Several studies have indicated that defense use is a function both of gender and of sexual orientation and that cross-gender role orientation or sexual identity is related to cross-gender use of defenses (e.g., Cramer, 1988; Cramer & Carter, 1978; Evans, 1982). Thus it seems likely that gender would interact with a gender-linked personality configuration in determining defense use. Moreover, one might expect different patterns of change in defense use following intensive treatment for patients whose predominant developmental preoccupations are congruent with their gender, as compared with patients whose predominant preoccupations are gender incongruent. It is the purpose of the present research to investigate these questions.

Method

Subjects

The 90 subjects in this study were inpatients (mean age = 21 years, range 18–29 years; 45 women, 45 men) admitted to a small, long-term, intensive, open, psychoanalytically oriented treatment facility. Approximately 30% of the sample were considered to be psychotic, 10% severely neurotic or depressed, and the remaining 60% severe character or borderline personality disorder. A full description of the background variables for this sample and method of diagnosis has been provided elsewhere (Blatt et al., 1988; Cramer et al., 1988).

All 90 patients were evaluated 6 weeks after admission and a detailed case record was prepared, including family background, developmental history, initial course in hospital, and psychodynamic formulation. A second detailed case record was prepared following an average of approximately 15 months of intensive treatment. At the same two times in the hospitalization, the patients were given an extensive psychological assessment battery. The study of these independently established clinical case records and psychological test protocols has provided information about the nature of change of these patients in the treatment process (Blatt et al., 1988).

On the basis of material available from the admission case records, two experienced judges separated the 90 patients into 42 considered to have a primarily anaclitic personality configuration and 48 who were considered to have a primarily introjective organization. Interrater reliability, based on a subset of 18 cases, was quite high, with the judges agreeing on 17 of the 18 cases. The anaclitic and introjective patients did not differ from one another on a large number of background and demographic variables, except for sex, as mentioned earlier (cf. Blatt et al., 1988).

Measures

From the material available at admission (time 1) and following, on average, 15 months of treatment (time 2), measures assessing the use of defense mechanisms, clinical symptoms, and interpersonal behavior were obtained. Information available in the case records provided the basis for two judges to rate the presence of clinical symptoms and the nature of the patients' interpersonal behaviors, using the rating scales described below. The case records of each patient at time 1 and at time 2 were scored by a different judge, each without knowledge of the other's ratings.

Information available from the Thematic Apperception Test (TAT) provided the basis for the assessment of defense mechanisms. These test data were scored by a judge who had no knowledge of the case record, including the patient's gender and anaclitic/introjective designation. In addition, the judge had no way of identifying whether a TAT protocol was from time 1 or time 2.

Defense Mechanisms

The use of the defenses of denial, projection, and identification was assessed from the patients' responses to three TAT cards (1, 14, and 13MF), administered both at time 1 and at time 2, according to a method developed by Cramer (1991). The categories of defense and example stories have been discussed, and adequate interrater reliability has been established on the present sample and numerous other samples (Cramer, 1991; Cramer et al., 1988). Change in defense use was determined by subtracting time 1 from time 2 scores.

Clinical Symptoms

From the detailed case records described earlier, judges rated the presence or absence, and severity, of 32 symptoms, using procedures developed by Strauss and Harder (1981). Interrater reliability was adequate (item alpha > .65). On the basis of previous work (Cramer et al., 1988), only the Bizarre-Disorganized scale was used. Symptoms rated included incomprehensibility, unkempt appearance, bizarre behavior, and labile affect. Change in symptoms was determined by subtracting time 1 from time 2 scores.

Interpersonal Behavior

Information in the case records regarding the patients' daily interactions with other patients and staff were used to rate interpersonal behavior, using a procedure developed by Fairweather et al. (1960). A high score is indicative of poor interpersonal relations. The two judges using this Fairweather Ward Behavior scale achieved an acceptable level of inter-rater reliability (item alpha > .65). Interpersonal behavior was also rated on five scales developed as part of the Menninger Psychotherapy Research Project (Harty, 1976). Based on a factor analysis, a summary measure, Menninger Factor I, was developed. This measure consisted of an assessment of the patient's motivation for treatment, the capacity for subliminatory activity, the quality of object relations, and the degree of superego integration. A high score on this measure is indicative of good personal relations. For each patient, scores on the Fairweather scale and on the Menninger Factor I scale were available for time 1 and time 2. Change in interpersonal behavior was determined by subtracting time 1 from time 2 scores.

Results

The Relationships Among Anaclitic/Introjective Personality Organization, Gender, and Defense Use

The defense scores obtained at time 1 were analyzed by a three-way analysis of variance (ANOVA): anaclitic/introjective (2) × gender (2) × defense (3), with the last variable a repeated measure (see Table 21.1). The results indicated a significant interaction between anaclitic/introjective group and gender, $F(1,86) = 8.73$, $p < .004$. Mean comparisons indicated that at time 1, anaclitic males had higher total defense scores than both anaclitic females, $t(40) = 3.27$, $p < .002$, and introjective males, $t(43) = 1.93$, $p < .06$. Furthermore, introjective females had higher total defense scores than anaclitic females, $t(43) = 2.41$, $p < .02$. Moreover, although the three-way interaction was not significant, planned comparisons indicated that the anaclitic males scored significantly higher on identification than did the introjective males, $t(43) = 2.58$, $p < .01$, and somewhat higher than anaclitic females, $t(40) = 1.84$, $p < .07$. Also, anaclitic males scored somewhat higher on denial than did anaclitic females, $t(40) = 1.66$, $p < .10$. Furthermore, introjective females, introjective males, and anaclitic males all had higher projection scores than anaclitic females, $t(43, 57, \text{ and } 40) = 2.26$, 1.94, and 2.60, $p < .03$, $.06$, and $.01$, respectively.

A similar ANOVA for the defense scores at time 2 indicated a significant interaction between anaclitic/introjective group and gender, $F(1,86) = 5.69$, $p < .02$. Again, anaclitic males had higher total defense scores

TABLE 21.1. Defense scores at time 1 and time 2 (T1, T2) for anaclitic and introjective male and female patients.

	Denial Mean (sd)		Projection Mean (sd)		Identification Mean (sd)		Total Mean (sd)	
Anaclitic males (N = 14)								
T1	2.64	(3.88)	3.14	(2.41)	3.21	(2.61)	9.00	(5.79)
T2	1.93	(1.59)	3.50	(3.06)	1.79	(1.58)	7.21	(4.41)
Introjective males (N = 31)								
T1	2.16	(1.86)	2.48	(2.03)	1.71	(1.32)	6.35	(3.38)
T2	1.16	(1.39)	1.87	(1.33)	1.84	(1.66)	4.87	(2.32)
Anaclitic females (N = 28)								
T1	1.32	(1.22)	1.57	(1.50)	2.04	(1.55)	4.93	(2.31)
T2	1.46	(1.29)	1.36	(1.70)	1.96	(1.82)	4.79	(3.01)
Introjective females (N = 17)								
T1	2.00	(1.94)	2.94	(2.58)	2.12	(1.05)	7.06	(3.63)
T2	2.35	(2.15)	1.94	(2.11)	1.53	(.87)	5.82	(3.64)

than anaclitic females, $t(40) = 2.10$, $p < .04$. In addition, the anaclitic/introjective group $\times$ gender $\times$ defense interaction was significant, $F(2,172) = 3.84$, $p < .02$. At time 2, anaclitic males used significantly more of the male-typed defense of projection than did anaclitic females, $t(40) = 2.93$, $p < .006$ or introjective males, $t(42) = 2.51$, $p < .02$. Also introjective females used more of the female-typed defense of denial than did Introjective males, $t(46) = 2.33$, $p < .02$ and somewhat more than anaclitic females, $t(43) = 1.74$, $p < .09$.

Change in Defenses Following Treatment

To assess changes in the use of defense mechanisms following 15 months of intensive treatment, the defense scores were analyzed by a four-way ANOVA: anaclitic/introjective (2) $\times$ gender (2) $\times$ time (2) $\times$ defense (3), with the last two variables as repeated measures (see Table 21.1). The results indicated a significant decrease in total defense use from time 1 to time 2, $F(1,86) = 5.19$, $p < .02$. There was also a significant main effect for gender, $F(1,86) = 4.62$, $p < .03$, which is best understood in terms of the highly significant interaction between anaclitic/introjective group and gender, $F(1,86) = 13.09$, $p < .0005$. As indicated in Table 21.1, the gender-incongruent patients, anaclitic males and introjective females, had higher total defense scores at both time 1 and time 2. The time $\times$ defense $\times$ gender interaction approached significance, $F(2,172) = 2.58$, $p < .08$, indicating that male patients showed a significant decrease in denial from time 1 to time 2, $t(44) = 2.14$, $p < .04$. Although the four-way interaction was not significant, $F(2,172) = 2.03$, $p < .14$, planned comparisons for the gender-incongruent groups (anaclitic males and introjective females), indicated a significant decrease in identification scores from time 1 to time 2, $t(13, 16) = 2.22$ and 2.42, $p < .05$, respectively. Also, male introjectives decreased their use of denial, $t(30) = 3.70$, $p < .001$.

This overall analysis indicated significant decreases in defense use after 15 months of intensive treatment. Moreover, gender-incongruent patients showed significant decreases in the use of identification, while male patients showed a significant decrease in the female-typed defense of denial.

The Relationship Between Change in Defense Scores and Change in Psychiatric Symptoms

Changes in defense scores from time 1 to time 2 were correlated with changes on the Strauss–Harder bizarre–disorganized symptom scale (see Tables 21.2 and 21.3). In three of the four patient groups, change in total defense use was positively correlated with changes on the symptom scale: anaclitic females, $r = .56$, $p < .001$; anaclitic males, $r = .55$, $p < .02$;

TABLE 21.2. Symptom and interpersonal behavior ratings time 1 and time 2 (T1, T2) for anaclitic and introjective, male and female patients.

	Straus–Harder bizarre–disorganized[a] Mean (sd)		Fairweather Mean (sd)		Menninger Factor I[a] Mean (sd)	
Anaclitic males (N = 14)						
T1	−.37	(0.95)	1.35	(0.25)	−1.44	(2.69)
T2	.20	(1.25)	1.16	(0.39)	0.14	(2.77)
Introjective males (N = 31)						
T1	−.12	(0.96)	1.34	(0.20)	−1.22	(2.68)
T2	−.42	(0.70)	1.14	(0.54)	1.12	(3.67)
Anaclitic females (N = 28)						
T1	.26	(1.01)	1.28	(0.22)	−0.90	(2.74)
T2	.38	(1.00)	1.34	(0.27)	0.20	(3.04)
Introjective females (N = 17)						
T1	.09	(1.27)	1.32	(0.23)	−0.42	(2.51)
T2	−.01	(0.78)	1.19	(0.38)	2.82	(4.68)

[a] Standarized scores.

introjective males, $r = .36$, $p < .02$ (one-tailed values). The correlation for the introjective females, however, was not significant. The correlations between the change scores (time 1 minus time 2) of the individual defenses of denial, projection, and identification and the Strauss–Harder bizarre-disorganized scale are presented in Table 21.3. For anaclitic females, changes in denial were positively correlated with changes in bizarre–disorganized behavior ($r = .47$, $p < .006$). For introjective males, a decrease in projection was associated with a decrease in bizarre–disorganized behavior ($r = .32$, $p < .04$). Also, for anaclitic and introjective females, changes in identification were positively related to changes in bizarre–disorganized scores ($r = .42$, $p < .01$ and $.05$, respectively).

The Relationship Between Change in Defense Scores and Change in Interpersonal Relationships

The correlations between changes in defense scores and changes on the interpersonal behavior rating scales (see Table 21.2) are presented in Table 21.3. For the gender-congruent patients (anaclitic females, introjective males), an increase in identification was associated with an improvement in interpersonal relationships. For anaclitic females, an increase in identification was correlated with an improvement in the Fairweather Ward Behavior scale ($r = -.33$, $p < .04$). For introjective males, change in identification was significantly correlated with change on the Menninger Factor I scale ($r = .31$, $p < .05$). On the other hand, for gender-incongruent patients, a decrease in identification was associated with improvement in interpersonal relationships. For anaclitic males, a decrease in identification was correlated with a decrease in the Fairweather scale (better interpersonal functioning) ($r = .54$, $p < .02$). For introjective females, there was a tendency for a decrease in identification to be correlated with an increase in the Menninger Factor I scale ($r = -.31$, $p < .11$). Also, for male patients, a decrease in the use of projection was related to an increased capacity for interpersonal relations, as seen in the correlation with lower Fairweather scores (better interpersonal functioning): introjective males, $r = .47$, $p < .004$; anaclitic males, $r = .41$, $p < .07$. Finally, for anaclitic males, a decrease in denial was associated with an increase on the Menninger Factor I scale ($r = -.46$, $p < .05$) (better interpersonal functioning).

Discussion

The results of this study show that following approximately one year of treatment, patients decreased in their overall use of defenses, and

TABLE 21.3. Correlations between changes in defense scores, bizarre–disorganized symptoms, and interpersonal behavior scales.

	Bizarre–disorganized	Fairweather	Menninger Factor I
Anaclitic males			
(N = 14)			
Denial	.43	−.10	−.46*
Projection	.27	.41	.04
Identification	.22	.54*	.23
Introjective males			
(N = 31)			
Denial	.23	−.16	−.01
Projection	.32*	.47**	−.03
Identification	.18	−.06	.31*
Anaclitic females			
(N = 28)			
Denial	.47**	.06	.03
Projection	.26	−.13	−.20
Identification	.42**	−.33*	−.06
Introjective females			
(N = 17)			
Denial	.33	.13	.10
Projection	−.23	−.16	.30
Identification	.42*	.16	−.31

NOTE: *$p < .05$, **$p < .01$.

this decrease was significantly correlated with a decrease in bizarre—disorganized symptoms in three of four patient groups. The measurement of defenses expressed in TAT stories also revealed significant differences between anaclitic and introjective patients, but as a function of gender. Patients with a gender-incongruent personality organization (introjective females, anaclitic males) had significantly higher total defense scores than gender-congruent patients (anaclitic females, introjective males). This finding supports our prediction that gender-incongruent patients would experience more conflict than gender-congruent patients. The importance of the issue of identity, as indicated by the significant decrease in the use of identification in gender-incongruent patients from time 1 to time 2, suggests that the conflict may be related to the unsatisfactory nature of their initial identification.

The findings also indicate that at the time of admission to the hospital, gender-incongruent patients utilized defenses that are consistent with their opposite gender. Accordingly, anaclitic males showed a tendency to use more denial (a feminine defense) than anaclitic females, and introjective females used more projection (a masculine defense) than anaclitic females. However, at time 2, gender-incongruent patients used more gender-consistent defenses: anaclitic males used more projection than anaclitic females or introjective males, while introjective females used more denial than introjective males or anaclitic females. Thus, after a year or so of treatment, those gender-incongruent patients shifted from gender-incongruent to gender-congruent defenses, consistent with the interpretation that the decrease from time 1 to time 2 in the identification scores of gender-incongruent patients reflects at least a partial discarding of a conflicted, inappropriate identity. The results also show that the significant changes in level of defense use were related to changes in clinical symptomatology and interpersonal relations, and that these relationships differed as a function of gender and anaclitic/introjective personality organization. For gender-incongruent anaclitic males, the significant decrease in the use of identification was associated with better interpersonal relations (Fairweather). The significant increase among anaclitic males in the gender-congruent defense of projection was associated with poorer interpersonal relations (Fairweather). Although the decrease in the anaclitic males' use of denial was not statistically significant, it was related significantly to improved interpersonal functioning (Menninger Factor I).

For introjective males, negative changes in the use of projection were related to decreases in clinical symptoms and better interpersonal relations (Fairweather). Also, positive changes in use of identification in this gender-congruent patient group were associated with improvement in interpersonal relations (Menninger Factor I). Among the anaclitic females, negative changes in the use of denial were related to decreases in clinical symptoms. Again, in this gender-congruent group, positive changes in the use of identification were associated with improved interpersonal relations (Fairweather). However, they were also associated with an increase in psychiatric symptoms. Finally, among gender-incongruent introjective females, the significant decrease in the use of identification was related to a decrease in psychiatric symptoms and improved interpersonal relations (Menninger Factor I). The significant increase in the use of denial was not associated with changes in the other variables.

These findings may be summarized as follows: an increase in identification among gender-congruent patients, but a decrease in identification among gender-incongruent patients, was generally related to better psychological functioning. Moreover, an increase in gender-congruent defenses among gender-incongruent patients was related to psychological improvement, while a decrease in gender-congruent defenses among gender-congruent patients was related to psychological improvement. Finally, for male patients, a decrease in the gender-incongruent defense of denial was related to improved functioning.

Two points are made in closing. First, investigations of personality variables must consider the issue of whether the variables are gender congruent or incongruent, which in the present study produced opposite effects on the manifestations of defense mechanisms. Second, the defense measure of identification, when used with individuals experiencing extreme disturbance, should be interpreted cautiously: high scores on identification may be indicative of a primitive, pathological identification that interferes with normal development, rather than indicating psychological strength.

References

Blatt, S.J., Ford, R.Q., Berman, W.R., Cook, B., & Meyer, R. (1988) The assessment of change during the intensive treatment of borderline and schizophrenic young adults. *Psychoanalytic Psychology*, *5*, 127–158.

Blatt, S.J. & Shichman, S. (1983) Two primary configurations of psychopathology. *Psychoanalysis and Contemporary Thought*, *6*, 187–254.

Cramer, P. (1988) The Defense Mechanism Inventory: A review of research and discussion of the scales. *Journal of Personality Assessment*, *52*, 142–164.

Cramer, P. (1991) *The development of defense mechanisms: Theory, research, and assessment*. New York: Springer Verlag.

Cramer, P., Blatt, S.J., & Ford, R.Q. (1988) Defense mechanisms in the anaclitic and introjective personality configuration. *Journal of Consulting and Clinical Psychology*, *56*, 610–616.

Cramer, P. & Carter, T. (1978) The relationship between sexual identification and the use of defense mechanisms. *Journal of Personality Assessment*, *42*, 63–73.

Fairweather, G., Simon, R., Gebhard, M., Weingarter, E., Holland, J., Sanders, R., Stone, C., & Reahl, J. (1960) Relative effectiveness of psychotherapeutic programs: A multicriteria comparison of four programs for three different patient groups. *Psychological Monographs, 74*(5, Whole No. 492).

Evans, R.G. (1982) Defense mechanisms in females as a function of sex-role orientation. *Journal of Clinical Psychology, 38,* 816–817.

Gilligan, C. (1982) *In a different voice.* Cambridge, MA: Harvard University Press.

Harty, M. (1976) A program to evaluate intensive psychiatric hospital treatment. *Journal of the National Association of Private Psychiatric Hospitals, 8,* 3.

Strauss, J.S. & Harder, D.W. (1981) The Case Record Rating Scale: A method for rating symptom and social function data from case records. *Psychology Research, 4,* 333–345.

22
Defense Mechanisms in Interaction with Intellectual Performance in Depressive Inpatients

Uwe Hentschel, Manfred Kießling, Heidi Teubner-Berg, and Herbert Dreier

Moodswings are an experience common to everyone, and to this experience also belong downward swings. Thus based on this common experience, diagnosing a depression should not be a major problem. A depressed mood is, however, very different from the clinical state of depression (cf. Willner, 1985), and here the criteria for a reliable diagnosis cannot always be derived from self-experience. In spite of a strong opposition to regarding psychiatric symptoms exclusively from a positivistic medical or biological point of view (Foucault, 1967; Szasz, 1972), there is a need for reliable diagnosis. Even if one does not adhere to Cattell's (1940) statement that nosology necessarily precedes etiology, the necessity of diagnosis is obvious when it comes to the evaluation of treatment, be it by psychopharmacopoeia or psychotherapy.

Without knowing the specific condition of the group who gets a specific treatment, the effects of such treatment cannot be assessed. The similarity of the phenomena related to depression, at least as it expresses itself in the Western world, has made it possible to derive a number of definitions with pretty much the same elements. Although since the introduction of the DSM in 1952 to DSM III-R, the diagnostic system as a whole as well as many categories have been changed, the core definition of depression remained rather stable. In 1968, for example, it was defined in a global form as "an emotional state with retardation of psychomotor and thought processes, a depressive emotional reaction, feelings of guilt or criticism and delusion of unworthiness" (American Psychiatric Association, 1968, p. 36). Also a broader list of symptoms connected with it is not so difficult to agree upon (cf. Table 22.1).

The problem here is rather that not all symptoms are exclusively related to depression, but that they show considerable overlap with other illnesses (cf. Clare & Blacker, 1986), as, for example, in the Chronic Fatigue Syndrome. Powell, Dolan, and Wessely (1990) could show that attribution of the illness and self-esteem can be used as differential diagnostic criteria, with true depressives showing more self-blame and lower self-esteem, together with an internal, stable, and global attri-

TABLE 22.1. List of typical symptoms of depressive disorders.

Dysphoric, apathetic mood
Negative self-image, hopelessness, anxieties
Feelings of shame and guilt
Social withdrawal
Suicidal thoughts
Somatic symptoms like:
Sleep difficulties
Loss of appetite
Loss of libido
Fatigue
Difficulties in concentration, loss of interest

SOURCE: Based on diagnostic criteria and evidence from empirical studies (cf. Brown & Haris, 1978; Feighner et al., 1972; Hentschel et al., 1976).

bution style characteristic for the helplessness–hopelessness syndrome (Abramson, Seligman, & Teasdale, 1978). This is at the same time, again, a good example of the need for a good diagnostic classification, since the two illnesses require different treatments. In the literature the relations of depression and pain also are discussed in many ways. Supported by empirical results, one possible conclusion is that pain could be a substitute for depression (Ahrens & Lamparter, 1989). Severe states of depression, on the other hand, seem to a large degree to exclude pain feelings (von Auersperg, 1963).

By extending the differential diagnostic endeavor, it should be possible also to diagnose different forms of depression. Differences to be considered here concern forms like unipolar–bipolar, primary–secondary, and endogenous–reactive. For a differential diagnosis of endogenous versus neurotic depression, the psychopathologic phenomena alone are not sufficient (Hentschel, Schubö, & von Zerssen, 1976; Schubö, Hentschel, von Zerssen, & Mombour, 1975).

One could say that the general agreement is quite good as long as the diagnostic endeavors are restricted to a phenomenological level and that it is considerably lower or even absent when it comes to attempts to explain the reasons for depression. Is it better understandable in purely behavioral terms, as a change in behavior frequencies, where avoidance and escape are augmented and other activities reduced (Ferster, 1974)? Are the purely cognitive and attributional variables the central ones that lead to a negative view of oneself and the outer world and the future, or is an approach that uses a combination of behavior and cognition like the revised learned helplessness–hopelessness theory the most appropriate? Or should an explanation comprise even more person-related aspects and elements from the personal history, like the psychoanalytic explanation for depression, focusing on the lack of narcissistic supplies and the struggle of an orally fixated person against an introjected ambivalent or unconsciously hated object (Fenichel, 1946)?

The differences in the theoretical explanations of the same phenomena are striking, but nevertheless probably would not have evoked so much attention if they were not linked with different approaches of treatment.

For several reasons, however, theory testing seems to be more promising in the field of diagnostics than in the field of treatment. Even here there are no clear-cut criteria for the best approach if one does not look for parsimony alone, for example. Moreover, within all the basic approaches—the behavioral, the cognitive, and the psychoanalytic—there are different points of view and changing concepts over time, with the result that it is not easy to define some generally acceptable requirements for a criterion-related validity test, but still it is easier here than in treatment, where other sets of variables are added.

Because this book is concerned with defense mechanisms, the reader may have guessed that our preference goes to the psychodynamic approach, in spite of its greater complexity, which covers implicit elements like developmental stages, with sensible phases, fixation to the oral stage due to some trauma, and a later regression to this stage following a similarly frustrating critical event, finally resulting in a structural conflict in the patient.

None of these assumptions could be tested in our study, but the concept of defense mechanisms is related to the structural conflict concept and covers a dynamic aspect that reaches farther than a mere phenomenological classification. Not too much is known about how and when certain defense mechanisms are "learned." Their basic roots may be inherited. Empirical studies show, however, that this development is embedded in the general cognitive and emotional development (Smith & Danielsson, 1980), so that theoretical links also are probable to other elements of the psychoanalytic view of depression, the elaboration of which is beyond the scope of this chapter. Here a more straightforward line is followed by referring to the general psychological impact of the concept of defense mechanisms (i.e., their reality relatedness). If one accepts the idea of putting defenses together in one dimension from immature to mature (Vaillant, 1974), including the concept of coping mechanisms, then all defense mechanisms at the lower immature end of this dimension should lead to a distortion of objective perception of reality. This is not true for the mature mechanisms like humor and sublimation, where something is added and/or transformed: Arieti (1976) speaks here of the magic synthesis of primary and secondary process thinking. At the lower (immature) end of the dimension, however, something is lacking (e.g., in repression, denial, regression, isolation) or transformed in such a way (reaction formation, turning against the self, projection) that an objective perception becomes impossible.

Psychoanalysis has never stated that there is a point-to-point relation between the diagnosis of symptoms on the one hand and defense mechanisms on the other, but it was always assumed that symptoms and diagnoses and clusters of defense would show some relation (A. Freud, 1936/1946).

In fact, explaining the resulting symptoms as a compromise in the structural conflict between the ego and the id or the superego, mediated by the functional construct of defense mechanisms, has added very much to a psychodynamic understanding of the psychic illnesses for which a basic phenomenological diagnostic system (Kraepelin, 1896) had already been created without the influence of psychoanalysis. Thus the assessment of defense mechanisms has an additional diagnostic value.

We wanted to regard defenses in relation to a field of reality-related performance (i.e., intellectual functioning). The basic hypothesis of our study was that depressive patients, in comparison to a control group, should show another pattern of intellectual functioning and defense mechanisms, that is, in a more concrete formulation, they would show a worse intellectual performance in interaction with more signs of defense. Originally, we wanted to test this with a mixed group of male and female depressive patients, and a corresponding control group, by means of an intelligence test, allowing for an estimation of the "intellectual potential" in comparison to the "actual performance."

For this purpose, we constructed an adapted German version of the Jastak test (Jastak, 1959). Defense mechanisms were measured by means of the Defense Mechanism Test (DMT, Kragh, 1969; see Chapter 7). The original design of the study calling for a mixed group of patients, and the rather simple, straightforward comparison of an experimental with a control group, had to be changed to accommodate the actual circumstances.

The hypothesis of an interaction of intellectual performance and defenses, however, could be kept.

Method

Subjects

Depressive inpatients were recruited from the Psychiatric University Hospital in Mainz. It soon became apparent that not enough male patients were admitted to the hospital during the planned period for the study, and the sample was restricted to female patients. This condition is in accordance with the clinical observation and results of epidemiologic studies that females prevail by far in the clinical group of unipolar depression (Weissman & Klerman, 1987), but at the same time it is a loss for the empirical study of defense mechanisms in depressive males. A matched control group of volunteers was formed to correspond to the

TABLE 22.2. Age ranges and education of the subjects in the study.

	Depressives (N = 29)	Original control group (N = 29)
Age	$M = 43.7; s = 9.9$; range, 22–67	$M = 46.3; s = 9.0$; range, 24–61
Education		
Elementary and middle school (Grundschule, Hauptschule)	21	15
Non-classical secondary school (Realschule)	5	9
Academic high school (Gymnasium)	1	3
University degree	2	2

29 female depressed patients, so that the whole sample comprised 58 women.

Table 22.2 gives the age ranges and educational levels of the two groups. The most important criterion for selection of the subjects in the control group was not being in psychiatric treatment.

Diagnosis of Depression

All patients were rated by a psychiatrist on the Hamilton Depression Scale (Hamilton, 1960), which can be regarded as one of the standard rating scales for the assessment of affective disorders. A cutoff point of 24 was used to allow the inclusion of one patient in the experimental group.

The Tests Used: The DMT and the Jastak Test

The DMT and its scoring procedures are described in greater detail in Chapter 7. The apparatus used in this study was a projection tachistoscope made by Zak (Simbach, Germany). The stimuli consisted of DMT slides from the 1969 manual (Kragh, 1969), including a distractor slide before, between, and after the two test series. The slides were projected on a mirror, so that a viewing device as in the original DMT apparatus could be used. All other circumstances were as similar as possible to the standard test situation. The scoring was done according to the manual (Kragh, 1969).

To overcome the problem of too low frequencies in some of the orginal scales and to avoid too many statistical analyses, the defense mechanisms were grouped into clusters of two (cf. Table 22.3), a strategy that can be defended on theoretical grounds and has been used before (Hentschel, Kießling, & Hosemann, 1991).

Jastak published his intelligence test (the Jastak Test of Potential Ability and Behavior Stability) in 1959. His aim was to evaluate retarded or

TABLE 22.3. Grouping of the DMT defense mechanisms as used in the analyses of variance.

Repression
Denial

Isolation
Reaction formation

Identification with the aggressor
Turning against the self

Introjection of the opposite sex
Introjection of another object

Projection
Regression

deviant children and adolescents by taking a measure of intellectual capacity (i.e., the highest subtest score). To say it the other way around, Jastak wanted to start from the idea of a homogeneous intelligence profile and from there determine where the greatest losses are. Even though the operationalization of the concept of capacity might not have been complex enough, the idea is fascinating and its application to the field of depression attractive.

Basically, we encountered two problems: the language problem (there is no German translation of the Jastak test) and a possible ceiling effect, since the original test was constructed for an age level up to 14.5 years. The language problem was solved by introducing subtests from other German intelligence tests that corresponded as much as possible to the respective original subtests. In a pretest with our new test, a ceiling effect did not occur.

Table 22.4 gives examples from the subtests of our adaptation of the Jastak test, together with the sources and their reliability estimates (Cronbach's alpha), achieved in this study.

Changes in the Original Design of the Study

The strategy of having a mixed sample had to be abandoned as a result of the actual base rates of male and female depressive patients admitted to the hospital. The other major change came from the consideration that the female patients tested differed in their actual state. The interval between diagnosis and testing was not a constant one. Also the use of a cutoff point of 24 in the Hamilton scale leaves enough space for considerable differences in the severity of depression. According to the basic psychodynamic assumption, the degree of disturbance and the number and severity of defense mechanisms should be related. An overall test for all defense mechanisms between the original patient and control groups showed no significant difference. Since there are no norms for the DMT available, it could not be learned whether this result should be ascribed to the experimental or the control group. The observation in the testing situation was that some of the patients who volunteered to be tested were not able to stand the 3–4 hours of testing and had to be sent back to their rooms without being tested, whereas others showed no obvious behavioral differences at all in comparison to the controls. This finding is in close correspondence to experimental research with depressive patients (Hentschel, 1980a,b), where in one study (Hentschel, 1980b) the time before leaving the hospital was used as a correction factor. These data were, however, not available in the present study. We therefore decided to cluster all subjects on the basis of their intellectual performance, giving up the idea of a clear-cut division of an experimental and a control group, and replacing it by the idea of different groups on a continuum from severely disturbed to normal, conserving at the same time the basic hypothesis of an interaction of defense mechanisms with intellectual functioning: that is, that the lower level of performance in the intelligence test is connected with more signs of combinations of defense mechanisms, or of one particular mechanism, in different phases. In this study, the actual level of functioning hypothesis is preferred to the hypothesis of a relatively close relation of percept-genesis to ontogenesis. In percept-genetic theory, Ulf Kragh especially has postulated a possible correspondence between ontogenetic phases and percept-genetic phases. He was also able to demonstrate this phenomenon convincingly in a number of case studies (e.g., Kragh, 1970, 1986). The combination of the ontogenesis–percept-genesis correspondence hypothesis with the psychodynamic fixation hypothesis would mean that in depressive patients, more and/or more severe signs for defense mechanisms should appear in the early phases of the DMT series. According to the actual level of functioning hypothesis, more signs for defense mechanisms are expected on a more conscious level (i.e., the later phases with longer exposure times in the DMT series). The latter hypothesis is simpler and stresses more the principle of a possible distortion of the objective reality. To make testable our expectation that a worse performance in the intelligence test will be accompanied by more signs of defense in the later phases of percept-genesis, we partitioned the whole DMT series into three thirds: an early, a middle, and a late one.

Results

Clustering on the Basis of the Jastak Test

The intelligence test was used to divide the whole group into subgroups, from better to worse performance. With all subtests of the Jastak test, a

TABLE 22.4. Contents of the German adaptation of the Jastak intelligence test.

Source	Subtest	Cronbach's alpha
Jastak (1959)	Arithmetic: test the four basic arithmetic operations	.85
LPS (Horn, 1962)	Spelling: words with printing errors must be corrected	.96
MWT (Lehrl, 1977)	Vocabulary: to find a correct word among nonsense words	.94
IST (Amthauer, 1970)	Verbal reasoning: to find a word that is not conceptually related to the others	.65
Jastak (1959)	Social concept: to find the picture that does not fit in	.64

Source	Subtest	Cronbach's alpha
Jastak (1959)	Picture reasoning: to put pictures in an ordered sequence (temporal, local, social, physical)	.68
CFT (Weiß, 1971)	Space series:	.69

a b c d e f

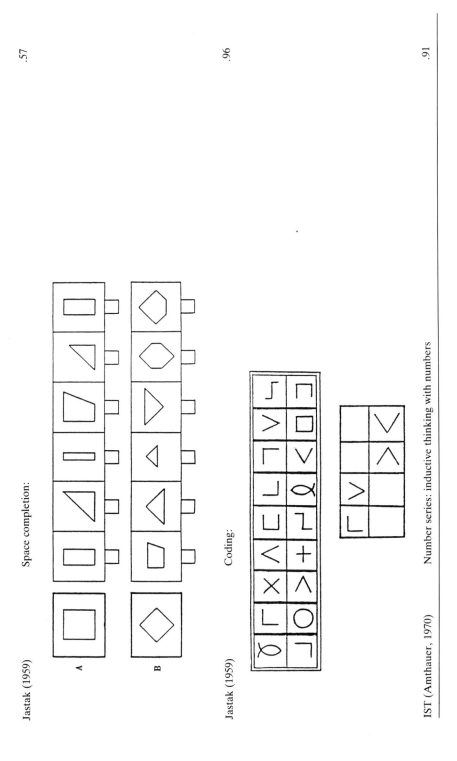

Space completion: .57

Jastak (1959)

Coding: .96

Jastak (1959)

Number series: inductive thinking with numbers   .91

IST (Amthauer, 1970)

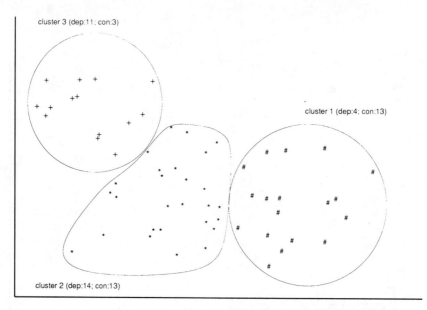

FIGURE 22.1. The three-person clusters based on the Jastak test: plane through the centers.

cluster analysis was calculated, resulting in three-person clusters, the differentiation of which by means of discriminant analysis resulted in a correct reclassification of the cases in 96.6%. These clusters are graphically presented in Fig. 22.1.

Cluster 1 is mostly a control group cluster, cluster 2 is mixed, and cluster 3 consists mostly of depressive patients. To check the possible differences of age between the clusters, an analysis of variance was calculated, showing no significant difference. Figure 22.2 gives three typical profiles from the different clusters, at the same time representing graphically the Jastak idea of varying discrepancies between the actual and the potential performance.

The respective profiles of the three clusters as a whole are given in form of a frequency polygon in Fig. 22.3. There is a clear difference in performance in all subtests, in most cases for the comparison of the three clusters, although in some cases only one cluster differs significantly from the other two. Differences that are not significant between all three clusters appear only in the subtests of arithmetic, space completion, and number series. To ensure that the main effects are not better explained in terms of a possible age and education effect in the specific subtest results, analyses of covariance were calculated for all subtests. In all cases, the reported main effects remained significant (cf. Table 22.4).

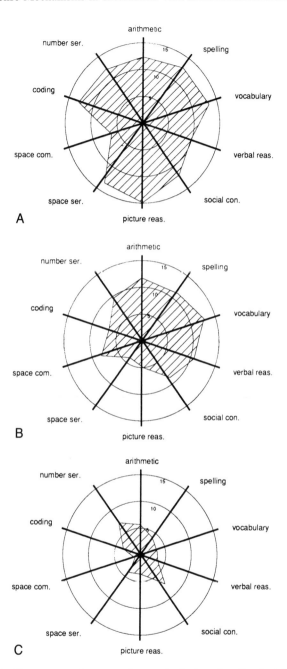

FIGURE 22.2. Three examples, one for each cluster, for the Jaṣtak Intelligence Profile. A. Cluster 1: Subject No. 25. B. Cluster 2: Subject No. 14. C. Cluster 3: Subject No. 9.

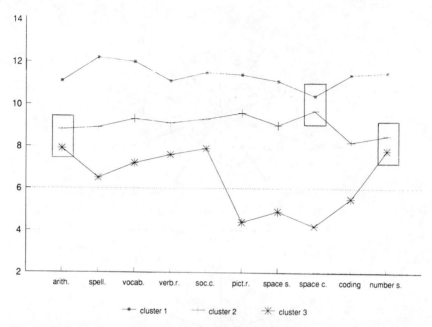

FIGURE 22.3. Performance differences of the three clusters in the 10 subtests of the Jastak test.

Defense in Interaction with Intellectual Performance

To test the interaction of defenses with intellectual performance, we chose to use analyses of variance, with the clusters as independent variables and the course of defenses in the three thirds of percept-genetic process as dependent variables (repeated measurement design). Of the five analyses, one showed a significant result (cf. Table 22.5). It is the isolation/reaction formation group of defenses that is significantly related to the clusters as presented in Fig. 22.4. There is no difference among the clusters in the first third in the DMT series; clusters 3 and 1 show a significant difference in the second third of the series, and in the last third cluster 1 again shows lower scores in isolation/reaction formation, this time in comparison with the two other clusters.

TABLE 22.5. Analysis of variance with isolation/reaction formation as dependent variable over the three parts of the DMT series (repeated measurements).

	F	df	p
Main effect clusters	1.68	2/55	n.s.
Repeated measurements	18.40	2/110	<.001
Repeated measurements × clusters	3.87	4/110	<.01

Discussion

Our results support the hypothesis of an interaction of defenses with intellectual functioning, clearly more related to the actual level of functioning in contrast to the also mentioned hypothesis of a possible parallelism between percept-genesis and ontogenesis. The conclusion would thus be that actual distortion of reality, to be inferred from the isolation/reaction formation combination, is greater for clusters 2 and 3 than for cluster 1. Through cluster 2 and the four persons each in clusters 3 and 1, there is considerable overlap between the patient group and the original normal control group, and this circumstance would seem to merit attention for further research.

Is it not possible to differentiate from depressive patients a certain subgroup of normal women, in a certain age range—most of them housewives—regarding their intellectual and emotional functioning, or were many of the depressive patients quite well recovered at the time of testing? The intellectual deficit visible from Fig. 22.3 seems to suggest that the question posed as the first alternative can be answered in the affirmative. The lowest performance is reached by subjects of cluster 3 in tasks that can be labeled as requiring fluid intelligence or speed (subtests 6, 7, 8, and 9).

In our basic hypothesis we did not specify which defense mechanism we expected to prevail in the more disturbed subjects. It is especially reaction

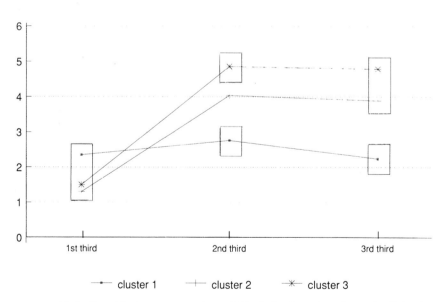

FIGURE 22.4. Graphical representation of "isolation/reaction formation" in the three clusters over the three parts of the DMT series.

formation as measured with the DMT that interferes with performance in high risk tasks, as piloting and diving (cf. Smith, Kragh, & Hentschel, 1980; Vaernes, 1982). The combination of isolation and reaction formation has been shown to be responsible for deficits in attention control under inadequate stimulation: that is, information underload and information overload (Hentschel et al., 1991). This effect, repeated now in depressive patients, requires some additional comments. A significant difference in the combination identification with the aggressor and turning against the self, which we did not find, would, according to psychodynamic theory, have been more self-evident. In an earlier study of Hentschel and Balint (1974) comparing psychopathological symptoms with defense ratings, depressive symptoms showed the strongest relation to ratings of introjection and turning against the self. We think that the result of our study in fact could have been influenced by a method effect. Isolation and especially reaction formation seem to have a very strong impact in many studies with the DMT, although it seems possible to differentiate clinical subgroups also by means of other signs of defenses in the DMT (Gitzinger, 1988).

From a psychodynamic point of view, it is plausible to differentiate depression into problems of dependency, self-criticism, and efficacy (Blatt, 1974; Blatt, D'Afflitti, & Quinlan, 1979). The interaction of intellectual deficits and defenses that we have found seems to mirror more the efficacy and dependency aspects. On the basis of our data, it is not possible to decide whether the lack of representation of the self-criticism aspect in the DMT defense mechanisms corresponds to a relative lack of these phenomena in our sample, or whether it could be due to a possible method effect, as mentioned above.

Zubin (1975) has criticized the dependence of most psychological testing for diagnostic purposes on motivation, attention, and interest, which usually leads to a mapping of deficits with largely unclear reasons for these deficits. He has proposed looking for more objective measures instead, also with the intention of finding performances in which the patients excel. This very interesting proposal should be given more support than it has so far enjoyed, probably because most clinical researchers do not think in that direction. A possible compromise also could be the search for physiological indicators in combination with motivational variables (e.g., Munz, Winkow, Kessler, & Traue, 1989).

The fact remains, however, that depression is an illness in which few social advantages can be seen, and those so labeled seem to be of doubtful value in daily life (cf. Mahendra, 1987).

The obvious deficits not only influence the test performance of these subjects, they have severe consequences for daily functioning too, which for the depressive patients in clusters 2 and 3 had led to a stay in the psychiatric hospital. We do not know any concrete details of the daily functioning of the control subjects in these two clusters, but we tend to infer that their performance also probably will be far from optimal. One can look at these results as only the reflection of deficits, or one can try to look for meaning and to see how the most severe symptoms are incorporated in the structure of the basic personality characteristics, of which Oliver Sacks (1982), for another group of patients, has given such impressing descriptions. He opted for an idiographic approach, but also from a nomothetic point of view, as in our case, one can focus on the obvious problems of the patients as meaning-related phenomena.

The defense combination that we have found to be significantly higher for cluster(s) 3 (and 2), in the later phases in the percept-genetic process, also can be interpreted as serving the purpose of preventing the intrusion of aggression into the subjective reality of these subjects by isolating it or turning it into the misperception of a friendly act.

The reality is distorted, but this also adds something to the world of these subjects, probably enabling them at least to keep their actual level of functioning as opposed to ending up in a completely empty experiential world. Interestingly enough, Berglund and Smith (1988) have found with another percept-genetic technique, the Meta-Contrast Technique (MCT) (see Chapter 7) that depressive patients without any defensive signs committed suicide significantly more often than those having a "protective shield" of defenses.

Seen from the point of view of optimal functioning and well-being, it is beyond any doubt that it is highly desirable to achieve some change in this part of the internal milieu of our depressive patients, and at the same time to reduce their intellectual deficits, which in some way interact with their defensive structure. The way of striving for harmony, already present on a subconscious level, in spite of the need for therapy to achieve a better level of adaptation, evokes respect for its deeply rooted human quality.

Acknowledgments. We thank a number of people for making this study possible: the director of the Psychiatric University Clinic in Mainz, Prof. O. Benkert, for giving permission to test the patients; U. Frommberger for his administrative support in selecting the patients; Dr. A. Westen for her helpful assistance in recruiting control subjects; and, of course, the patients and the control persons for their participation.

References

Abramson, L.Y., Seligman, M.E.P., & Teasdale, J.D. (1978) Learned helplessness in humans: critique and reformulation. *Journal of Abnormal Psychology*, 87, 49–74.

Ahrens, S. & Lamparter, U. (1989) Objektale Funktion des Schmerzes und Depressivität [The function of pain as an object and depression]. *Psychotherapie Psychosomatik Medizinische Psychologie, 39*, 219–222.

American Psychiatric Association (1952) *Diagnostic and statistical manual of mental disorders* (1st ed.). Washington, DC: Author.

American Psychiatric Association (1968) *Diagnostic and statistical manual of mental disorders* (2nd ed.). Washington, DC: Author.

American Psychiatric Association (1987) *Diagnostic and statistical manual of mental disorders* (3rd ed. rev.). Washington, DC: Author.

Amthauer, R. (1970) IST, Intelligenz-Struktur-Test [*IST, Intelligence Structure Test*]. Göttingen: Hogrefe.

Arieti, S. (1976) *Creativity: The magic synthesis*. New York: Basic Books.

Auersperg, A. von (1963) Schmerz und Schmerzhaftigkeit [Pain and painfulness]. Berlin: Springer.

Berglund, M. & Smith, G. (1988) Postdiction of suicide in a group of depression patients. *Acta Psychiatrica Scandinavica*, 77, 504–510.

Blatt, S.J. (1974) Levels of object representation in anaclitic and introjective depression. *Psychoanalytic Study of the Child*, 29, 107–157.

Blatt, S.J., D'Afflitti, J.P., & Quinlan, D.M. (1979) *Depressive Experiences Questionnaire*. Yale University, New Haven, CT.

Brown, G.W. & Harris, T. (1978) *Social origins of depression: A study of psychiatric disorder in women*. London: Tavistock.

Cattell, R.B. (1940) The description of personality: 1. Foundation of trait measurement. *Psychological Review*, 50, 559–594.

Clare, A.W. & Blacker, R. (1986) Some problems affecting diagnosis and classification of depressive disorders in primary care. In M. Shepherd, G. Wilkinson, & P. Williams (Eds.), *Mental illness in primary care settings* (pp. 7–26). London: Tavistock.

Feighner, J.P., Robins, E., Guze, S.B., Woodruff, R.A., Jr., Winokur, G., & Munoz, R. (1972) Diagnostic criteria for use in psychiatric research. *Archives of General Psychiatry*, 26, 56–73.

Fenichel, O. (1946) *The psychoanalytic theory of neurosis*. London: Routledge & Kegan Paul.

Ferster, C.B. (1974) Behavioral approaches to depression. In R.Y. Friedman & M.M. Kate (Eds.), *The psychology of depression* (pp. 29–53). New York: Wiley.

Foucault, M. (1967) *Madness and civilisation*. London: Tavistock.

Freud, A. (1946) *The ego and the mechanisms of defense*. Madison CT: International Universities Press. (Original work published 1936)

Gitzinger, I. (1988) *Operationalisierung von Abwehrmechanismen: Wahrnehmungsabwehr und Einstellungsmessung Psychoanalytischer Abwehrkonzepte* [Operationalization of defense mechanisms: Perceptual defense and measurement of attitude in psychoanalytic defense concepts]. Unpublished thesis, Freiburg.

Hamilton, M. (1960) A rating scale for depression. *Journal of Neurology, Neurosurgery, and Psychiatry*, 23, 56–62.

Hentschel, U. (1980a) Kognitive Kontrollprinzipien und Neuroseformen [Cognitive styles and types of neurosis]. In U. Hentschel & G. Smith (Eds.), *Experimentelle Persönlichkeitspsychologie* [*Experimental personality psychology*] (pp. 227– 321). Wiesbaden: Akademische Verlagsgesellschaft.

Hentschel, U. (1980b) Zur Validität serial ausgewerteter Interferenztests [On the validity of serially scored interference tests]. In U. Hentschel & G. Smith (Eds.), *Experimentelle Persönlichkeitspsychologie* [*Experimental personality psychology*] (pp. 337–349). Wiesbaden: Akademische Verlagsgesellschaft.

Hentschel, U. & Bálint, S. (1974) Plausible diagnostic taxonomy in the field of neurosis. *Psychological Research Bulletin. Lund University*, *14*, No. 2. Monograph Series.

Hentschel, U., Kießling, M. & Hosemann, A. (1991) Anxiety, defense and attention control. In R.E. Hanlon (Ed.), *Cognitive microgenesis: A neuropsychological perspective* (pp. 262–285). New York: Springer.

Hentschel, U., Schubö, W., & Zerssen, D. v. (1976) Diagnostische Klassifikationsversuche mit zwei standardisierten psychiatrischen Schätzskalen [Attempts at a nosological classification with two standardized psychiatric rating scales]. *Archiv für Psychiatrie und Nervenkrankheiten*, *221*, 283–301.

Horn, W. (1962) *Das Leistungsprüfsystem* [*The performance test system*]. Göttingen: Hogrefe.

Jastak, J.F. (1959) *The Jastak Test* (*Junior Highschool Level*). Minneapolis: Educational Publishers.

Kraepelin, E. (1896) *Psychiatrie* (5. Auflage) [Psychiatry (5th ed.)]. Leipzig: Barth.

Kragh, U. (1969) *Manual till DMT—Defense Mechanism Test* [Manual for the DMT—Defense Mechanism Test]. Stockholm: Skandinaviska Testförlaget.

Kragh, U. (1970) Pathogenesis in dipsomania. In U. Kragh & G. Smith (Eds.), *Perceptgenetic analysis* (pp. 160–178). Lund: Gleerup.

Kragh, U. (1986) Life panorama under the microscope: A paradigmatic case study. In U. Hentschel, G. Smith, & J.G. Draguns (Eds.), *The roots of perception* (pp. 145–159). Amsterdam: North-Holland.

Lehrl, S. (1977) *Mehrfachwahl-Wortschatz-Intelligenztest* (*MWT-B*) [*Multiple choice vocabulary intelligence test* (*MWT-B*)]. Erlangen: Straube.

Mahendra, B. (1987) *Depression: The disorder and its associations*. Lancaster, PA: MTP Press.

Munz, D., Winkow, E., Kessler, M., & Traue, H.C. (1989) *The moderating effect of motivation and attribution on the behavior of depressives*. Paper presented at the 3rd European Conference on Psychotherapy Research, September, Bern.

Powell, R. Dolan, R., & Wessely, S. (1990) Attributions and self-esteem in depression and chronic fatigue syndromes. *Journal of Psychosomatic Research*, *34*, 665–673.

Sacks, O. (1982) *Awakenings*. London: Pan Books.

Schubö, W., Hentschel, U., Zerssen, D. v., & Mombour, M. (1975) Psychiatrische Klassifikation durch diskriminanzanalytische Anwendung der Q-Faktorenanalyse [Psychiatric classification by means of a discriminatory application of Q-factor analysis]. *Archiv für Psychiatrie und Nervenkrankheiten*, *220*, 187–200.

Smith, G. & Danielsson, A. (1980) Ideenreichtum, Ich-Beteiligung und Effektivität bei einer Gruppe von Natur- und Geisteswissenschaftlern (Richness in ideas, ego-involvement and efficiency in a group of scientists and humanists). In U. Hentschel & G. Smith (Eds.), *Experimentelle Persönlichkeitspsychologie* [Experimental personality psychology]. Wiesbaden: Akademische Verlagsgesellschaft.

Smith, G., Kragh, U., & Hentschel, U. (1980) Perceptgenetische Verfahren: Historische und methodologische Übersicht [Perceptgenetic techniques: Historical and methodological overview]. In U. Hentschel & G. Smith (Eds.),

Experimentelle Persönlichkeitspsychologie [Experimental personality psychology] (pp. 31–63). Wiesbaden: Akademische Verlagsgesellschaft.

Szasz, T. (1972) *The myth of mental illness*. London: Paladin.

Vaernes, R. (1982) The Defense Mechanism Test predicts inadequate performance under stress. *Scandinavian Journal of Psychology*, *23*, 37–43.

Vaillant, G.E. (1974) *Adaptation* to life. Boston, Little, Brown.

Weiß, R.H. (1971) *Grundintelligenztest CFT 3 Skala 3* [*Basic intelligence test CFT 3 scale 3*]. Braunschweig: Westermann.

Weissman, M.M. & Klerman, G. (1987) Gender and depression. In R. Formanek & A. Gurian (Eds.), *Women and depression: A lifespan perspective* (pp. 3–15). New York: Springer.

Willner, P. (1985) *Depression: A psychobiological synthesis*. New York: Wiley.

Zubin, J. (1975) A biometric approach to diagnosis and evaluation of therapeutic intervention in schizophrenia. In G. Usdin (Ed.), *Overview of the psychotherapies* (pp. 153–204). New York: Brunner & Mazel.

23
Defense Mechanisms and Hope as Protective Factors in Physical and Mental Disorders

Louis A. Gottschalk and Janny Fronczek

Whether defense mechanisms may serve as markers of increased vulnerability or resistance to illness is an issue that merits being more clearly and definitively addressed and investigated. Anna Freud (1936/1946) focused on defense mechanisms as tools used to relieve anxiety and their presence might, hence, be seen as clues to some underlying psychopathological process. The ways in which defense mechanisms function to influence the course of illness have been rarely studied. On the other hand, hope is a state or trait that has been examined over many years in empirical studies to determine whether it is capable of influencing the onset or course of illness. French (1952) and Frank (1968) regarded hope as a personal incentive toward encouraging a person to cope better with inner psychological conflicts. Perley, Winget, and Placci (1971) found that elevated hopefulness predicted patients who followed up recommendations that they seek psychiatric treatment. Gottschalk, Kunkel, Wohl, Saenger, and Winget (1960) found that hope scores derived from verbal samples predicted the duration of survival of patients with terminal cancer receiving irradiation treatment. Gottschalk, Mayerson, and Gottlieb (1967) and Gottschalk, Fox, and Bates (1973), moreover, found that high measures of hopefulness pointed to relatively favorable outcome in psychotherapy. Udelman and Udelman (1986) reported a significant correlation between hope scores and indicators of immune competence, namely mitogenic stimulation by concanavalin A and percentage of B cells. Gottschalk and Hoigaard-Martin (1986) found significantly higher affect denial scores and positive hope scores, derived from the content analysis of speech (Gottschalk 1979; Gottschalk & Gleser, 1969; Gottschalk, Lolas, & Viney 1986), for a group of women ($N = 123$) experiencing a mastectomy as compared to groups of women having a cholecystectomy ($N = 74$), women having a normal breast biopsy ($N = 63$), and physically healthy women. These findings prevailed, although the severity of the emotional impact, as adjudged from the anxiety and hostility scores from these women derived from their speech samples and the Symptom Checklist 90 Analogue (Derogatis, Lipman, Rickels, Uhlenhuth, & Covi, 1964) and

TABLE 23.1. Intercorrelations of Hope scale scores and other psychological states or traits.

Subjects	Anxiety	Hostility Out	Hostility In	Hostility Ambivalent	Social Alienation–Personal Disorganization
		Content analysis measures			
Normative adult group (N = 91)	−.19	−.26*	−.14	−.22*	−.30*
Normative children's gourp (N = 109)	−.46*	−.45*	−.36*	−.38*	−.61*
Crisis clinic outpatients (N = 55)	—	—	—	—	−.63*
Medical inpatients (N = 36)	—	—	—	—	−.75*

Subjects	Content analysis measures of human relations	Patient improvement	Anant Belong-ingness Scale	Barron Ego Strength Scale
Normative children's group (N = 109)	+.51*	—	—	—
Crisis clinic outpatients (N = 54)	+.68*	+.26*	+.29*	+.21*
Medical inpatients (N = 25)	+.75*	—	—	—

NOTES: * = statistically significant (two-tailed test) $p < .05$.
— = correlation not carried out because data not available.

the Global Assessment Scale (Endicott, Spitzer, Fleiss, & Cohen, 1976), revealed a stepwise increase in emotional disturbance going from measures obtained from the healthy through noncancerous to cancerous women.

Studies involving the Hope scale by Gottschalk (1974) have demonstrated that hope scores, derived from the content analysis of speech, correlate positively with content-analysis-derived markers of personal competence, such as good human relations and object relations, and negatively with markers of vulnerability or psychopathological problems, such as anxiety, hostility out, hostility in, depression, and social alienation–personal disorganization (see Table 23.1). These hope scores also correlate significantly positively with other measures of emotional well-being, such as, scores from the Anant Belongingness Scale (1967) and the Barron Ego Strength Scale (1953). Other empirical evidence that hope functions to strengthen tolerance to life stress (see also Table 23.1) is suggested by the finding that pretreatment hope scores—from outpatients receiving crisis intervention psychotherapy—correlated significantly negatively with measures of psychiatric morbidity 6–10 weeks later (Gottschalk et al., 1973). And in a group of acute schizophrenic patients ($N = 24$), 48 hours after being given oral thioridazine (4 mg/kg)—a major tranquilizer—hope scores improved significantly (1.79, $p < .05$) and total hostility outward (-1.73, $p < .05$), social alienation–personal disorganization (-2.27, $p < .05$), and depression scores (-1.83, $p < .05$) decreased significantly, all scores being obtained from the content analysis of 5-minute speech samples (Gottschalk, 1974; Gottschalk, Biener, Noble, Birch, Wilbert, & Heiser, 1975).

To pursue these issues, the following series of studies was undertaken to look at the relationships between the defense mechanisms of displacements, denial, and hope with illness behavior and mental disorder. Many of the Gottschalk–Gleser scales for measuring the magnitude of psychological states through the content analysis of verbal behavior (Gottschalk, 1979; Gottschalk & Gleser, 1969) include counting verbal references not only to the self having or experiencing an emotional state (e.g., I am scared), but also verbal references to others (animate or inanimate) having the emotional condition (e.g., he is afraid; the auto's engine died.). Other defenses or coping mechanisms in these scales include verbal references denying the state (e.g., I am not frightened) or assertions of hopefulness in the face of stressors (e.g., I am sure everything will come out satisfactorily; God will certainly protect me).

Methods and Procedures

Content analysis scores obtained from earlier studies were reexamined focusing on the frequency of use of the verbal categories of the Gottschalk–Gleser Anxiety and three Hostility scales (Gottschalk, Hoigaard, Birch, & Rickels, 1979) involving displacement and denial (Gottschalk, 1976; Gottschalk & Gleser, 1969; Gottschalk et al., 1973, 1975, 1976). Of interest was how the percentage use of those verbal categories, such as displacement and denial, by different psychiatric groups compares to the frequency of use of direct verbal statements of experiencing affects (e.g., I am anxious). The effect of demographic factors, such as sex, age, and intelligence quotients, was also examined, as well as how the frequency of use of these various verbal categories designating anxiety varies with scores from the same subjects on the three Gottschalk–Gleser Hostility scales (Gottschalk et al., 1963; Gottschalk & Gleser, 1969), namely, Hostility Outward, Hostility Inward, and Ambivalent Hostility (which under certain circumstances appear to function as defense mechanisms against, e.g., anxiety, rather than merely expressions of solitary emotions of hostility: Gleser & Ihilevich, 1969; Ihilevich & Gleser, 1986).

Another approach was to determine the relative cerebral glucose meta-bolic rates associated with anxiety and hope scores during three states of consciousness, namely, during silent wakeful mentation, REM dreaming, and NONREM mentation, using Positron Emission Tomography (PET). The procedures and rationale used in these latter studies have been described more fully elsewhere (Gottschalk, Buchsbaum, Gillin, Wu, Reynolds, & Herrera, 1992). Briefly, 48 normal male subjects were screened by medical and psychiatric interviews, physical examinations, laboratory measures, normal sleep habits, and the absence of the use of medication for participation in PET studies to compare cerebral glucose metabolic rates during the states of sleep and wakefulness. The subjects were studied during the waking state, Rapid-Eye-Movement (REM), and Non-Rapid-Eye-Movement (NONREM) sleep, each state being con-firmed by standard EEG and other criteria. Intravenous infusion with 18-F D-deoxyglyucose (FDG) was started when all the criteria indicated that the subjects were awake or in REM or NONREM sleep. Thirty-two minutes after the FDG injection, each subject was aroused and asked to give 5-minute tape-recorded reports of their dreams or mental events as well as free-associations to the content of these mental experiences.

Other investigators have reported (Huang, Phelps, Hoffman, Sideris, Selin, & Kuhl, 1980; Sokoloff, Reivich, Kennedy, Des Rosiers, Patlak, Pettigrew, Sakurada, & Shinohara, 1977) that 30 minutes after a single intravenous injection of FDG, there is negligible error in estimates of localized cerebral glucose consumption, for most of the free desoxyglucose has been fixed and converted in the brain tissues to desoxyglucose-6–phosphate, the relative amounts of which can be detected 45–120 minutes later by the PET scanner. The typescripts of these reports were blindly content analyzed by the senior author using the Gottschalk–Gleser Anxiety and Hostility scales (Gottschalk & Gleser, 1969) and the Gotts-chalk Hope scale (1974).

Subjects

Six groups of subjects were involved in these investigations.

1. A group of normal young males, average age 25.3 + 6.6 to 26.2 + 5.8, consisting of three subgroups of sleeping or wakeful subjects (Gottschalk et al., 1991): the REM group ($N = 10$), the NONREM group ($N = 10$), and wakeful group ($N = 10$). In the collection of this group, clinical examinations and tests were done to exclude subjects with detect-able mental or physical disorders.

2. One group was comprised of normative adult subjects of ages ranging from 20 to 50, gainfully employed and without known physical or mental disorders (Gottschalk & Gleser, 1969, pp. 71–72), consisting of 15 males (low IQ, 80–100, $N = 6$; medium IQ, 101–115, $N = 3$; high IQ,

116 and up, $N = 6$; IQ determined by the Wonderlic test [1945]) and 15 females (low IQ, $N = 6$; medium IQ, $N = 3$; high IQ, $N = 6$). Clinical examinations and tests were not carried out to exclude mental or physical disorders.

3. Another group consisted of normative school children (Gottschalk, 1976), that is, children without known physical or mental disorders, ranging in age from 6 to 16 years, both boys ($N = 15$) and girls ($N = 15$). For this group, clinical examinations and tests were not done to rule out the presence of mental or physical disorders.

4. A group of adult patients with psychoneuroses (Gottschalk et al., 1979, p. 41 f) and consisting of males ($N = 10$) and females ($N = 10$).

5. A group of emotionally disturbed criminal offenders imprisoned in Patuxent Institution in Patuxent, Maryland (Gottschalk, Covi, Uliana, & Bates, 1973), consisting of 44 males, average age 25.6 + 6.15 and average educational level 8.25 + 1.90 years.

6. A group of acute schizophrenic patients ranging in age from 21 to 55 years (Gottschalk et al., 1975) and consisting of males ($N = 10$) and females ($N = 12$).

Measurement of Emotions and Defenses

Scores on the Gottschalk–Gleser affect scales are corrected for number of words spoken by deriving a score per 100 words spoken (Gottschalk & Gottschalk, 1969; Gottschalk, Winget, & Gleser, 1969), for discontinuity of frequency distributions of scores due to zero scores by adding .5 to the raw score, and for nonparametric frequency distribution of scores by square-rooting the adjusted score (see Tables 23.2–23.5, indicating the Anxiety, Hostility Outward, Hostility Inward, and Ambivalent Hostility scales). These mathematical transformations of the scores permit comparisons of such scores across different occasions and individuals and lead to a frequency distribution of scores approximating a parametric distribution. The Gottschalk Hope scale also corrects for the number of words spoken by deriving a score per 100 words (Gottschalk, 1974) and in the present study .5 was added to raw zero scores, but the final hope scores are not square-rooted (see Table 23.6, illustrating the verbal categories for the Hope scale). A minimum of 70 words has been recommended for a reliable sample (Gottschalk et al., 1969, p. 15).

Statistical Procedures

The statistical procedures applied to testing the hypotheses put forward included nonparametric tests (e.g., Spearman, Kendall tau, etc.) to examine the intercorrelations between the frequency of occurrence of verbal category references involving the self and verbal category statements involving others (displacement) or denials across the different

TABLE 23.2. Anxiety scale.[a]

1. Death anxiety: references to death, dying, threat of death, or anxiety about death experienced by or occurring to:
   a. Self (3)
   b. Animate others (2)
   c. Inanimate objects destroyed (1)
   d. Denial of death anxiety (1)
2. Mutilation (castration) anxiety: references to injury, tissue or physical damage, or anxiety about injury or threat of such experienced by or occurring to:
   a. Self (3)
   b. Animate others (2)
   c. Inanimate objects (1)
   d. Denial (1)
3. Separation anxiety: references to desertion, abandonment, loneliness, ostracism, loss of support, falling, loss of love object, or threat of such experienced by or occurring to:
   a. Self (3)
   b. Animate others (2)
   c. Inanimate objects (1)
   d. Denial (1)
4. Guilt anxiety: references to adverse criticism, abuse, condemnation, moral disapproval, guilt, or threat of such experienced by:
   a. Self (3)
   b. Animate others (2)
   c. Denial (1)
5. Shame anxiety: references to ridicule, inadequacy, shame, embarrassment, humiliation, overexposure of deficiencies or private details, or threat of such experienced by:
   a. Self (3)
   b. Animate others (2)
   c. Denial (1)
6. Diffuse of nonspecific anxiety: references by word or in phrases to anxiety and/or fear without distinguishing type of source of anxiety:
   a. Self (3)
   b. Animate others (2)
   c. Denial (1)

[a] Numbers in parentheses are weights.

groups listed above. Analysis of variance was employed to determine whether sex, intelligence, or age influenced the average patterns of occurrence of displacements or denials in verbal behavior among the groups studied. These statistical tests were run by SPSS computer programs (SPSS, 1990).

Results

No significant effects of sex, age, or intelligence were found on the frequency of occurrence of the phenomena of displacements and denials in the spoken language of the six groups of subjects. Nor were there any significant effects of the state of consciousness—namely when the mental

TABLE 23.3. Hostility directed outward scale: Thematic categories of destructive, injurious, critical thoughts and actions directed to others.

I. Hostility outward—overt[a]	II. Hostility outward—covert[a]
a 3 Self killing, fighting, injuring other individuals or threatening to do so.	a 3 Others (human) killing, fighting, injuring other individuals or threatening to do so.
b 3 Self robbing or abandoning other individuals, causing suffering or anguish to others, or threatening to do so.	b 3 Others (human) robbing or abandoning other individuals, causing suffering or anguish to others, or threatening to do so.
c 3 Self adversely criticizing, depreciating, blaming, expressing anger, dislike of other human beings.	c 3 Others (human) adversely criticizing, depreciating, blaming, expressing anger, dislike of other human beings.
a 2 Self killing, injuring, or destroying domestic animals, pets, or threatening to do so.	a 2 Others (human) killing, injuring or destroying domestic animals, pets, or threatening to do so.
b 2 Self abandoning, robbing domestic animals, pets, or threatening to do so.	b 2 Others (human) abandoning, robbing domestic animals, pets, or threatening to do so.
c 2 Self criticizing or depreciating others in a vague or mild manner.	c 3 Others (human) criticizing or depreciating other individuals in a vague or mild manner.
d 2 Self depriving or disappointing other human beings.	d 2 Others (human) depriving or disappointing other human beings.
	e 2 Others (human or domestic animals) dying or killing violently in death-dealing situation or threatening with such.
	f 2 Bodies (human or domestic animals) mutilated, depreciated, defiled.
a 1 Self killing, injuring, destroying, robbing wildlife, flora, inanimate objects, or threatening to do so.	a 1 Wildlife flora, inanimate objects, injured, broken, robbed, destroyed, or threatening with such (with or without mention of agent).
b 1 Self adversely criticizing, depreciating, blaming, expressing anger or dislike of subhumans, inanimate objects, places, situations.	b 1 Others (human) adversely criticizing, depreciating, expressing anger or dislike of subhumans, inanimate objects, places, situations.
c 1 Self using hostile words, cursing, mention of anger or rage without referent.	c 1 Others angry, cursing without reference to cause or direction of anger. Also instruments of destruction not used threateningly.
	d 1 Others (human, domestic animals) injured, robbed, dead, abandoned, or threatened with such from any source including subhuman, inanimate objects, situations (storms, floods, etc.).
	e 1 Subhumans killing, fighting, injuring, robbing, destroying each other or threatening to do so.
	f 1 Denial of anger, dislike, hatred, cruelty, and intent to harm.

[a] Numbers serve to give weight as well as to identify category; letters also help to identify category.

TABLE 23.4. Hostility directed inward scale: Thematic categories of self-destructive, self-critical thoughts and actions.

I. Hostility inward[a]	
a 4	References to self (speaker) attempting to kill self, with or without conscious intent.
b 4	References to self wanting to die, needing or deserving to die.
a 3	References to self injuring, mutilating, disfiguring self or threats to do so, with or without conscious intent.
b 3	Self blaming, expressing anger or hatred to self, considering self worthless or of no value, causing oneself grief or trouble, or threatening to do so.
c 3	References to feelings of discouragement, giving up hope, despairing, feeling grieved or depressed, having no purpose in life.
a 2	References to self needing or deserving punishment, paying for one's sins, needing to atone or do penance.
b 2	Self adversely criticizing, depreciating self; references to regretting, being sorry or ashamed for what one says or does; references to self mistaken or in error.
c 2	References to feeling of deprivation, disappointment, lonesomeness.
a 1	References to feeling disappointed in self; unable to meet expectations of self or others.
b 1	Denial of anger, dislike, hatred, blame, destructive impulses from self to self.
c 1	References to feeling painfully driven or obliged to meet one's own expectations and standards.

[a] Numbers serve to give weight as well as to identify category; letters also help to identify category.

TABLE 23.5. Ambivalent hostility scale: Thematic categories of destructive, injurious, critical thoughts and actions of others to self.

II. Ambivalent hostility[a]	
a 3	Others (human) killing or threatening to kill self.
b 3	Others (human) physically injuring, mutilating, disfiguring self or threatening to do so.
c 3	Others (human) adversely criticizing, blaming, expressing anger or dislike toward self or threatening to do so.
d 3	Others (human) abandoning, robbing self, causing suffering, anguish, or threatening to do so.
a 2	Others (human) depriving, disappointing, misunderstanding self or threatening to do so.
b 2	Self threatened with death from subhuman or inanimate object, or death-dealing situation.
a 1	Others (subhuman, inanimate, or situation), injuring, abandoning, robbing self, causing suffering, anguish.
b 1	Denial of blame.

[a] Numbers serve to give weight as well as to identify category; letters also help to identify category.

TABLE 23.6. Hope scale.

Weight		Content category
+1	H 1.	References to self or others getting or receiving help, advice, support, sustenance, confidence, esteem (a) from others; (b) from self.
+1	H 2.	References to feelings of optimism about the present of future by (a) others; (b) self.
+1	H 3.	References to being or wanting to be or seeking to be the recipient of good fortune, good luck, God's favor or blessing by (a) others; (b) self.
+1	H 4.	References to any kinds of hope that lead to a constructive outcome, to survival, to longevity, to smooth-going interpersonal relationships (this category can be scored only if the word "hope" or "wish" or a close synonym is used).
−1	H 5.	References to not being or not wanting to be or not seeking to be the recipient of good fortune, good luck, God's favor or blessing.
−1	H 6.	References to self or others not getting or receiving help, advice, support, sustenance, confidence, esteem (a) from others; (b) from self.
−1	H 7.	References to feelings of hopelessness, losing hope, despair, lack of confidence, lack of ambition, lack of interest; feelings of pessimism, discouragement by (a) others; (b) self.

experiences reported and recorded from each subject while awake actually occurred when the individual was having REM dreaming, NONREM thoughts and feelings, or silent waking fantasies and reveries.

1. In the group of normal male adults, the frequency of occurrence of verbal statements referring to the self being anxious, displacements of anxiety, and denials of anxiety were significantly and positively inter-correlated. In the group of normative adults, the frequency of occurrence of verbal references to the self being anxious and denials of anxiety were significantly positively correlated. The group of psychoneurotic adults showed a significant negative correlation between the occurrence of verbal references to the self being anxious and denials of anxiety ($r = -.48$, $p < .03$) and a negative nonsignificant correlation ($r = -.30$, $p < .15$) between verbal references to the self and verbal displacements of anxiety to others. The groups of normative children, emotionally disordered criminals, and schizophrenic patients had no significant intercorrelations of any of these kinds (see Table 23.7).

Hence, the phenomena of (verbal) displacements and denials of anxiety, particularly when they are not intense or of great magnitude, are associated with mental health, especially in adults, and are linked statistically (as adjudged from significant positive correlations) and psychodynamically (on the basis of observations with individual subjects or patients) with diverse hostile affects (Gottschalk, Fronczek, & Abel,

TABLE 23.7. Intercorrelations between verbal statements referring to the self being anxious (a), others being anxious (b + c), denial of anxiousness (d), and their p-values.

Group 1. Normal male adults			Group 2. Normative adults		
Categories	a	b + c	Categories	a	b + c
b + c	.45		b + c	−.01	
	(.007)			(.472)	
d	.42	.65	d	.42	.23
	(.010)	(.000)		(.010)	(.107)

Group 3. Normative children			Group 4. Neurotic patients		
Categories	a	b +c	Categories	a	b + c
b + c	.17		b + c	−.30	
	(.182)			(.150)	
d	.10	.02	d	−.48	.16
	(.305)	(.448)		(.016)	(.256)

Group 5. Emotionally disturbed criminals			Group 6. Schizophrenics		
Categories	a	b + c	Categories	a	b + c
b + c	−.08		b + c	.09	
	(.303)			(.349)	
d	.16	.18	d	−.01	.08
	(.153)	(.115)		(.499)	(.371)

1993a). In patients with neuroses, the verbal denials and displacements tend to substitute for verbal statements concerning the self being anxious; hence, these variables are negatively intercorrelated, which illustrates and confirms that denial and displacement are used as defense mechanisms in the neuroses.

2. Among normative children (from age 6 to 16), probably for developmental reasons, (verbal) displacements and denials of anxiety are not linked in any clear way, statistically, with other affects. How displacement and denial are linked with hostility and other affects apparently needs to be determined in each single case.

3. In mentally disordered groups of adults, (verbal) displacements and denials may serve a defensive or coping function and substitute, to some extent, for disturbing affects (as adjudged from their relative infrequent significant positive intercorrelations).

4. In schizophrenic patients, the personal disorganization of the schizophrenic syndrome may serve to obscure the possible usefulness as a defense or coping mechanism of the expression of anxiety or hostility in various forms. In this connection, clinicians have uniformly observed that frequently the affects expressed by acute schizophrenic patients are driven by the content of their delusions and hallucinations (see Figs. 23.1 and 23.2).

5. The state of consciousness—namely, wakefulness, REM dreaming, and NONREM mentation—influences the intercorrelations between anxiety and hostility and localized cerebral glucose metabolic rates (Gottschalk et al., 1991a,b, 1992, 1993a,b). Furthermore, the same states of consciousness influence the cerebral areas, where significant inter-correlations occur between positive hope scores, negative hope scores, and total hope scores (the sum of positive and negative hope scores) with cerebral glucose metabolic rates (Gottschalk, Fronczek, Abel, & Buchsbaum, 1993b).

6. The direction of lateralization—right-sided versus left-sided hemispheric dominance—and the ratios of positive to negative significant correlations between cerebral glucose metabolic rates and total anxiety (a+b+c+d), self-anxiety (a), anxiety displacements (b+c), and anxiety denials (d) varies with the brain areas examined: that is, whole brain, medial and subcortical gray areas, and lateral cortical regions (see Table 23.8).

7. Based on the location of the largest number of significant correlations (positive or negative), there is left-sided lateralization for total anxiety during wakeful (silent) mentation in whole brain and right-sided

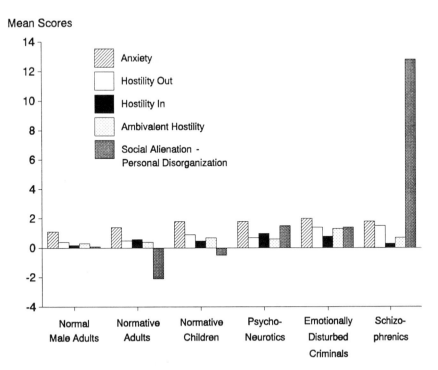

FIGURE 23.1. Comparisons of mean affect and social alienation–personal disorganization scores for six groups of subjects.

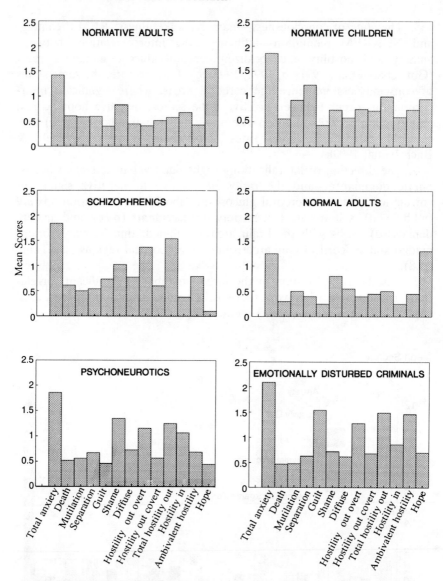

FIGURE 23.2. Comparison of anxiety, anxiety subscales, and hostility scores for six groups of subjects.

lateralization for total anxiety, self references, and displacements in medial and subcortical gray regions and left-sided lateralization for anxiety denials in these brain regions. In lateral cortical cerebral regions, the lateralization differs in that there is left-sided dominance for total anxiety scores and self references, right-sided dominance for displacements, and no definite lateralization for denials of anxiety.

8. Denials of anxiety tend to have an opposite cerebral hemispheric dominance (or no lateralization, depending on the brain region) than affirmations of anxiety, which suggests a yes–no function for the two cerebral hemispheres.

9. The findings with respect to the intercorrelations of localized cerebral glucose metabolic rates with total anxiety, self-anxiety, anxiety displacement, and anxiety denial clearly indicate that the cerebral neurobiological representations of these anxiety variables have largely distinct and separate cerebral localizations. (For full details, see Gottschalk et al., 1991b,c,e.) Moreover, the significant increases or decreases in cerebral energy consumption (in the form of localized glucose metabolic rates) associated with changes in the verbal measures of anxiety involve brain areas known from other animal and human studies to subserve the functions of cognition, reasoning, memory, audition, vision, and emotions.

10. Positive hope and negative hope scores tend to have significant correlations with glucose metabolic rates in opposite cerebral hemispheres in medial cortical and subcortical gray as well as lateral cortical areas (see Table 23.8). And when these correlations involve similar identical cerebral locations, the significant correlations between positive and negative hope with glucose metabolic rate are in opposite directions (Gottschalk et al., 1991d,e).

Figure 23.3 illustrates the brain areas targeted for glucose metabolic rates based on the neuroanatomical atlas of Matsui and Hirano (1987).

TABLE 23.8. Hemispheric lateralization and number of significant positive (+) and negative (−) correlations between anxiety and hope scores during silent mentation with cerebral glucose metabolic rates.

Scores	Whole brain				Medial cortical and subcortical gray				Lateral cortical				Sums			
	Left		Right		Left		Right		Left		Right		Left		Right	
	+	−	+	−	+	−	+	−	+	−	+	−	+	−	+	−
Anxiety																
Total scores	1				1	2	2	3		1			2	3	2	3
Self references (verbal)	1			1	1	3	2	3		1			2	4	2	4
Displacements	1	1	1	1	1	2	1	4	1		2		3	3	4	5
Denials	2	1		1	3	9	2	3	1	1		2	6	11	2	6
Hope																
Total hope	1	2	1	1	1	2	4	1				1	2	4	5	3
Positive hope	1	1	1			3	2	2	1			1	2	4	3	3
Negative hope	2				2	1	1	1		2			4	3	1	1

NOTES: Left = significant correlations ($p < .05$, two-tailed) in left cerebral hemisphere; Right = significant correlations ($p < .05$, two-tailed) in right cerebral hemisphere.

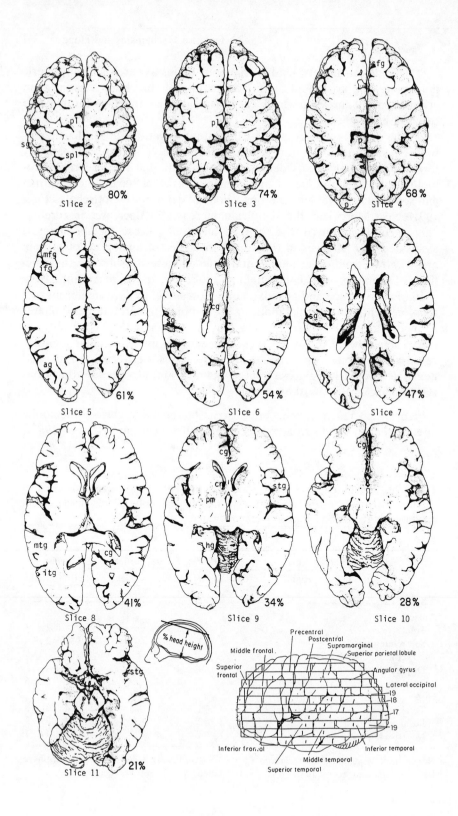

Table 23.8 aims to summarize the tendencies for hemispheric lateralization, based on the criterion of the largest number of significant intercorrelations (positive or negative), between anxiety and hope scores with localized cerebral glucose metabolic rates.

During wakeful silent mentation in whole brain, positive hope scores correlate positively with glucose metabolic rates in the parietal lobe, left temporal cortex, occipital cortex, and right occipital cortex and negatively with glucose metabolic rate in the left temporal lobe. Negative hope scores correlate positively with glucose metabolic rate in the left frontal lobe and left temporal lobe (Gottschalk et al., 1991b). The precise significant correlations between cerebral glucose metabolic rates with anxiety and hope scores are reported in detail elsewhere (Gottschalk et al., 1991a,b, 1992, 1993b).

Discussion

These findings, using the objective method of verbal behavior content analysis and the noninvasive method of measuring localized energy consumption in the living human brain by recording the relative cerebral glucose metabolic rates via positron emission tomography, provide novel perspectives on psychological defense and coping mechanisms and how these relate to psychopathological and neurobiological processes. At the same time, an introduction is given to the cerebral locations associated with the alerting and usually negative emotions of anxiety, hostility, and hopelessness and the positive emotion of hope. Our findings with respect to these psychological mechanisms and psychopathological processes can be easily discussed and possibly integrated with other bodies of knowledge on the subject.

Our findings, however, with regard to these psychological mechanisms and their ongoing neurobiological substrates as represented by cerebral

←——————————————————————————————

FIGURE 23.3. Brain slices and locations: drawing of brain levels from atlas of Matsui and Hirano showing slice number, percentage of head height above canthomeatal line, and location of statistically significant correlations with anxiety. Regions on cortical surface were assessed with the radial cortical peel computer algorithm (Buchsbaum, Gillin, Wu, Hazlett, Prager, Sicotte, & Dupont, 1989) and regions in the medial areas of the brain with square, stereotaxically placed regions of interest. All correlations with $p < .05$, two-tailed, of this exploratory analysis are given in Table 23.8. Abbreviations: spl = superior parietal lobule, sg = supramarginal gyrus, ifg = inferior frontal gyrus, sfg = superior frontal gyrus, pl = paracentral lobule, p = precuneus, cg = cingulate gyrus, ag = angular gyrus, ol = occipital lobe.

glucose metabolic correlates, since they constitute a first look at such interrelationships, are almost beyond lengthy intelligent discussion. As with the first explorers of a new continent or of the Earth's moon, the easiest and most natural communication to others is to describe what one sees and, then, to wait for others to corroborate the existence of the initial phenomena observed. Along that approach, our initial observations regarding cerebral glucose metabolic correlates with the verbal-behavior-derived scores for anxiety, hostility, hope, and some of their defenses provide a new map of unexplored land that bears checking and replication. Since there is no extant empirical body of knowledge throwing light on the cerebral correlates of emotions and their defenses, our findings at this time need further scrutiny, reflection, and cautious assimilation. It is perhaps permissible to go one step beyond that position and with modest certainty claim that apparently brain circuits record yes-and-no matters, such as anxious thoughts and denials of anxious thoughts, in opposite cerebral hemispheres. And though not quite as uniformly, hopeful thoughts are more often processed in the opposite cerebral hemisphere than unhopeful thoughts. Moreover, the cerebral neurobiological representations—as adjudged from the locations of significant correlations with cerebral glucose metabolic rates—of total anxiety, self-anxiety, anxiety displacement, anxiety denial, hopefulness, and hopelessness have largely discrete and separate cerebral localizations. Beyond these observations, there is no more to say except to be prepared for new hypothesis generating on the relationships of brain functioning and psychological functioning.

With regard to emotions, defenses, and psychopathological processes, the findings in this study support the viewpoint that (verbal) displacements and denials of anxiety, when they are not of great magnitude, are associated with mental health, especially in adults, and are highly positively correlated in their frequency of occurrence with direct statements of the self being anxious. As the severity of the psychopathological processes increases, significant intercorrelations between assertions of the self being anxious and denials of anxiety become significantly negative in patients with neuroses. And as the psychopathological processes become even more severe—for example, in emotionally disordered criminals and in acute schizophrenic patients—such intercorrelations disappear entirely. Since the frequency of occurrence of verbal statements concerning the self being anxious and displacements and denials of anxiety all tend to increase with the severity of emotional and mental impairment, the magnitude of self-anxiety or displacements or denials of anxiety can all serve as signs of the severity of mental incapacity (see also Gottschalk et al., 1993a).

Hope scores, derived from the content analysis of speech, appear to serve a protective function in mental health. The greater the mental health of individuals, the higher their hope scores. This observation (see

Table 23.1) is backed up by current findings that our group of normal young males, during wakefulness, had mean hope scores of +0.43 ± 1.02, our group of normative adults had mean hope scores of +0.73 ± 1.03, our normative children had mean hope scores of +.04 ± 1.25l, our emotionally disordered criminals had average hope scores of −.49 ± 1.49, and our group of acute schizophrenic patients had average hope scores of −.78 ± 1.64.

With regard to the cerebral lateralization of positive and negative emotions, Tucker (1981) has reported that negative emotions, such as anxiety, are more often lateralized to the left cerebral hemisphere, whereas Sackeim, Greenberg, Weiman, Gur, Hungerbuhler, and Geschwind (1982) and Campbell (1982) observe that the left hemisphere is more frequently associated with positive emotions and the right hemisphere is more frequently associated with negative emotions. These conflicting hypotheses may be explainable by our own findings in that we find slight left-sided cerebral lateralization for total anxiety in the whole brain and right-sided lateralization for total anxiety, self-anxiety, and displaced anxiety in medial cortical and subcortical gray areas and left-sided lateralization for total anxiety in lateral cortical areas (see Table 23.8). We suggest that the determination of cerebral lateralization is influenced by the methods and criteria used for assessing such cerebral localization and, certainly, by the range and completeness of brain regions examined. Our use of positron emission tomography has allowed us to survey the whole brain as well as cortical and subcortical areas of interest, and our criterion of ascertaining lateralization by locating the brain areas where the majority of significant correlations are found between the magnitude of the emotions and localized cerebral glucose metabolic rates would seem to be more reliable than other methods used heretofore. Looking at the cerebral lateralization associated with positive and negative hope scores derived from verbal reports during wakeful silent mentation would tend to favor the hypothesis that negative hope scores (feelings and thoughts of hopelessness) are localized in the left cerebral hemisphere if one considers whole brain and lateral gray areas, but that there is less clear lateralization if one focuses on the medial cortical and subcortical gray areas. And if one considers the state of consciousness—that is, whether the subject is awake or asleep during the experiencing of these emotions— the constancy of cerebral lateralization during emotions disappears. Obviously, further studies to clarify these issues are in order.

Finally, we recommend the use of the content analysis of natural language as a very specific and reliable method of determining the occurrence of psychological defense mechanisms, such as displacements, denials, and hopefulness. No inferences are necessary to establish when such psychological dimensions are being used, for their occurrence is manifestly observable in the content of verbal behavior itself. Furthermore, other studies we have cited provide construct validation.

Summary and Conclusions

This is a study examining, through the content analysis of verbal behavior, the extent to which the verbalization of an emotion, such as anxiety, correlates significantly with the frequency of verbalization of "defenses" against anxiety, such as displacements and denials of anxiety, across different groups of subjects, ranging from mentally and physically healthy individuals to emotionally disturbed criminals and schizophrenic patients. With the availability of positron emission tomography at our Brain Imaging Center, the opportunity was presented to examine, also, the relationship of verbalizations of anxiety, anxiety displacements, and anxiety denials as well as verbalizations of hopefulness and hopelessness to localized cerebral glucose metabolic rates. Since hope is often regarded as a defensive or protective state or trait against mental or physical disorders the exploration of its cerebral neurobiology with respect to glucose metabolic rate appeared to be a relevant undertaking.

With the exception of children, the more mentally healthy the group of subjects, the more likely were there to be significant intercorrelations between verbal statements of the self being anxious and displacements and denials of anxiety. Sex, intelligence, and age had no significant effects on the frequency of occurrence of the phenomena of displacements and denials in the spoken language of six groups of subjects.

Opposite cerebral hemispheres had significant intercorrelations between measures of the self being anxious and denials of such anxiety with cerebral glucose metabolic rates, and less consistently, measures of hopefulness and hopelessness revealed a similar phenomenon. There are quite different cerebral representations for verbalized self-anxiety, anxiety displacements, anxiety denials, hopefulness, and hopelessness during the same and different states of consciousness, specifically, silent wakeful mentation, REM dreaming, and NONREM mentation.

A discussion is offered of the bearings our findings have on the issues of cerebral lateralization of positive and negative emotions. We believe our findings provide more stringent criteria for determining such lateralization than previous studies in this area. Moreover, positron emission tomography provides an opportunity to survey all brain regions, instead of omitting possibly crucial areas, and it affords occasions for noninvasive cerebral neurobiochemical assessments in the living human subject.

References

Anant, S.S. (1967) Belongingness, anxiety, and self-sufficiency. *Psychological Reports, 20,* 1137–1138.

Barron, F. (1953) An ego strength scale which predicts response to psychotherapy. *Journal of Consulting and Clinical Psychology, 17,* 327–333.

Buchsbaum, M.S., Gillin, J.C., Wu, J., Hazlett, E., Prager, L., Sicotte, N., & Dupont, R. (1989) Regional cerebral metabolic rate in human sleep assessed by positron emission tomography. *Life Sciences*, *45*, 1349–1356.

Campbell, R. (1982) The lateralization of emotion: A critical review. *International Journal of Psychology*, *17*, 211–229.

Derogatis, L.R., Lipman, Rr., Rickels, K., Uhlenhuth, E.H., & Covi, L. (1974) The Hopkins Symptom Checklist (HSCL): A measure of primary symptom dimensions. In P. Pichat (Ed.), *Psychological measurements in psychopharmacology: Vol. 7* (pp. 79–110). Basel: Karger.

Endicott, J., Spitzer, R., Fleiss, J., & Cohen, J. (1976) The global assessment scale. *Archives of General Psychiatry*, *33*, 766–771.

Frank, J. (1968) The role of hope in psychotherapy. *International Journal of Psychiatry*, *5*, 383–395.

French, T.M. (1952) *The integration of behavior: Vol. 1*. Chicago: University of Chicago Press.

Freud, A. (1946) *The ego and the mechanisms of defense*. New York: International Universities Press. (Original work published 1936)

Gleser, G.C. & Ihilevich, D. (1969) An objective instrument for measuring defense mechanisms. *Journal of Consulting and Clinical Psychology*, *33*, 51–60.

Gottschalk, L.A. (1976) Children's speech as a source of data towards the measurement of psychological states. *Journal of Youth and Adolescence*, *5*, 11–36.

Gottschalk, L.A. (1974) A hope scale applicable to verbal samples. *Archives of General Psychiatry*, *30*, 779–785.

Gottschalk, L.A., Biener, R., Noble, E.P., Birch, H., Wilbert, D.E., & Heiser, J.F. (1975) Thioridazine plasma levels and clinical response. *Comprehensive Psychiatry*, *16*, 323–337.

Gottschalk, L.A., Buchsbaum, M., Gillin, J.R., Wu, J., Reynolds, C., & Herrera, D.B. (1991a) Anxiety levels in dreams: Relation to localized cerebral glucose metabolic rate. *Brain Research*, *538*, 107–110.

Gottschalk, L.A., Buchsbaum, M., Gillin, J.R., Wu, J., Reynolds, C., & Herrera, D.B. (1991b) Positron emission tomographic studies of the relationship of cerebral glucose metabolism and the magnitude of anxiety and hostility experienced during dreaming and waking. *Journal of Neuropsychiatry and Clinical Neuroscience*, *31*, 131–142.

Gottschalk, L.A., Buchsbaum, M., Gillin, J.R., Wu, J., Reynolds, C., & Herrera, D.B. (1992c) The effect of silent mentation on cerebral glucose metabolic rate. *Comprehensive Psychiatry*, *33*, 52–59.

Gottschalk, L.A., Covi, L., Uliana, R., & Bates, D.E. (1973) Effects of diphenylhydantoin on anxiety and hostility in institutionalized prisoners. *Comprehensive Psychiatry*, *14*, 503–511.

Gottschalk, L.A., Fox, R.A., & Bates, D.E. (1973) A study of prediction and outcome in a Mental Health Crisis Clinic. *American Journal of Psychiatry*, *190*, 1107–1111.

Gottschalk, L.A., Fronczek, J., & Abel, L. (1993a) Emotions, defenses, coping mechanisms, and symptoms (In press). *Psychoanalytic Psychology*.

Gottschalk, L.A., Fronczek, J., Abel, L., & Buchsbaum, M. (1993b) The cerebral neurobiology of hope and hopelessness (In press). *Psychiatry*.

Gottschalk, L.A. & Gleser, G.C. (1969) *The measurement of psychological states through the content analysis of verbal behavior*. Berkeley, Los Angeles: University of California Press.

Gottschalk, L.A., Gleser, G.C., & Springer, K.J. (1963) Three hostility scales applicable to verbal samples. *Archives of General Psychiatry, 9*, 254–279.

Gottschalk, L.A. & Hoigaard-Martin, J. (1986) The emotional impact of mastectomy. *Psychiatry Research, 17*, 153–167.

Gottschalk, L.A., Hoigaard, J.C., Birch, H., & Rickels, K. (1979) The measurement of psychological states: Relationships between Gottschalk–Gleser content analyses scores and Hamilton Anxiety Rating Scales score, Physician Questionnaire Rating Scales scores, and Hopkins Symptom Checklist scores. In L.A. Gottschalk (Ed.), *Content analysis of verbal behavior: Further studies* (pp. 41–94). New York: Spectrum.

Gottschalk, L.A., Kunkel, R.L., Wohl, T., Saenger, E., & Winget, C.N. (1969) Total and half body irradiation. Effect on cognitive and emotional processes. *Archives of General Psychiatry, 21*, 574–580.

Gottschalk, L.A., Lolas, F., & Viney, L.L. (Eds.) (1986) *Content analysis of verbal behavior. Significance in clinical medicine and psychiatry* (pp. 249–256). Heidelberg, Germany: Springer-Verlag.

Gottschalk, L.A., Mayerson, P., & Gottlieb, A. (1967) The prediction and evaluation of outcome in an emergency brief psychotherapy clinic. *Journal of Nervous and Mental Disease, 144*, 77–96.

Gottschalk, L.A., Winget, C.N., & Gleser, G.C. (1969) *Manual of instructions for using the Gottschalk–Gleser Content Analysis Scales: Anxiety, Hostility, and Social Alienation–Personal Disorganization.* Berkeley, Los Angeles: University of California Press.

Huang, S.C., Phelps, M.E., Hoffman, E.J., Sideris, K., Selin, C.J., & Kuhl, D.E. (1980) Noninvasive determination of local cerebral metabolic rate of glucose in man. *American Journal of Physiology, 238*, E69–E82.

Ihilevich, D. & Gleser, G.C. (1986) *Defense mechanisms. Their classification, correlates, and measurement with the defense mechanisms inventory.* Owosso, MI: DMT Associates.

Matsui, T. & Hirano, A. (1987) *An atlas of the human brain for computerized tomography.* Tokyo: Igaku-Shoin.

Perley, J., Winget, C.N., & Placci, C. (1971) Hope and discomfort as factors influencing treatment continuance. *Comprehensive Psychiatry, 12*, 557–563.

Sackeim, H.A., Greenberg, M.S., Weiman, A.L., Gur, R.C., Hungerbuhler, J.P., & Geschwind, N. (1982) Hemispheric asymmetry in the social expression of positive and negative emotions: Neurological evidence. *Archives of Neurology, 39*, 210–218.

Sokoloff, L., Reivich, M., Kennedy, C., Des Rosiers, M.S., Patlak, D.S., Pettigrew, K.D., Sakurada, O., & Shinohara, M. (1977) The [^{14}C] deoxyglucose method for the measurement of local cerebral glucose utilization: Theory, procedure, and normal values in the conscious and anesthetized albino rat. *Journal of Neurochemistry, 28*, 897–916.

SPSS (1990) *SPSS reference guide.* Chicago: SPSS, Inc.

Tucker, D.M. (1981) Lateral brain function, emotion, and conceptualization. *Psychological Bulletin, 89*, 19–46.

Udelman, D.L. & Udelman, H.D. (1986) A preliminary report on antidepressant therapy and its effect on hope and immunity. In L.A. Gottschalk, F. Lolas, L. L. Viney (Eds.). (1986) *Content analysis of verbal behavior. Significance in clinical medicine and psychiatry.* (pp. 249–256). Heidelberg, Germany: Springer-Verlag.

Uliana, R.L. (1979) Measurement of black children's affective states and the effect of interviewer's race on affective states as measured through language behavior. In L.A. Gottschalk (Ed.), *Content analysis of verbal behavior: Further studies* (pp. 175–233). New York: Spectrum.

Winget, C., Seligman, R., Rauh, J.L., & Gleser, G.C. (1979) Alienation–Personal Disorganization assessment in disturbed and normal adolescents. *Journal of Nervous and Mental Disease, 167*, 282–287.

Wonderlic, E.F. (1945) *Wonderlic Personnel Test Manual.* Norfield, IL: Wonderlic and Associates.

24
Defense Mechanisms in Patients with Bone Marrow Transplantation: A Retrospective Study

CHRISTINA SCHWILK, DANIELA AESCHELMANN, HORST KÄCHELE, CLAUDIA SIMONS, and RENATE ARNOLD

Theoretical Considerations and Guiding Questions

The impact of defense processes on coping with life-threatening diseases has been shown in many studies, especially with regard to cancer, chronic hemodialysis, and after myocardial infarction (Gaus & Köhle, 1986). However, systematic studies on patients after bone marrow transplantation (bmt) rarely focus on defense mechanisms influencing the adaptation process.

Brown and Kelly (1976) describe psychological problems in six adolescent and six adult bmt patients during eight phases of the treatment. Being confronted with the anxiety-inducing decision to bmt, they reacted with denial and displacement. Patenaude and Rappeport (1982) report on several defense mechanisms occurring in four patients after bmt, such as minimalization, withdrawal, and denial after death of the patient "in the other bed." These retrospective studies with small groups of patients discover defense mechanisms as side effects.

The patients of our study, being confronted with the diagnosis of a hematological disease such as leukemia and an aggressive medical treatment (for a detailed description of the bmt treatment at University Hospital, Ulm, see Arnold et al., 1986) like bmt must cope with the following unspecific stress situations comparable to other cancer diseases: sudden confrontation with a life-threatening diagnosis; short time period between first symptoms, diagnosis, and treatment; overstraining side effects due to the medical treatment (pain, loss of hair, infections); invasive diagnostic and therapeutic operations; uncertainty concerning the success of the therapy; and necessity of an adaptive organization of the patient's daily life. In addition, the patients are confronted with bmt-specific stress situations (Beutel, 1988): germ-free isolation in the tent, physical inactivity, and the waiting period for the taking of the new bone marrow (several weeks). Finally, the graft-versus-host disease puts success at risk. The bmt is the patient's only hope. Because of advancing developments in bmt, the treatment conditions had been changing during the period (1978–1986) we retrospectively investigated.

The aim of our study is to identify which defense mechanisms are occurring and to explore whether the defense organization changes during the different treatment phases.

Our theoretical understanding of defense processes is characterized by a detachment of drive-related foundations of the psychoanalytic concept; we conceptualize defense as a major tool of the regulation of self- and object relation (Steffens and Kächele, 1988). By means of defense, the ego masters internal conflicts aroused by the external trauma. The stress caused by disease and therapy may well reactivate past unconscious conflicts as well as stir up new dangerous and painful affects, which by themselves initiate defense maneuvers. The ego must balance between intrapsychic object-related needs and wishes and the external demands of the disease and its treatment consequences. The defense mechanisms lead to a distorted perception of reality and to the exclusion of conflicting self-aspects. This influences the cognitions, emotions, actions, and social relations of the patient, possibly resulting in a less optimal adaptation to the therapeutic situation or even weakening the tolerance for unbearable situations. On the other side, the defense operations may conserve the functioning of the ego in a situation of overwhelming anxiety and impending fragmentation of the self.

Since the material of the study consisted of retrospective interviews, it is evident that a host of factors are operating that counteract the ecological validity of this pilot study. What we in fact are investigating are defense mechanisms as they are operating when patients retrospectively describe their experience. However, this approach seems suitable to gain first experiences in a new field of research. The results may support the generation of hypotheses and the development of appropriate methods for the assessment of defense mechanisms in a prospective study.[1]

Method

With the exception of instruments for measuring denial, methods for the assessment of defense mechanisms are scarcely available (Beutel, 1985a,b). Since defense mechanisms are conceptualized as an unconscious process, ratings by expert observers may be more congruent with the logic of the object than procedures for self-rating. The verbatim transcripts of 34 retrospective semistructured interviews with patients after bmt provided the basic information for the two raters in this investigation.

---

[1] Since January 1990 there has been an interdisciplinary prospective long-time study concerning somatic and psychosocial rehabilitation in bmt patients at the Ulm University Hosptial (Departments of Internal Medicine and Psychotherapy.

The interviewer and the two raters were not identical. Our approach entails that defense mechanisms not only be a stable part of personality development, which to a certain extent may be the case, but also show a certain amount of reactivity to situational factors. Therefore we differentiated three phases in the patients' descriptions:

Phase a: acute confrontation of the patient with the diagnosis, the vital threat by the disease itself, and the suggested treatment.

Phase b: ongoing crisis, with extreme somatic and psychic stress during the procedure of bmt (radiation, chemotherapy, isolation in Life Island beds, transplantation).

Phase c: stabilization and consolidation after discharge from inpatient treatment, with diminishing danger of somatic complications and adaptation to changes in somatic, cognitive–emotional, and social aspects.

To achieve at least what Luborsky (1984) calls a guided clinical rating, we decided to work with a defense mechanism rating scale called Clinical Assessment of Defense Mechanisms (CADM, German: KBAM, Ehlers & Czogalik, 1984). We shall report on results with a slightly modified version of the CADM adapted to the specific situation of our patients. The original CADM contains 26 categories that can be rated on a five-point intensity scale. The rating is directed toward the probability of the presence of a given defense mechanism. The categories cover the classical defense mechanisms as described by A. Freud (1936), some of M. Klein's early defense formations (1948), as well as some symptoms that are thought of as products of defense activity. The Ulm version of the CADM contains 21 categories, because of the exclusion of some defenses that were unlikely to turn up in our material.

The symptom formations were dropped. Some of the categories of the CADM were condensed into one (e.g., reaction formation and turning into the opposite). However, we added the category "sublimation" to cover creative solutions of perceived dangerous situations and the category "symbiotic alliance" as an interpersonal defense mechanism (Mentzos, 1976) occurring in the face of severe threat. Most of the other categories have been revised only slightly; however, we have given up the drive-related aspects describing the transformation of wishes, ideas, affects, and imagined or real dangers (Bibring, Dwyer, Huntington, & Valenstein, 1961; Ehlers, 1983; A. Freud, 1936; S. Freud, 1926, 1968; Laplanche & Pontalis, 1967/1986).

The identification of the defense mechanisms is hardly possible without some detailed knowledge of a patient's general makeup; therefore the phase of identifying relevant text passages also served the useful purpose of familiarizing us with the particularities of each of the patients. The following examples give an impression of the text material:

Example 1: avoidance ". . . I don't know if anybody supported me, but I believe that this is my fault, I rejected everybody—not intentionally,

TABLE 24.1. Clinical–hematological characteristics of 34 patients.

Age	17–50 years; M = 23 (at time of bmt)
Sex	16 women
	18 men
Diagnosis	21 acute lymphatic and myeloic leukemia
	7 chronic myeloic leukemia
	3 severe aplastic anemia
	3 myelodysplastic syndrome
Time lag between bmt and interviews	7–96 months

but I said I didn't want to see anybody, or I didn't like that, but I didn't want to talk to anybody . . ."

Example 2: regression ". . . it was impossible at home and it was so extreme, that I didn't do anything without help, neither getting up or washing myself or taking my medicine, I was totally dependent . . ."

Example 3: reaction formation/turning into the opposite ". . . and then I've found it very exciting that I'm here, and also, the operation for the Hickman catheter just recently, suddenly the thought occurred to me, my school mates they've got to work hard and I'm lying here leisurely . . ."

Example 4: projection " . . . it really was a hard blow for my mother, the illness, I think she's grown older, it seems to me . . . "

Results

The clinical-hematological characteristics of the sample are presented in Table 24.1.

The estimation of reliability of highly inferential codings, as is the case with defense mechanisms, must allow some ambiguity. However, it is important to know about the details of how both raters worked. Since rater x did not use score 2 and rater y only scarcely, the matrix can be simplified into yes or no decisions, where scores of 1 or 2 indicate no and scores of 3 to 4 indicate yes decisions (Table 24.2). As it turns out, the interrater reliability of the defense rating is not overwhelming ($\kappa = .42$, $p < .001$). Although there is significant agreement, still it indicates considerable differences between the judgments. The differences occur

TABLE 24.2. Yes or no interrater reliability.

	y1,2 (no)	y3,4,5 (yes)	Total
x1,2 (no)	1318	387	1705
x3,4,5 (yes)	156	323	479
Total	1474	710	2184

TABLE 24.3. Mean intensity of defense mechanisms.

Defense mechanism	Mean intensity
1. Denial	3.45
2. Avoidance	2.57
3. Minimalization	2.55
4. Repression	2.42
5. Isolation	2.39
6. Reaction formation	2.26
7. Rationalization	2.18
8. Displacement	2.14
9. Projection	2.02
10. Regression	1.92
11. Resignation	1.76
12. Identification	1.66
13. Undoing	1.52
14. Idealization	1.50
15. Sublimation	1.47
16. Symbiotic alliance	1.41
17. Omnipotence fantasies	1.39
18. Somatization	1.36
19. Turning against self	1.27
20. Devaluation	1.20
21. Splitting	1.12

mainly because rater y favors the occurrence of defense mechanisms whereas rater x does not see one.

The next step consisted of calculating the mean intensity of defense mechanisms in the sample (Table 24.3). These intensity measures are mean values, which were averaged over all patients and phases.

Cluster analysis of the defense mechanisms reveals some interesting interconnections of defenses, which on the level of simple correlation (similarity measure) match clinical presuppositions.[2] In Table 24.4 the first pair of defense mechanisms is correlated to higher degree than the second, the second than the third, and so on.

TABLE 24.4. Correlating defense mechanisms.

1. Idealization	Omnipotence fantasies
2. Regression	Resignation
3. Resignation	Avoidance
4. Somatization	Devaluation
5. Reaction formation	Minimalization

---

[2] Cluster analysis on variables was used here. Amalgamation was done by complete linkage. The similarity measure used was the correlation found between defense mechanism values.

[3] The analysis of variance model was used here with repeated measurements (*t*-test), four-linked random tests, and assessed with nonparametric techniques.

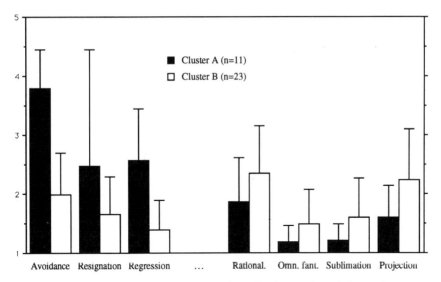

FIGURE 24.1. Defense mechanisms by patients in cluster A and cluster B: means and standard deviations.

Next we tried to find subgroups of patients having same or similar configurations of defense mechanisms. For this purpose a nonhierarchical cluster analysis of cases was applied.[3] A two-cluster solution was suitable for a clinically meaningful interpretation (Fig. 24.1):

Cluster A, consisting of 11 patients: their "typical" constellation of defenses includes avoidance, resignation, and regression. "Typical" means that these defense mechanisms are significantly higher in this patient group than in the other group.
Cluster B, consisting of 23 patients: their typical constellation of defenses includes projection, sublimation, and fantasies of omnipotence.

By applying discriminant analysis between the two clusters, we intended to find some "extremely typical" patients representing their cluster and being as far removed as possible from the other cluster. We were looking for extreme cases, so called "super A" and "super B" patients. In this way we wanted to recombine our statistical results with the clinical experience. Gradual discriminant analysis confirmed that with help of defense mechanism values it is possible to discriminate patients between cluster A and cluster B. The discriminant function used for this classification is positive for cluster A and negative for cluster B. Four patients with the highest positive value were classified as "super A" and two patients with extreme negative value as "super B" (Fig. 24.2).

By factor analysis of the defense mechanisms we find the first three factors explaining 37% of the complete variance. Factor 1 subsumes

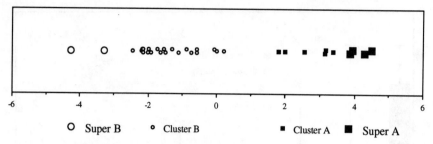

FIGURE 24.2. Defense types (discriminant analysis).

cluster A and cluster B completely and explains 15% of the complete variance. Therefore we see small groups of defense mechanisms contributing to more various factors. Factor 2 subsumes a group of denying defense mechanisms (displacement, repression, denial). Since complete interpretation of factor analysis results would be rather complicated, we confined ourselves to the interpretation of the first unrotated factor.

Relating the analysis of defense mechanisms to the three phases of the treatment, we found no systematical differences.

Case Reports

As an illustration of the significant difference between cluster A and cluster B, we describe the course the illness and the rehabilitation took in two typical patients.

Ms. A. ("Super A")

The main defense mechanisms in the super A case are denial and projection in phase a, and avoidance, resignation, and repression, in phase b and c.

When Ms. A. was 27 years old an acute myelonic leukemia was diagnosed; 9 months later the bmt was done. Being a single woman without children, she lived with a girl friend. After bmt she started to work in the same factory as before but changed from the assembly line to quality control. She was told the diagnosis after visiting different hospitals. Obviously shocked by the diagnosis, she remembered her aunt dying of leukemia. But she emphasized her family's shock at the diagnosis. In the tent phase she became depressive and withdrew into herself. She was afraid of losing her sister, the bone marrow donor, by an accident before the bmt. After discharge her physical condition was good. She was able to do sports, and 9 months after bmt she held a full-time job. She retired from social contacts with her peer group more than before; whereas the relationship to the family members became closer. She was no longer interested in men because her medical treatment caused sterility. Future perspectives seemed to be restricted by her tendencies to resign and to avoid contacts.

Mr. B. ("Super B")

The main defense mechanisms in the super B case are denial in phase a, followed by isolation, rationalization, and fantasies of omnipotence in phases b and c.

Mr. B. was 22 years old when an acute lymphatic leukemia was diagnosed. One year later after a second relapse he was transplanted. The donor was his twin brother. The retrospective interview took place 24 months after bmt. He still lived with his parents and was quite satisfied with his job. Upon being told the diagnosis, he first refused to realize it. The bmt was the great chance that had to work. In the interview he explicitly described the physical stress in the tent phase. In times of impending crisis and resignation he became angry. The relationship with his symbiotically allied twin brother helped him to enter into struggles with the treating physicians. In the tent phase he refused the medicine, criticizing the "high" dose. After discharge, somatic rehabilitation was excellent. Doing physical exercises he felt no physical impediments. After 9 months he went back to work. He had discontinued the relationship with his girl friend at the beginning of the disease, because he felt she did not appreciate how serious things were. He did not get involved in a close relationship but was increasing his social activities. His psychic status seemed to him much better after the bmt experience than before. He felt more able to enjoy life; depressive thoughts could be mastered by training. He solved the problems connected with his sterility by an imagined identification with his twin brother, who would procreate the children for him.

Discussion

In agreement with other studies concerning defense mechanisms in severe diseases (Beutel, 1988; Gaus & Köhle, 1986) denial was most prominent. Whether denial favors or inhibits successful coping with diseases and rehabilitation is the subject of controversy. According to Vaillant (1971), denial in psychological disturbances is seen as an immature defense mechanism. In situations of immense external danger, which rarely can be minimized by a specific behavior, denial seems to increase the individual capacity to act. We agree with Battegay (1989), who points out that if defense allows an active life, a severe disease has a better prognosis. If denial persists as the strongest and most important defense mechanism in the rehabilitation phase, the adaptation process may be inhibited (A. Freud, 1936) by the distorted perception of reality.

The cluster analysis generated clinically interesting groups. Elsewhere we presented the results of our investigation on the emotional vocabulary in this text material supporting the validity of our findings. (Kächele, Hölzer & Schwilk, 1989).

The "Affective Dictionary," developed and presented by Hölzer, Scheytt, Pokorny, and Kächele (1989) according to the theory of emotions of Dahl (1978), subsumes and classifies the emotional vocabulary into the following categories: positive object emotions (love, attraction), positive self emotions (contentment, joy), negative object emotions (anger, fear), and negative self emotions (depression, anxiety). The correlation between the intensity of defense mechanisms and the frequency of affective labels yielded some interesting results. There was a negative correlation between overall intensity of defense and affective labeling (−.34). Closer inspection of the correlation matrix shows avoidance and resignation correlating strongly negatively, omnipotence positively. Although this is not significant for most mechanisms, the intensity of 15 defense mechanisms (out of 21) is negatively correlated with negative self emotions; the exceptions in somatization and turning against self were to be expected. These negative correlations may highlight the primary function of defense: to secure positive feelings for the individual. Hence the predominance of positive correlations between intensity of defense and positive emotions is understandable. The highly positive correlation between omnipotence and positive self feelings seems to be particularly noticeable. The highly negative correlation between "avoidance" and the emotional vocabulary of the category "anger" (−.79) and between "avoidance" and the verbal activity (−.65) reflect the clinical impression that these patients avoid not only conflictual content but also talking itself.

These results help us to generate some hypotheses. The main defense mechanisms in cluster A (avoidance, resignation, regression) may lead to a withdrawal from vital interests. The sequels seem to be minimized self-esteem, and less satisfaction, and less activity concerning the patient's life and life perspective. The main defense mechanisms in cluster B (projection, sublimation, fantasies of omnipotence) may lead to self-esteem and satisfying activity in life. Whether they improve the rehabilitation results and the disease prognosis, we can only speculate. Temporarily this group seems to experience a higher quality of life. In this context the reference to the results of coping strategies in the only prospective study concerning distress of bmt patients during transplantation phase (Neuser, 1989) is interesting. By means of patient self-rating, active problem-oriented coping (fighting against the disease, believing in the treating physicians, intending to live more intensively) was regarded as the most helpful behavior.

Because of the retrospective character of the interviews, we did not find specific defense patterns related to the three phases of the disease. Further investigation must be done within our prospective study. To improve interrater reliability, we decided to intensify the training of the raters, cataloguing typical text examples and specifying situation-related definitions. The prospective investigation should answer some important questions:

What is successful defense and how does it interact with a successful coping and adaptation process?
Do defensive maneuvers depend on situational factors?
Do they change during the different phases of treatment and rehabilitation?
Does defensive organization influence prognosis of the psychic and social rehabilitation process after bmt?

References

Arnold, R., Schmeiser, T., Friedrich, W., Carbonell, F., Goldman, S.F., Heit, W., Kohne, E., Kurrle, E., Kleihauer, E., Heimpel, H., & Kubanek, B. (1986) Knochenmarktransplantation; Ergebnisse der Ulmer Transplantationsgruppe [Bone marrow transplantation; results of the Ulm transplantation group]. *Klinische Wochenschrift, 62,* 577–585.

Battegay, R. (1989) Das Ich—Abwehrmechanismen und Coping [The ego—Defense mechanisms and coping]. *Psychosomatic Medicine, 35,* 220–240.

Beutel, M. (1985a) Approaches to taxonomy and measurement of adaptation in chronic disease. *Psychotherapy and Psychosomatics, 43,* 177–185.

Beutel, M. (1985b) Zur Erforschung der Verarbeitung chronischer Krankheit. Konzeptualisierung, Operationalisierung und Adaptivität von Abwehrprozessen am Beispiel von Verleugnung [Chronic illness. Conceptualization, operationalization and adaptivity of defense mechanisms; by the example of denial]. *Psychotherapie Psychosomatik Medizinische Psychologie, 35,* 295–302.

Beutel, M. (1988) *Bewältigungsprozesse bei chronischen Erkrankungen* [Coping processes in chronic diseases]. Weinheim: Edition Medizin, VCH.

Bibring, G.L., Dwyer, T.F., Huntington, D.S., & Valenstein, A.F. (1961) A study of the psychological process in pregnancy and the earliest mother–child relationship. *Psychoanalytic Study of the Child, 16,* 9–72.

Brown, H.N. & Kelly, M.J. (1976) Stages of bone marrow transplantation. A psychiatric prospective. *Psychosomatic Medicine, 38,* 439–446.

Dahl, H. (1978) A new psychoanalytic model of motivation. *Psychoanalysis and Contemporary Thought, 1,* 373–408.

Ehlers, W. (1983) Die Abwehrmechanismen. Definition und Beispiele [The defense mechanisms; definition and examples]. *Praxis der Psychotherapie und Psychosomatik, 28,* 55–56.

Ehlers, W. & Czogalik, D. (1984) Dimensionen der klinischen Beurteilung von Abwehrmechanismen [Dimensions of clinical assessment of defense mechanisms]. *Praxis der Psychotherapie und Psychosomatik, 29,* 129–138.

Freud, A. (1936) *Das Ich und die Abwehrmechanismen* [The ego and the mechanisms of defense]. Vienna: Internationaler Psychoanalytischer Verlag.

Freud, S. (1926/1968) *Hemmung, Symptom und Angst* [Inhibitions, symptoms and anxiety. In *The Standard edition of the complete psychological works of Sigmund Freud: Vol. 20* (pp. 77–172). London: Hogarth Press.

Gaus, E. & Köhle, K. (1986) Psychische Anpassungs- und Abwehrprozesse bei körperlichen Erkrankungen [Psychic adaptation and defense mechanisms in somatic diseases]. In T. von Uexküll (Ed.), *Lehrbuch der psychosomatischen Medizin* [Textbook of psychosomatic medicine] (3rd. ed.). Munich: Urban & Schwarzenberg.

Hölzer, M., Scheytt, N., Pokorny, D., & Kächele, H. (1989) *A comparative study of emotional vocabulary in 2 cases.* Paper presented at the 20th Annual Meeting of the Society of Psychotherapy Research, Toronto.

Kächele, H., Hölzer, M., & Schwilk, C. (1989) *Defense mechanisms during severe illness and how they are reflected by vocabulary measures.* Paper presented at the 20th Annual Meeting of the Society of Psychotherapy Research, Toronto.

Klein, M. (1948) *Contributions to psychoanalysis 1921–1945.* London: Hogarth Press.

Laplanche, J. & Pontalis, J.B. (1986) *Das Vokabular der Psychoanalyse* [The vocabulary of psychoanalysis]. Frankfurt: Suhrkamp. (Original work published 1967).

Luborsky, L. (1984) Principles of psychoanalytic psychotherapy. A manual for supportive-expressive treatment. New York: Basic Books.

Mentzos, S. (1976) Interpersonale und institutionalisierte Abwehr [Interpersonal and institutionalized defense]. Frankfurt: Suhrkamp.

Neuser, J. (1989) *Psychische Belastungen unter Knochenmarktransplantation: Empirische Verlaufsstudien an erwachsenen Leukämiepatienten* [Psychological stressors accompanying bone marrow transplantation: Empirical longitudinal studies on adult leukemia patients]. Frankfurt: Europäische Hochschulschriften, Reihe 6, Psychologie Bd. 294.

Patenaude, A. & Rappeport, J.M. (1982) Surviving bone marrow transplantation: The patient in the other bed. *Annals of Internal Medicine*, *97*, 915–918.

Steffens, W. & Kächele, H. (1988) Abwehr und Bewältigung—Mechanismen und Strategien. Wie ist eine Integration möglich? [Defense and coping: Mechanisms and strategies. How is an integration possible?]. In H. Kächele & W. Steffens (Eds.), *Bewältigung und Abwehr. Beiträge zur Psychologie und Psychotherapie schwerer Krankheiten* [Coping and defense. Contributions on psychology and psychotherapy of severe diseases]. New York: Springer.

Vaillant, G.E. (1971) Theoretical hierarchy of adaptive ego mechanisms. *Archives of General Psychiatry*, *24*, 107–118.

Part V
Psychosomatics

25
Attitudes Towards Illness and Health and Defense Mechanisms in Psychosomatic Patients

Frits J. Bekker, Uwe Hentschel, and Marion Reinsch

Von Uexküll and Wesiack (1990), in their theory on a biopsychosocial model of psychosomatic medicine, state that the human being can be seen as an organism living in a circular interaction with its environment. This interaction serves to maintain a well-balanced homeostasis within the unity formed by the organism and its own world (*Umwelt*) on two levels:

1. The level of biological needs and supplies: the functional circle (*Funktionskreis*).
2. The level of psychological needs and cues: the situational circle (*Situationskreis*).

In the maintenance of equilibrium in the relationship between the organism and its environment and within the organism itself, perception (interpretation of sensory signals) and information processing (concept and attitude formation) play an important role. As long as the results of perception and information processing stay within the boundaries set by pragmatic and the communicative reality criteria, it is possible to speak of a well-adapted person. This means among other things that temporary disruptions of equilibrium—for example, by conflicts or frustrations—are restored by the normally functioning individual in such a way that the disturbed arousal levels within the organism return to their normal values. According to the theory, this is possible only if the perception of the conflict and the information processing with regard to the solving of the conflict meet the usual criteria of reality. If this is not the case, the solutions are not real, but at best fantasized solutions, with the effect that the internal arousal levels may be chronically disturbed. Von Uexküll theorizes that the psychological problem behind psychosomatic complaints is one of chronically disturbed perception and information processing. Because of this, psychosomatic patients never reach a realistic scope on all, or a certain kind of conflicts they meet in life. Consequently, they will never come to realistic solutions, and the result will be a chronically disturbed arousal level in the neurological and endocrinological systems, which may lead to tissue damage in the end. The nature of the distortions in perception and information processing may differ from one kind of psychosomatic complaint to the other. Thus the perspective on life and the way in which they handle information may be distorted in one way in patients suffering from colitis ulcerosa, while in patients suffering from essential hypertension they may vary in another way. Hermann, Rassek, Schäfer, Schmidt, and von Uexküll (1990) draw attention to the impact of emotions in the process of perception, and they give a survey of the literature regarding the relationship between emotions and hypertension. The following findings are borrowed from their survey.

Emotions play an important role in the way in which the individual interprets his environment. Each situation has a specific emotional meaning for the subject; there are no neutral situations. Many authors have stressed the impact of emotional factors on blood pressure levels and on the pathogenesis of essential hypertension. Alexander (1939) found in his hypertensive patients something he regarded psychoanalytically as an "unspecific conflict" between aggressive tendencies and feelings of dependence toward the objects on which the aggression was directed. In such a conflict, feelings of anger, jealousy, and hate toward the person on whom one feels dependent are seen as dangerous. They elicit fears of object loss and feelings of guilt. Gaus, Klingenberg, and Köhle (1983) found during their investigations a typical conflict theme consisting of aggression versus submission and endurance versus giving up. Furthermore they found conflicts with regard to self-esteem, as well as ambivalences resulting from pathological reactions to actual object losses. In earlier publications on these conflicts the role of the authoritarian father has been stressed. Perini, Amann, Bolli, and Bühler (1982), however, found that hypertensive patients showing characteristics of the above-mentioned conflicts also may have been brought up in overprotective families, which suggests a disturbed mother–child relationship. Both situations seem to induce the development of a strict and rigid superego, which prevents aggressive feelings from being brought out into the open. This means that not only the destructive aspects of aggression are inhibited, but also the positive ones, which guarantee the development of independence and self-reliance and sustain the action potential necessary to achieve benign results. Bastiaans (1963) in this respect speaks of a "Law-and-Order Superego." This kind of superego can be recognized in behavior in general as well as in perception.

Many authors (Aresin, 1960; Enke & Gercken, 1955; Michaelis, 1966; Pflanz & Von Uexküll, 1962; Stern, 1958; Wyss, 1955) in their descriptions of hypertensive patients have mentioned the unrealistic, compulsive and perfectionist attitude towards their own performances. Often they are unable to objectively judge the merits of their own actions. They see their actions more as duties imposed by some authority than as attempts to satisfy their own desires. These characteristics are to a high degree in accordance with the observations made by Rosenman and Friedman (1970, 1975) with respect to type-A behavior. The alterations in perception, still following Herrmann et al. (1990), were demonstrated in an experiment by Sapira, Eileent, Heib, Moriarty, and Shapiro (1973). Hypertensive patients, in contrast to normotensive subjects, did not recognize certain differences in a doctor's behavior in two otherwise identical situations, which were presented to them in a film. Cochrane (1973) and Ostfeld (1973), especially, doubt whether the observations regarding psychodynamics and personality in hypertensive patients are valid for all patients in the same way.

More recent investigations by Esler, Julius, Randall, De Quattio, and Zweifler (1976) and Perini, Amann, Bolli, and Bühler (1982) distinguish between hypertensives with high plasmarenin levels and hypertensives with normal levels. The Rosenzweig Picture Frustration Test (Rosenzweig, 1950) did not differentiate between the latter group and a group of normotensive subjects. The hypertensives with high plasmarenin levels, however, reacted in a significantly different way: they did not recognize frustrations and they did not withstand them well; they were less aggressive and more inclined to submission. There was a trend toward a strong need to solve conflicts immediately, together with a tendency to deny them, an inability to express feelings, and tendencies to passively submit to a situation and to introject aggression. These differences could be demonstrated in mild hypertensive patients as well as in patients with clear essential hypertension. Therefore they seem to contribute in a causal way to the development of essential hypertension with a high renin level rather than to be its sequel (Perini et al., 1982). These results underline a physiological and a psychological differentiation of the two groups. The evidence from the literature as represented in the recent overview by Herrmann et al. thus seems to support the value of the biopsychosocial approach also for empirical research with hypertensives.

Distortion of reality can also take place as a result of an exaggerated use of defense mechanisms. Defense mechanisms may play an acceptable role as long as they serve the maintenance of an adequate interaction between the individual and his environment. As soon as the person uses too many defense mechanisms or some defense mechanisms too intensively, his perception of reality may become seriously distorted and may no longer serve an adequate adaptation. Supporting evidence for this can be found in many contributions to this volume. In particular, conflict solving and dealing with frustrations may become inadequate. But defense mechanisms play a role not only in conflicts; they also affect the way in which the individual looks upon and deals with life situations in general, such as family relations, social relations outside the family, and the vocational situation.

Aim and Method

The present study is concerned with the question of whether there is a relationship between the psychosomatic illness, the use of defenses, and the attitudes toward five different aspects of life, as well as an interaction of illness and defenses in regard to these attitudes. Two areas were studied in which distortions in perception and information processing might show up in hypertensive patients:

1. The use of defense mechanisms in the handling of conflicts.
2. The attitudes and concepts used with regard to five different aspects of life.

The following methods were used: 37 outpatients diagnosed as suffering from essential hypertension (stage 1 or 2; systolic >140 mm Hg; diastolic 90–115 mm Hg), were examined by means of the Dutch Version of an inventory on conflict-solving strategies (FKBS: Hentschel & Bekker, in preparation; Hentschel, Kießling, & Wiemers, in press; cf. also Chapter 5), and they were extensively interviewed on their attitudes and feelings with regard to many different aspects of life (family, job situation, health care, etc.). These data were statistically processed and compared to the data from a group of 120 randomly chosen control subjects.

The FKBS

The FKBS (cf. Chapter 5) yields three different scores, one for reactions on the feeling level, one for reactions on the action level, and one total score, in which both scores are summarized. Since earlier results had shown that the scores on the feeling level are often more valid, only these were used in this study. From the personality characteristics of essential hypertension patients as mentioned in the literature, a number of hypotheses can be formulated with regard to their use of defense mechanisms. If their potential level of aggression is high, while at the same time they repress their aggression instead of openly showing it, their score on the defense mechanism of Turning of Aggression Against Object (TAO) can be expected to be low.

For the same reason, combined with the observation that hypertensive patients tend to introject their aggressive feelings and to submit passively to a situation, their scores on the defense mechanism of Turning of Aggression Against Self (TAS) can be expected to be high. As usually assumed for hypertensive patients in the literature, suppression of aggression means that not only the destructive aspects of aggression are inhibited, but also the positive ones from which independence and self-reliance are derived. This could be translated into the hypothesis that the Defense Mechanism of Reversal (REV) also may prevail in the hypertensives. Finally, a rigid superego structure in hypertensive patients, together with a compulsive and perfectionist attitude, may mean that the hypertensives will score high on the Defense Mechanism of Principalization (PRN): that is, rationalization, intellectualization, isolation.

The Interview

The interview was originally developed at the University of Mainz in Germany and consists of a set of open, closed, and scaled questions. Furthermore a few projective situations are presented to the interviewees

TABLE 25.1. The five factors and the items with high loadings on each factor.

Factor 1:	Health and medical care	
	The following are important in keeping fit:	
	.64	vacation
	.61	hygiene
	.60	conventional medical care (vs. alternative ways of healing)
	.53	entertainment
	.52	sports
Factor 2:	Social relations (outside the family)	
	The following are important in the vocational setting:	
	.71	nice friends
	.60	interesting work
	.60	a good boss
	The following also are important in keeping fit:	
	.56	socializing with friends
	.49	being able to relax
Factor 3:	Family and family life	
	In keeping fit it is important:	
	.57	to have hobbies
	.55	to have good housing
	When suffering from a stomach ulcer it may help:	
	.53	to change your life style
	It is important in the vocational setting to have:	
	.52	shorter working hours
	An important goal in life is:	
	.44	to raise children
	Thinking about my death I become anxious because:	
	.44	it could cause grief to my family and friends
Factor 4:	Fear of death and dying	
	.81	I feel fear of death
	.80	I feel fear of dying
	.39	I have dreams about death
Factor 5:	Social status	
	Important aspects of the vocational setting are:	
	.75	social status
	.63	possibilities for promotion
	In keeping fit it is important:	
	.51	to have sex

(Hentschel, 1989; Hentschel & Bekker, 1987; Hentschel & Kießling, 1986).

The questions ask for the opinion of the interviewee on a great number of topics pertaining to the health care system, the professional competence of doctors, the use of medicines, the vocational situation, social relations, fear of death and dying, and so on (some of the topics included in the interview can be deduced from the factor loadings presented in Table 25.1). The verbal answers to the questions are put into numerical categories, which are processed together with the scores on the different scales. Since not all interview data have been processed yet, the present results are based on a selection from the total interview. Up to now not very much is known with respect to the attitudes and concepts of hypertensive patients regarding everyday life topics. Hence the study must be considered to be explorative, with the consequence that no specific hypotheses could be formulated regarding the results of the interview, with the exception of a general expectation that the subjects' attitudes would differ from those of the control group.

Results

The FKBS data (Fig. 25.1) show that with regard to their mean defense mechanism scores, the hypertensive patients differ from the control subjects in the following areas: the hypertensive patients score significantly lower on TAO and significantly higher on TAS, REV, and especially PRN. In the use of the defense mechanism of PRO, the two groups do not differ. This indicates that in conflict situations the hypertensive patients tend to direct their aggression not against others, but against themselves. Furthermore they ascribe positive characteristics to the frustrating person (reversal), and they use rationalizations (principalization) to "solve" the conflict. Summarizing these results, it can be said that the hypertensive patients, as expected, use three defense mechanisms more and one less intensely than the control subjects do.

In relation to the basic theoretical framework, the foregoing results mean that this group of psychosomatic patients perceive their environment and process information from the environment in a manner that clearly differs from the control group at least in frustrating conflict situations. If this holds true for their way of information processing in general as well, the hypertensive patients should, as mentioned before, also differ in their views on health and life in general. On the basis of a frequency analysis and the results of several exploratory factor analyses, 24 variables were selected from the total of almost 600 variables that resulted from the total interview. These 24 variables from the control group were factor analyzed together with those from the hypertensive group, using a PCA with Varimax rotation. Five factors with an eigenvalue

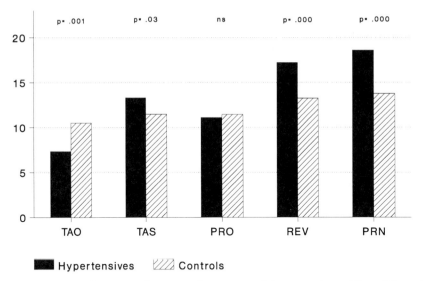

FIGURE 25.1. Differences between the scores of hypertensives ($N = 37$) and controls ($N = 120$) on each of the five defense mechanisms.

greater than 1 could be extracted, together explaining 40% of the total variance. On the basis of the variables with higher loadings, these factors could be named as follows (cf. Table 25.1):

1. Health and conventional medical care.
2. Social relations outside the family.
3. Family and family life.
4. Fear of death and dying.
5. Social status.

For each subject the factor scores on each of the five factors were computed. The two groups were compared with regard to the differences between the mean factor scores per factor, by means of t-tests. The hypertensive patients show significantly higher mean factor scores on the factors 1 (health and conventional medical care) and 3 (family and family life), than the control subjects do. According to the significant results, the hypertensive patients feel health and conventional medical care as well as family and family life to be significantly more important than the controls do. On factors 3 (social relations outside the family), 4 (fear of death and dying), and 5 (social status), no significant differences occurred in the mean factor scores of the two groups (cf. Table 25.2).

Finally, the study asked whether any interactions would occur between the groups and the use of defenses with respect to attitudes toward the five specific aspects of life. Five two-way analyses of variance were carried out for each of the five factors, with the groups (experimental and

TABLE 25.2. Differences between the mean factor scores of the hypertensive patients (HP) (*N* = 37) and the control subjects (C) (*N* = 120) on each of the factors.

Factor	Group	Mean	*t*-value	*p*
1	C	−.15	−3.97	.000
	HP	.47		
2	C	.07	1.32	n.s.
	HP	−.24		
3	C	−.17	−3.89	.000
	HP	.54		
4	C	.04	.86	n.s.
	HP	−.12		
5	C	−.04	−.80	n.s.
	HP	.12		

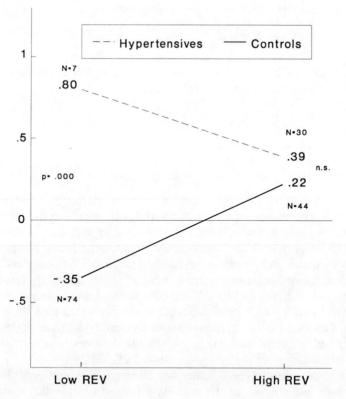

FIGURE 25.2. Factor 1: Difference between hypertensives and controls with regard to use of REV and attitude toward health and medical care.

control group) and the defense mechanisms (divided at the median and classified as high or low) as independent variables and the factor scores as dependent variables. On factor 1 (health and medical care), a significant interaction was found with respect to the defense mechanism of reversal ($p = .03$)(cf. Fig. 25.2).

The control subjects with a low REV score do not attach any importance to health and medical care. If the defensive attitude is high, the control subjects attribute at least some value to these matters. The hypertensives behave in just the opposite way. In the case of a low REV score they strongly emphasize the importance of health and conventional medical care, whereas the hypertensives with a high defensive attitude do this much less, roughly to the same degree as the control group with high REV scores. The interaction between the scores on the health and medical care factor (factor 1) and those for the defense mechanism of PRN (principalization) are not significant but very similar to that of the pattern for the REV scores (cf. Figs. 25.2 and 25.3).

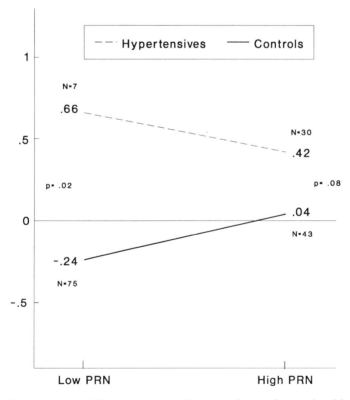

FIGURE 25.3. Factor 1: Difference between hypertensives and controls with regard to use of PRN and attitude toward health and medical care.

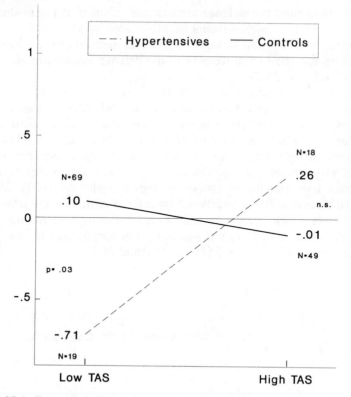

FIGURE 25.4. Factor 2: Difference between hypertensives and controls with regard to use of TAS and attitude toward social relationships outside the family.

The main effect for the difference between the hypertensives and the controls regarding the importance they attach to health and medical care has already been mentioned (cf. Table 25.2). According to the standard comparisons as given in Figs. 25.2 and 25.3, it seems to come mainly from the groups with low REV and/or PRN scores. Hypertensives with low scores on these scales value health and medical care more than the low-scoring controls do. For factor 2 (social relationships outside the family), one significant interaction was found with the use of the defense mechanism of TAS ($p = .004$; cf. Fig. 25.4).

In the control group, the value attached to social relationships outside the family does not change very much with high or low TAS. The hypertensive patients having a low defensive attitude (in the sense of TAS), on the contrary, attach significantly less importance to these relations than do the controls who are low on TAS. The

highly defensive hypertensives stress the importance of these relations much more and in doing so, they do not differ significantly from
the highly defensive controls in this respect. On the third factor (family
and family life), one tendency toward an interaction (p = .09) was
established in the sense that the hypertensive patients, in contrast
with the control subjects, seem to attribute less importance to family
life when their defensive attitude (TAO) is high than when it is low
(cf. Fig. 25.5).

The remaining interactions between the strength of the defensive attitude and the opinions on the family in the hypertension group do not
differ from those in the control group. The only significant main effect,
which is already known from the t-tests on the factor scores, is that
whether the defensive attitude is high or low, the hypertensive patients
always put more stress upon the importance of family life than the control
subjects do (cf. Fig. 25.6). On factors 4 (fear of death and dying) and 5
(social status), no significant results occurred.

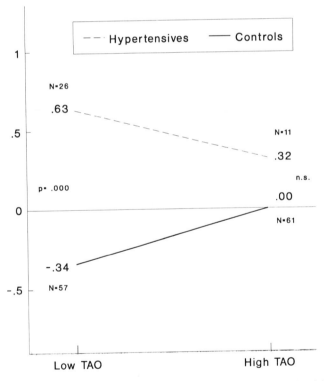

FIGURE 25.5. Factor 3: Difference between hypertensives and controls with regard
to use of TAO and attitude toward the family and family life.

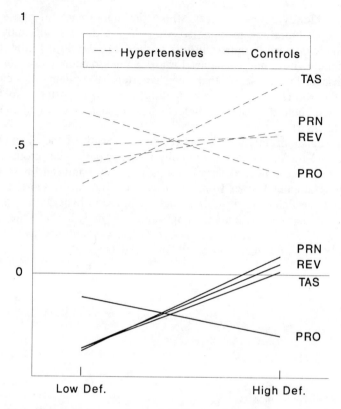

FIGURE 25.6. Factor 3: Comparison of the interactions between attitudes toward family life and the defense mechanisms of TAS, PRO, REV, and PRN, respectively, of the control group and the hypertensive group.

Discussion

Hypothetical differences between hypertensives and the control group were checked in three ways: with respect to the differences in the defense measures, in the attitudes toward different aspects of life, and in the interactions between groups and defenses with respect to the attitudes. The explicitly formulated hypotheses regarding the differences between the hypertensive patients and the control subjects with regard to the way in which they make use of defense mechanisms were supported. In accordance with the findings from other studies, hypertensives, when confronted with a conflict, are significantly less inclined to behave in an openly aggressive way (TAO). Instead they show a significantly stronger disposition than the control subjects to direct aggression inward and to put the blame on themselves (TAS). Hypertensives also use reaction formation significantly more often than control subjects do, in the sense that they attribute positive characteristics to the frustrating person (REV). Finally hypertensives make significantly more use of rationalizations to avoid real clashes in conflict situations (PRN) than control subjects. These results support the descriptions from others according to which hypertensive patients are aggression-repressing, submissive, rather rigid, and seemingly friendly persons. The hypertensives differ from the control subjects with respect to their attitudes toward health and the family also. The hypertensive patients attach significantly more value to health and conventional medical care as well as to the family and family life. With regard to social relations outside the family, fear of death, and the appraisal of social status, no significant differences could be shown between the hypertensives and the controls. Thus in certain specific aspects of life that could be hypothetically related to the illness, the hypertensive patients seem to differ from the control subjects in their attitudes, whereas in other also hypothetically important aspects, they do not.

From the results as given in Figs. 25.2 and 25.3, the following tentative conclusions can be drawn. The control subjects who use the defense mechanisms of Reversal (REV) and Principalization (PRN) to a low degree, thus those who do not feel they should please frustrating others and those who do not rationalize, do not emphasize the importance of health and conventional medical care. It looks as if they "normally" do not care too much about these topics. The controls with high REV scores, however, look on these topics as having at least some importance. They may admit that these topics should be important, particularly since the interviewer asks questions about them. On the other hand, the hypertensives who make a minor use of Reversal (REV) and rationalization (PRN) stress the importance of health and medical care significantly more than the controls with low scores on these defenses. Hypertensives with high REV scores do not differ with respect to attitude toward health and health care compared to the controls with high REV scores. For the two high-PRN groups, there is a tendency of a difference. It seems that the low-defensive (in the sense of REV and PRN) hypertensives feel free to express that health and medical care are important to them, whereas the highly defensive hypertensives pretend that these topics are of less interest. This may mean that the latter patients try to avoid being conspicuous in this respect, to be rational, and to reassure themselves, and maybe even to please the interviewer ("do not worry, nothing is wrong with me").

The effect of being chronically ill may be that attention is focused on health and medical care and that these topics therefore become very important, unless defense mechanisms are used that make it possible to "convince" oneself and others that nothing is really wrong and that thus health and medical care are not very important. This interaction implicitly comprises the danger of a neglecting attitude toward the illness. As mentioned before, it seems that the controls behave in just the opposite way. The strength of the tendency to direct aggression toward oneself (TAS) influences the attitude of the hypertensives toward the importance of social relationships outside the family. A weak tendency to put the blame on oneself goes together with a strong denial of the importance of such relationships, and for those with a high TAS score the involvement in social relations outside the family could possibly be a conflictual one based on thoughts like "I have to . . ." or "It is my fault if this does not run smoothly." Hypertensives with a low TAO score seem to be very family-bound and thus restricted in their social relations, those with high TAO scores are comparable to the control group. We do not know yet whether these results reflect a rather general tendency of a relation between the direction of the aggression (inward vs. outward) and the importance given to social relationships (inside and outside the family) or a specific conflict-related pattern, typical for special subgroups of hypertensive patients, with their general tendency to restrict their experiential world to events in the family (Platteel, 1988) and to give greater importance to the actual social relationships there. To what degree these family relations are relatively conflict-free or problematic seems to be an interesting question for further research.

Concluding Remarks

The patients suffering from mild essential hypertension who were examined in this study differ significantly from the randomly chosen control subjects in a number of areas. These differences apply to the use of four different defense mechanisms (Turning Against Object, Turning Against Self, Reversal, and Principalization), as well as to the attitudes toward two different dimensions of aspects of life (health and medical care, family and family life). Moreover, significant interactions between the groups (hypertensives and controls) and the use of defense mechanisms (REV, TAO, and TAS) with respect to the attitudes toward different aspects of life (health and medical care; family and family life) were revealed.

These promising results seem to indicate that further research into psychosomatic conditions from a biopsychosocial viewpoint, simultaneously aiming at analysis of group-specific information processing characteristics, might be fruitful.

References

Alexander, F. (1939) Emotional factors in essential hypertension. *Psychosomatic Medicine, 1*, 173–179.

Aresin, L. (1960) *Über Korrelationen zwischen Persönlichkeit, Lebensgeschichte und Herzkrankheit* [On correlations between personality, life-history, and heart disease]. Leipzig: VEB Fischer.

Bastiaans, J. (1963) Emotiogene Aspekte der essentiellen Hypertonie [Emotiogenic aspects of primary hypertension]. *Verhandlungen Deutsche Gesellschaft für Innere Medizin, 69, 7*, 510–522.

Cochrane, R. (1973) Hostility and neuroticism among unselected essential hypertensives. *Journal of Psychosomatic Research, 17*, 215– 218.

Enke, H. & Gercken, G. (1955) Der seelische Befund bei essentiellen Hypertonikern. Psychodiagnostisch-statistische Untersuchungen [The psychological status of patients with primary hypertension]. *Klinische Wochenschrift, 33, 23/24*, 551–556.

Esler, M., Julius, D., Randall, O., DeQuattro, V., & Zweifler, A. (1976) High-renin essential hypertension: Adrenergic cardiovascular correlates. *Clinical Science and Molecular Medicine, 51* (Suppl. 3), 181–184.

Gaus, E., Klingenberg, M., & Köhle, K. (1983) Psychosomatische Gesichtspunkte in der Behandlung von Hypertoniepatienten—Möglichkeiten eines integrierten internistisch-psychosomatischen Ambulanzkonzeptes [Psychosomatic aspects in the treatment of hypertensives—Possibilities of an integrated internal-psychosomatic polyclinical concept]. *Psychotherapie Psychosomatik Medizinische Psychologie, 33*, 53–60.

Hentschel, U. (1989) *Expectations in the health care system from a crosscultural and group-specific perspective*. Paper presented at the symposium "Comparative Perspectives in Bio-Psycho-Social Health" at the 10th World Congress of the International College of Psychosomatic Medicine, Madrid, October.

Hentschel, U. & Bekker, F. (in preparation) *Vragenlijst voor konfliktoplossingsstrategieën—FKBS* [Conflict-solving strategy inventory]. University of Leiden.

Hentschel, U. & Bekker, F. (1987) *Interview: Ziekte en gezondheid* [Interview: Illness and health]. University of Leiden.

Hentschel, U. & Kießling, M. (1986) *Interview: Krankheit und Gesundheit* [Interview: Illness and health]. University of Mainz.

Hentschel, U., Kießling, M., & Wiemers, M. (in press) *Fragebogen zu Konfliktbewältigungsstrategien—FKBS* [Conflict-solving strategy inventory]. University of Leiden.

Herrmann, J.M., Rassek, M., Schäfer, N., Schmidt, T.H., & von Uexküll, T. (1990) Essentielle Hypertonie [Primary hypertension]. In R. Adler, J.M. Herrmann, K. Köhle, O.W. Schonecke, T. von Uexküll, & W. Wesiack (Eds.), *Psychosomatische Medizin* [Psychosomatic medicine] (pp. 719–744). Munich: Urban & Schwarzenberg.

Michaelis, R. (1966) Beitrag zur Kenntnis ätiologisch-pathogenetischer Faktoren der essentiellen juvenilen Hypertonie [Contribution to the knowledge of the etiologic–pathogenic factors of primary hypertension in adolescents]. *Zeitschrift für Psychosomatische Medizin und Psychoanalyse, 12*, 1.

Ostfeld, A.M. (1973) What's the payoff in hypertension research? *Psychosomatic Medicine, 35*, 1–3.

Perini, C., Amann, F.W., Bolli, P., & Bühler, F.R. (1982) Personality and adrenergic factors in essential hypertension. *Contr. Nephrol., 30*, 64–69.

Pflanz, M. & von Uexküll, T. (1962) Psychosomatische Untersuchungen an Hochdruckkranken [Psychosomatic investigations with hypertensive patients]. *Medizinische Klinik, 57*, 345–351.

Platteel, D. (1988) *De bloeddrukmeter als psychologische test?* [The blood pressure instrument as a psychological test?]. Unpublished academic thesis, University of Leiden.

Rosenman, R.H., Friedman, M., et al. (1970) Coronary heart disease in the Western Collaborative Group Study. A follow-up experience of 4.5 years. *Journal of Chronic Diseases, 23*, 173–190.

Rosenman, R.H. & Friedman, M. (1975) Neurogenic factors in pathogenesis of coronary heart disease. *Medical Clinics of North America, 58*, 259–269.

Rosenzweig, S. (1950) Levels of behavior in psychodiagnosis with special reference to the Picture Frustration Study. *American Journal of Orthopsychiatry, 20*, 23–29.

Sapira, J.D., Eileent, S., Heib, B.A., Moriarty, R., & Shapiro, A.P. (1971) Differences in perception between hypertensive and normotensive populations. *Psychosomatic Medicine, 33*, 239–250.

Stern, E. (1958) Zum Problem der Spezifität der Persönlichkeitstypen und der Konflikte in der psycho-somatischen Medizin [On the problem of the specificity of personality types and the conflicts in psychosomatic medicine]. *Zeitschrift für Psychosomatische Medizin und Psychoanalyse, 4*, 153–168.

Uexküll, T. von & Wesiack, W. (1990) Wissenschaftstheorie und Psychosomatische Medizin, ein bio-psycho-soziales Modell [Theory of science and psychosomatic medicine, a bio-psycho-social model]. In R. Adler, J.M. Herrmann, K. Köhle, O.W. Schonecke, T. von Uexküll, & W. Wesiack (Eds.), *Psychosomatische Medizin* [Psychosomatic medicine] (pp. 5–38). Munich: Urban & Schwarzenberg.

Wyss, D. (1955) Psychosomatische Aspekte der juvenilen Hypertonie [Psychosomatic aspects of hypertension in adolescents]. *Nervenarzt, 26*, 197–210.

26
Anorexics and Bulimics Compared Vis-à-Vis Defense, Proximity, and Separation

PER JOHNSSON

Anorexia nervosa and bulimia nervosa are psychosomatic disorders of manifest life-threatening nature. They have been described in various reports as diseases with a variety of psychopathological backgrounds, ranging from neurosis to psychosis and schizophrenia (Johnsson, 1989). The past decade has seen growing interest in performing empirical studies of psychopathology in these disorders, though only in a few studies have the two entities been compared. Where comparison has been made, bulimics have been found to have a more distorted body image (Button, Fransella, & Slade, 1977), a more depressive symptomatology (Casper, Eckert, Halmi, Goldberg, & Davis, 1980; Russel, 1979; Stonehill & Crisp, 1977; Strober, 1981), poorer impulse control (Casper et al., 1980), more family conflicts (Strober, 1981), and poorer prognosis than anorexics (Garfinkel, Moldofsky, & Garner, 1980).

For many years patients with anorexia nervosa were considered to be a homogenous group. From 1914, for a period of about 30 years, anorexia nervosa was known as Simmond's disease and was considered to be primarily an endocrine disorder. In early psychoanalytic descriptions, anorexia nervosa was seen as an expression of fear of becoming pregnant, or self-starvation as an expression of depression (Fenichel, 1946). Hilde Bruch (1973) viewed anorexia nervosa as having both primary and secondary phases. Primarily there is a drive for thinness, a strongly distorted body image, inability to recognize and interpret somatic and emotional signals, and a pervasive feeling of inability to influence one's surroundings and run one's own life. In the secondary, nonspecific phase, loss of weight is of subordinate import because it is usually the result of symbolical misinterpretations of eating function. This was the first real division of anorexia nervosa into two entities. In a paper published in 1977, Beumont distinguished between cases of self-starvation (i.e., anorexia nervosa) and of induced vomiting, the former where patients controlled their weight by not eating, the latter where they did so by vomiting and the use of laxatives. Garfinkel et al. (1980) describe the same heterogeneity in anorexia nervosa, and in an analysis of patients with eating disorders clearly distinguished those who were bulimics. Boskind-Lodahl (1976) differentiated between anorexics and anorexics with bulimia, referring to the latter as being bulimarexic, the sole difference being that bulimarexics controlled their weight not by eating little but by vomiting. Etiological theories concerning anorexia nervosa have predominantly stressed the involvement of ego weakness and interpersonal factors (Bruch, 1973). More recently attempts have been made to explain anorexia in terms of object relations (Chediak, 1977; Masterson, 1977; Sours, 1974). These theorists have tried to identify the problems anorexics have had during early development. Masterson (1977) views anorexia nervosa as of borderline pathology. This means that he traces the disorder to the earlier part of the separation–individuation phase, when self- and object representations are assigned to a good or a bad constellation, splitting, projection, and denial being the predominant modes of defense. Masterson also suggests that if the child relinquishes the control function, which was the mother's during the symbiotic phase but which the child subsequently takes over, a fixation can develop whereby the child is trapped in a constant struggle to assume control vis-à-vis intake of food.

Theorizing as to the cause of bulimia nervosa has been less comprehensive. Sugarman and Kurash (1982) explain bulimia on the basis of Margaret Mahler's theories (Mahler, Pine, & Bergman, 1975). They suggest that the error in development probably occurs in the practicing period of the separation–individuation process. In turn, the error results in a narcissistic fixation with the body, which comes to be considered as a transitional object (Winnicott, 1971). Sugarman and Kurash view the eating/swallowing in bulimia as an attempt to reexperience the original symbiotic relationship with the mother, and vomiting as an attempt at individuation from the mother. The bulimic's need to resolve the conflict between symbiosis and separation has also been proposed by Swift and Letven (1984). Depression as a factor of eating disorders has been discussed in recent years (Hinz & Williamson, 1987). Of a group of 30 female anorexics, whose case data they compiled from hospital records and therapists, Rollins and Piazza (1978) found 77% to suffer from depression. In a number of published reports, depression has been seen as a component in borderline pathology (Sours, 1981; Sugarman & Quinlan, 1981), while others have seen it rather as a neurotic manifestation (Cantwell, Sturzenberger, Burroughs, Salkin, & Green, 1977; Eckert, Goldberg, Halmi, Casper, & Davis, 1982). In reports by Herzog (1982) and by Pope and Hudson (1985), the biological components in bulimic depression have been discussed, the conclusion being drawn that they are similar in character to those in most affective disorders.

Sugarman and Quinlan (1981) view anorexia as a defense against anaclitic depression, the primary feelings in which are of hopelessness, emptiness, and of being unloved. There is also a strong need to be taken care of, helped, and being fed and protected. People in the anorexic's surroundings are evaluated solely in terms of their ability to satisfy the anorexics's needs (Blatt, 1974). Anaclitic depression must be considered in relation to introjective depression, which is primarily linked to the oedipal situation. The predominant feeling in introjective depression is of having erred or failed to live up to expectations. Feelings toward others in their environment are contradictory and aggressive, and often hard to express for fear of losing their love (Blatt, 1974).

In the study presented here, percept-genetic methods have been used to delineate intrapsychic events in anorexics and bulimics. In a large number of studies of children, with or without psychiatric symptoms, the Meta-Contrast Technique (MCT) has been capable of elucidating the development of their defense strategies (Smith & Danielsson, 1982). Moreover, the MCT has been shown to be an effective instrument for shedding light on a patient's ability to deal with threat and threatening situations (Smith & Westerlundh, 1980). The aim has been to attempt to measure defense strategies in anorexics and bulimics, and to ascertain whether these patients' defense strategies are more neurotic or more primitive than those of other psychiatric patient groups or healthy people. The attempt was also made, with the help of thematic pictures, to identify any differences in response patterns between anorexics and bulimics. Thematic pictures have been used successfully in percept-genetic research (Hansson, Rydén, & Johnsson, 1985; Nilsson, 1983; Smith et al., 1980)— for instance, in distinguishing between patients with primitive hysteria and those with obsessive–compulsive neurosis (Nilsson, 1983). On the basis of previous findings, bulimics might be expected to respond more depressively to thematic pictures representing separation or proximity, whereas anorexics would be likely to deny separation content and to recognize proximity content. Finally, the study was intended to confirm reported differences between anorexics and bulimics on psychological and behavior dimensions, as measured with Eating Disorder Inventory (EDI) (Garner, Olmsted, & Polivy, 1982/83).

Method

Subjects

The subjects comprised 54 female patients with a mean age of 19.4 years (range, 15–25 years), of whom 48 had been in contact with the adult psychiatric clinic and 6 with the child and youth psychiatry clinic, both at University Hospital, Lund Sweden. All patients studied had been diagnosed as having either anorexia nervosa or bulimia nervosa.

Diagnostic Criteria

At both clinics diagnosis had been made on the basis of DSM-III-R criteria (American Psychiatric Association, 1987) for anorexia nervosa and bulimia nervosa, as outlined below.

Criteria for a Diagnosis of anorexia nervosa:

1. Refusal to maintain body weight over a minimal weight for age and height (e.g., weight loss leading to maintenance of body weight 15% below that expected).
2. Intense fear of gaining weight or becoming fat, even though underweight.
3. Disturbance in the way in which one's body weight, size, or shape is experienced (e.g., the person claims to "feel fat" even when emaciated, believes that one area of the body is "too fat" even when obviously underweight.)
4. In females, absence of at least three consecutive menstrual cycles when otherwise expected to occur (primary or secondary amenorrhea).

Criteria for a diagnosis of bulimia nervosa:

1. Recurrent episodes of binge-eating (rapid consumption of a large amount of food in a discrete period of time).
2. A feeling of lack of control over eating behavior during the eating binges.
3. The person regularly engages in self-induced vomiting, use of laxatives or diuretics, strict dieting or fasting, or vigorous exercise to prevent weight gain.
4. A minimum average of two binge-eating episodes a week for at least 3 months.
5. Persistent overconcern with body shape and weight.

Of the 54 patients, 25 fulfilled criteria for anorexia nervosa and 29 those for bulimia nervosa.

Control Group

The control group comprised 56 female university students, with a mean age of 21.2 years (s = 5.31), drawn in equal proportions from the departments of biology, psychology, and art history at Lund University.

Psychological Methods

This study constitutes a small part of a larger project concerning anorexia nervosa and bulimia nervosa, where the following instruments have been used: MCT (Meta-Contrast Technique), RFT (Rod-and-Frame Test), separation and proximity pictures presented with percept-genetic techniques, self-rating scale ("I think," "I am"; Birgerstam, 1984), and the Eating Disorder Inventory (EDI) of Norring and Sohlberg (1988).

In addition, subjects underwent two interviews, at the first of which object relations, affect, adaptability, self-confidence, reality, etc., were investigated. At the second, the disorder was traced in greater detail as to when and how it began.

Test Instruments

The MCT is described in detail by Kragh and Smith (1970) and in the manual (Smith, Johnsson, & Almgren, 1989). It is based on percept-genetic and psychoanalytic theories of how anxiety-provoked defense mechanisms are expressed in perceptual processes. The MCT consists of the tachistoscopic projection of a pair of pictures (stimuli A and B). Stimulus A is sometimes incongruent with stimulus B or directed at B (B being a boy—the hero figure—who is seated at a table with a narrow window behind him). Stimulus B is projected at exposures of increasing duration starting with .01 second and lengthened in geometric progression by a factor of 2. When the subject has reported B correctly, exposure time is reduced again to .06 second, where it is held constant. Stimulus A is now shown immediately preceding stimulus B, starting with an exposure time of .01 second, which is increased gradually until both A and B have been reported correctly in two consecutive trials. Subjects are asked to report every detail they see on the screen each time. Before correct recognition of the picture, it is often misinterpreted in a variety of ways, which can be assigned to different defense categories listed in the manual (Smith et al., 1989). The categories adopted for the present study were anxiety, repression, isolation, sensitivity, and depression, and the exposure time at which the subject correctly identified the picture. The test has been evaluated against psychiatric criteria in clinical groups, and is of well-documented reliability and validity (Smith & Danielsson, 1982; Smith & Westerlundh, 1980). The theoretical basis for the test has been described in detail by Westerlundh and Smith (1983).

Thematic Pictures

Separation Theme. The method is the same as that used for MCT (see above). The subject is seated 1.5 m (5 ft) from a screen on which the picture is projected. The picture is projected once for each step on the scale, starting with an exposure time of .01 second. Subjects are requested to report everything they see at each exposure. The trial is ended when the subject has reported the picture content correctly twice in a row (C-phase). The subject's verbal description is noted by the experimenter each time. The separation theme used consisted of a women with a bag in one hand coming out of the doorway to a room at the right in the background. She is half turned toward a child of about 12 months in the

TABLE 26.1. Separation theme: Distribution of various interpretations among anorexics (A), bulimics (B), and controls (C), and junctures at which correct identification was made of the picture as a whole.

Interpretation	A (N = 25)	B (N = 29)	C (N = 56)		p		
Mother identified correctly	10.1	10.6	11.0				
Child identified correctly	10.38	11.76	10.75				
Child an animal	3	5	7				
Mother an animal	0	2	0				
Child someone familiar	0	0	2				
Mother someone familiar	2	1	0				
Mother/child a plant	1	3	5				
Picture shows a room	13	12	19				
Mother/child a doll	1	2	0				
Picture a cheerful one	1	4	3				
Some dead thing in the picture	3	3	2				
Picture a sad one	10	16	5	B × C	.001		
Child screaming	0	1	4				
Child stretching out its hand	12	13	26				
Picture "muted"	7	5	4				
Child crawling toward the mother	7	7	17				
Mother approaching child	0	2	1				
Mother leaving child	13	14	32	A × B	.01;	A × C	.002
Child demanding something of the mother	13	5	9				
Child wants comforting	9	3	0	A × B	.05;	A × C	.001
Child afraid of something	3	4	3				
Child showing anger	1	3	0				
Details of mother's face described	13	2	7	A × B	.001;	A × C	.001
Details of picture described	16	3	5	A × B	001;	A × C	.001
Picture identified correctly	14.0	13.9	13.9				

foreground, who is in a crawling posture with one hand stretched out toward the woman. There are a few toys on the floor close to the child. No coding categories were used in the present study, only the subjects' interpretations are categorized (see Table 26.1).

Proximity Theme. Again the same method was used as for the MCT. The picture showed a woman seated in the foreground with her legs stretched out. In front of her is a small child in a crawling posture. The woman is patting the child on the back and smiling. The child's facial expression is neutral. The subjects' interpretations were categorized in the same manner as those for the separation theme (see Table 26.2).

EDI (Eating Disorder Inventory)

The EDI is a questionnaire consisting of eight subscales: drive for thinness, bulimia, body dissatisfaction, interpersonal distrust, ineffectiveness, perfectionism, interoceptive awareness, and maturity fears. These subscales are related to specific psychological and behavioral dimensions considered to be of significance in anorexia nervosa and bulimia nervosa (Garner et al., 1982/83; Norring & Sohlberg, 1988).

Test Reliability

The MCT and both the separation and proximity themes of the thematic test have been evaluated by two independent judges. Agreement was almost complete, assessments differing in only a couple of cases.

Results

Table 26.3 shows specific details for the anorexics and bulimics. A noteworthy finding was that the two groups did not differ with regard to age at onset, duration of disease, or Body Mass Index (BMI). The result of the EDI show two significant differences between anorexics and bulimics, the latter having higher scores for the variable drive for thinness (df = 46, t = 2.21), and for bulimia (df = 51, t = 3.00).

TABLE 26.2. Proximity theme: Distribution of various interpretations among anorexics (A), bulimics (B), and controls (C), and junctures at which correct identification was made of the picture as a whole.

Interpretation	A (N = 25)	B (N = 29)	C (N = 56)	P		
Mother identified correctly	8.6	8.97	8.50			
Child identified correctly	10.41	10.23	9.37	A × C	.01; B × C	.01
Child an animal	7	1	6	A × B	.03	
Mother an animal	2	2	7			
Mother/child a doll	0	1	0			
Picture a cheerful one	8	4	8			
Some thing dead in the picture	2	9	9			
Child sad	6	16	6	A × B	.04; B × C	.04
Child screaming	1	2	3			
Child showing anger	1	2	2			
Mother is taking care of the child	10	3	28	A × B	.01; B × C	.01
Child being smacked by mother	3	1	4			
Picture a pleasant one	11	3	24	A × B	.01; B × C .01	
Picture empty	3	1	0			
Mother sad	0	9	0	A × B	.01; B × C	.01
Details of mother's face described	17	1	7	A × B	.001; A × C	.001
Picture identified correctly	14.1	14.3	13.4			

TABLE 26.3. Particulars of 54 female patients with eating disorders: anorexics (A), and bulimics (B).

	A (N = 25)	B (N = 25)	p
Age at onset	15.9	16.4	
Duration of disease	4.1	4.6	
Body Mass Index	19.1	21.5	
Binge eating frequency (days/week)	0	5.6	.01
Eating Disorder Inventory			
Drive for thinness	8.9	12.3	.03
Bulimia	3.3	7.6	.01
Body dissatisfaction	11.3	13.3	
Ineffectiveness	12.4	11.6	
Perfectionism	6.5	5.5	
Interpersonal distrust	6.9	7.0	
Interoceptive awareness	11.1	11.5	
Maturity fears	8.0	5.0	

MCT (Meta-Contrast Technique)

The distribution of defense categories in MCT results is shown in Table 26.4. Depression was more common among bulimics than among controls or among anorexics. The bulimics differ from controls with regard to scores for the item isolation. A high frequency of sensitivity was characteristic of the anorectic group, which differed in this respect from controls and from bulimics. On the item repression, anorexics had significantly lower scores than had controls; there was a similar but nonsignificant difference between bulimics and controls. The MCT included some items

TABLE 26.4. Distribution of items in the MCT among anorexics, bulimics, and controls.

	Anorexia (N = 25) A	Bulimia (N = 29) B	Control group (N = 56) C	p	
Repression	5 (20%)	11 (38%)	32 (57%)	A × C	.01
Isolation	4 (16%)	9 (31%)	7 (13%)	B × C	.05
Depression	6 (24%)	18 (62%)	8 (14%)	A × B	.01
				B × C	.01
Sensitivity	17 (68%)	10 (34%)	9 (16%)	A × B	.02
				A × C	.01
Anxiety	4 (16%)	0 (0%)	6 (11%)		
Narcissism	2 (8%)	0 (0%)	3 (5%)		
Sad hero reported	0 (0%)	8 (28%)	0 (0%)	A × B	.01
				B × C	.01
Reports of food in the picture	0 (0%)	6 (21%)	0 (0%)	A × C	.01
				B × C	.01
C-phase	14.35	14.78	16.71	A × C	.01
				B × C	.01

that, though not included in the manual, would nonetheless seem to be of interest in the context. Reports of a "sad hero" were significantly more common among bulimics than among anorexics or among controls. Reports of food present in the picture were also more frequent among bulimics than among anorexics or among controls. Controls had higher thresholds vis-à-vis correct identification than either anorexics or bulimics.

Separation Theme

The various interpretations are listed in Table 26.1, which also shows their distribution among the three groups. Interpretations of the atmosphere in the picture as "sad" occurred more frequently among bulimics than among controls. Anorexics reported the child as demanding something of the mother more often than either the bulimics or the controls; they also paid more attention to mother's facial expression and noted more details in the picture than either of the other two groups.

Proximity Theme

The various interpretations are listed in Table 26.2, which also shows their distribution among the three groups. Controls identified the child figure sooner than did either anorexics or bulimics. The anorexics reported the child as being an animal significantly more often than bulimics or controls and paid significantly more attention to the mother's facial expression than either of the other two groups. The child and the mother were described as being sad by a larger proportion of the bulimic group than of either the anorectic group or the control group; and there were fewer reports of the picture as being pleasant among the bulimics, who also more rarely reported the mother to be taking care of the child.

EDI and MCT

There were no relationships between defense mechanisms (as defined by the MCT) and psychological or behavioral dimensions (as defined by the EDI). There was, however, a noteworthy relationship between the item repression on the MCT and the number of admissions to hospital; of 16 subjects with repression in the eating disorder population as a whole, only one had been hospitalized more than once at the psychiatric clinic.

Discussion

During recent years, research on anorexia nervosa and bulimia nervosa has been focused on the issue of whether differences exist between the two categories, and if so what they are. The present findings suggest that certain significant differences do exist between the two groups, but that similarities are also to be found. The groups did not differ with regard to age at onset, duration of disease, and body mass index. On the self-rating Eating Disorder Inventory, bulimics scored higher than anorexics on the items drive for thinness and bulimia. The low scores of anorexics for the item bulimia show that at testing they were free from bulimic symptoms, and that diagnosis according to the DSM-III-R criteria had been correct. The higher scores of the bulimics on the item drive for thinness are at variance with findings of previous studies (Garner et al., 1983). Garner et al. (1983) also found differences between anorexics and bulimics with regard to the items bulimia and body dissatisfaction.

In the present study, there were no differences between anorexics and bulimics on any of the other psychological or behavioral dimensions, which suggests that the superficial symptoms of these disorders camouflage more important problems requiring investigation. Meta-Contrast Technique results showed bulimics to be more depressive than anorexics or controls. In studies by Casper et al. (1980) and by Garfinkel et al. (1980), the same trend was found, namely for bulimics to be more depressive than anorexics. The MCT records reactions to a preconscious threat to the hero figure, and as the hero figure represents the ego, the self, it is the ego that is being threatened. The mode of ego defense varies depending on the subject's level of maturity, of course; the more mature mode of defense, the further the subject has progressed in development (Gedo & Goldberg, 1973). When the bulimic's hero figure is threatened, her response is depressive. The type of response common to bulimics (stereotyped repetitions) resembles that noted by Berglund and Smith (1988) in a group of depressive patients who subsequently committed suicide. In a significantly greater proportion of cases, the depressive tendency is reinforced by seeing a sad hero.

In the present study, bulimics manifested immature isolation to a greater extent than did controls: with few exceptions, in previous studies it has been possible to distinguish anorexics from bulimics with reference to the items isolation and obsession/compulsion; both Rosen and Leitenberg (1982) and Williamson, Kelley, Davis, Ruggiero, and Blouin (1985) found bulimics to be more preoccupied with obsessive thoughts than anorexics, and more prone to compulsive behavior in attempting to overcome their anxiety. In the MCT anorexics differed both from bulimics and controls primarily in their scores for the item sensitivity; as a group they also manifested a lower frequency of repression than did controls or bulimics. A high score for the item sensitivity on the MCT has been found to be an indicator of poor prognosis in obese subjects (Rydén & Sörbris, 1986) and to be associated with a greater degree of psychological vulnerability, which makes it hard for such patients to endure diet regimes. Sensitivity is related to projection, which is an immature defense strategy according to psychoanalytic theory. In particular, sensitivity in combination with lack of repression would seem to be an immature response probably indicative of a borderline personality. That the repressive response was combined with greater adaptive capacity in the present study is suggested by the fact that of 16 subjects who employed repression, only one had been hospitalized at the psychiatry department more than once. The sensitivity scores of the anorexics are also reflected in their lower thresholds with regard to correct identification of the picture, compared with controls.

In the separation theme, bulimics described the picture in depressive terms more often than did controls. In the proximity theme too, they interpreted the mother and child as being sad more often than did anorexics or controls, and in significantly more cases they found the theme less pleasant than did the other two groups and more often interpreted the mother as taking care of the child. Goodsitt (1984) describes the question of eating disorders as a battlefield in the separation–individuation process. This notion derives support from findings of Sugarman and Kurash (1982), who regard the eating in bulimia as an attempt to reexperience the earlier relationship to the mother and vomiting as an attempt at separation from her.

In thematic pictures particularly, the proximity theme aroused depressive responses in bulimics, which suggests that in their introjected view the mother is sad, or in Kohuts's terms (1971) the mirror reflected in the mother is a sad one. A number of workers have seen bulimia as a tension-regulating device (Johnson, 1984; Swift & Letven, 1984), a reasonable interpretation being that it is an attempt to reduce tension between conflicting desires of separation versus proximity vis-à-vis the mother. The bulimics' depressive interpretations of the thematic picture are in accord with their depressive responses in MCT testing. Craig Johnson (1984) stresses the importance of distinguishing between introjective and anaclitic depression; the bulimics' interpretations in thematic testing and their responses in MCT testing indicate that they suffer from anaclitic depression.

As compared both with bulimics and controls, the anorectic group is characterized primarily by greater attention to the mother's facial expression in both thematic pictures, and the greater detail in which they describe it in the separation theme. Anorexics reported seeing an animal in the proximity theme more often than did either bulimics or controls. The intensity and detail of anorexics' interpretations of separation and proximity themes might be viewed as a defense of a more projective nature. Masterson (1977) suggested that one of the predominant defenses in anorexia is projection. Sensitivity scores in the MCT were remarkably high among anorexics, which may be seen as being related to the degree of their attention to detail in the thematic picture test. Since sensitivity does not result in distortion of the pictures to be interpreted but in heightened attention to detail, it would seem more reasonable to view it as "coping" rather than as a defense mechanism. In anorexics, this may have developed at an early stage owing to complete separation from the mother; to avoid being overwhelmed by affect, perhaps they are constantly forced to interpret and adapt themselves to the mother's intentions. Presumably anorexics from an all-too-early stage have been obliged to adapt themselves to their surroundings rather than permitting their own wishes and feelings to be expressed. Such an interpretation is in accord with the conclusion of Krystal (1975) that certain children fail to develop a satisfactory degree of self-care and consider certain parts of their bodies still to "belong" to the mother. The anorexics' obedience and complaisance vis-à-vis their parents becomes self-destructive because it involves bottling up feelings that thus never find expression. The constant suppression of affect finally forces them to take over control of some aspect of themselves, to save themselves from drowning in a multiplicity of repressed feelings. Their rigid discipline with regard to diet enhances the anorexics' self-esteem. They develop a false independence as a defense against helplessness and impotence with respect to the flood of affects over which they have no control and which they fear. In the present study no relationship was found between the defense strategies elicited with the MCT and the psychological and behavioral dimensions uncovered with EDI. This suggests that the gravity of the symptoms is unrelated to the underlying pathology. This finding constitutes support for the view that the trends both in anorexia and bulimia are not only to be found in serious cases, but also in "normally neurotic" and healthy groups, where dieting and overeating constitute transient or mild problems.

In conclusion, the present findings show bulimics to have greater drive for thinness than anorexics and to manifest more bulimic behavior; they also report more depressive interpretations, both in the thematic picture test and in MCT. Anorexics, on the other hand, are more sensitive and lack repression in MCT testing, and they show a greater attention to detail with regard to the mother and situation in thematic picture test. Further study of the etiology in anorexia nervosa and bulimia nervosa should focus on the underlying depression, which may be either introjective or anaclitic.

References

American Psychiatric Association. (1987) *Diagnostic and statistical manual of mental disorders* (3rd ed., rev.). Washington, DC: Author.

Berglund, M. & Smith, G.J.W. (1988) Postdiction of suicide in a group of depressive patients. *Acta Psychiatrica Scandinavica*, 77, 504–510.

Beumont, P.J. (1977) Further categorization of patients with anorexia nervosa. *Australian and New Zealand Journal of Psychiatry*, 11, 321–325.

Birgerstam, P. (1984) *Jag-tycker-jag-är*. ["I think", "I am"]. *En metod för studie av barns och ungdomars självuppfatning*. [A method for studying childrens' and adolescents attitudes toward themselves]. Manual. Stockholm: Psykologiförlaget.

Blatt, S.J. (1974) Levels of object representation in anaclitic and introjective depression. *Psychoanalytic Study of the Child*, *29*, 107–157.

Boskind-Lodahl, M. (1976) Cinderella's stepsisters: A feminist perspective on anorexia nervosa and bulimia. *Journal of Women in Culture and Society*, *2*, 342–356.

Bruch, H. (1965) The psychiatric differential diagnosis of anorexia nervosa. In J.E. Meyer & H. Feldman (Eds.), *Anorexia nervosa-symposium in Göttingen*. Stuttgart: Thieme.

Bruch, H. (1973) *Eating disorders. Obesity, anorexia nervosa and the person within*. New York: Basic Books.

Button, E., Fransella, F., & Slade, P. (1977) A reappraisal of body perception disturbance in anorexia nervosa. *Psychological Medicine*, *7*, 235.

Cantwell, D.P., Sturzenberger, S., Burroughs, J., Salkin, B., & Green, J.K. (1977) Anorexia nervosa: An affective disorder? *Archives of General Psychiatry*, *34*, 1087–1093.

Casper, R., Eckert, E., Halmi, K., Goldberg, S.C., & Davis, J.M. (1980) Bulimia: Its incidence and clinical importance in patients with anorexia nervosa. *Archives of General Psychiatry*, *37*, 1030–1035.

Chediak, C. (1977) The so-called anorexia nervosa: Diagnostic and treatment considerations. *Bulletin of the Menninger Clinic*, *41*, 453–474.

Eckert, E., Goldberg, S.C., Halmi, K., Casper, R., & Davis, J.M. (1982) Depression in anorexia nervosa. *Psychological Medicine*, *12*, 115–122.

Fenichel, O. (1946) *The psychoanalytic theory of neurosis*. London: Routledge & Kegan Paul.

Garfinkel, P.E., Moldofsky, H., & Garner, D.M. (1980) The heterogeneity of anorexia nervosa: Bulimia as a distinct subgroup. *Archives of General Psychiatry*, *37*, 1036–1040.

Garner, D.M., Olmsted, M.P., & Polivy, J. (1982/1983) Development and validation of a multidimensional Eating Disorder Inventory for anorexia nervosa and bulimia. *International Journal of Eating Disorders*, *2*, 15–34.

Gedo, J. & Goldberg, A. (1973) *Models of the mind*. Chicago: University of Chicago Press.

Goodsitt, A. (1984) Self psychology and the treatment of anorexia nervosa. In I.D.M Garner & P.E Garfinkel (Eds.), *Handbook of psychotherapy for anorexia nervosa and bulimia* (pp. 55–82). New York: Guilford Press.

Hansson, S.B., Rydén, O., & Johnsson, P. (1985) Perceptgenetic correlates of field-independence in a group of young women. *Psychological Research Bulletin*, *8*, 1–21.

Herzog, D.P. (1982) Bulimia: The secretive syndrome. *Psychosomatics*, *23*, 481–487.

Hinz, L.D., & Williamson, D.A. (1987) Bulimia and depression: A review of the affective variant hypothesis. *Psychological Bulletin*, *1*, 150–158.

Johnson, C. (1984) Initial consultation for patients with bulimia and anorexia nervosa. In D.M. Garner & P.E. Garfinkel (Eds.), *Handbook of psychotherapy for anorexia nervosa and bulimia* (pp. 19–51). New York: Guildford Press.

Johnsson, P. (1989) Psykopatologi och ätsjukdomar [Psychopathology and eating disorders]. *Psykisk Hälsa*, *1*, 34–44.

Kohut, H. (1971) The analysis of the self. *The Psychoanalytic Study of the Child: Monogr. 4*. Madison, CT: International Universities Press.

Kragh, U. & Smith, G.J.W. (1970) *Percept-genetic analyses.* Lund: Gleerup.

Krystal, H. (1975) Affect tolerance. *Annuals of Psychoanalysis, 3,* 179–219.

Mahler, M., Pine, F., & Bergman, A. (1975) *The psychological birth of the human infant.* New York: Basic Books.

Masterson, J.F. (1977) Primary anorexia nervosa in borderline adolescents—An object-relations view. In I.P. Hartocollis (Ed.), *Borderline personality disorders* (pp. 475–494). Madison, CT: International Universities Press.

Nilsson, A. (1983) Application of a perceptgenetic approach to separation and oedipal conflict problems in primitive hysteria and obsessive-compulsive neurosis. In G.J.W. Smith, W.D. Fröhlich, & U. Hentschel (Eds.), *From private to public reality. Meaning and adaptation in perceptual processing* (pp. 135–148). Bonn: Bouvier.

Norring, C. & Sohlberg, S. (1988) Eating Disorders Inventory with Swedish patients, recovered patients, and controls: Description, crosscultural comparison and clinical utility. *Acta Psychiatrica Scandinavica, 78,* 567–575.

Pope, H.G., Jr. & Hudson, J.I. (1985) Biological treatments of eating disorders. In S.W. Emmett (Ed.), *Theory and treatment of anorexia nervosa and bulimia: Biomedical, sociocultural, and psychosocial perspectives* (pp. 73–92). New York: Brunner/Mazel.

Rollins, N. & Piazza, E. (1978) Diagnosis of anorexia nervosa: A critical reappraisal. *Journal of American Academy of Child Psychiatry, 17,* 126–137.

Rosen, J.C. & Leitenberg, H. (1982) Bulimia nervosa: Treatment with exposure and response prevention. *Behavior Therapy, 13,* 117–124.

Russel, G.F.M. (1979) Bulimia nervosa: An ominous variant of anorexia nervosa. *Psychological Medicine, 9,* 429–448.

Rydén, O. & Sörbris, R. (1986) Weight maintenance after fasting: A look at somatic and psychological parameters. *Journal of Obesity and Weight Regulation, 3,* 166–180.

Sjöbäck, H. (1973) *The psychoanalytic theory of defensive processes.* Lund: Gleerup.

Smith, G.J.W., Almgren, P.E., Andersson, A.L., Engelsson I., Smith, M., & Uddenberg, G. (1980) The Mother–Child Picture Test: Presentation of a new method for the evaluation of mother–child relations. *International Journal of Behavioral Development, 3,* 365–380.

Smith, G.J.W. & Danielsson, A. (1982) Anxiety and defensive strategies in childhood and adolescence. *Psychological Issues: Monogr. 52.* Madison, CT: International Universities Press.

Smith, G.J.W., Johnsson, G., & Almgren, P.E. (1989) *MCT—Meta Contrast Technique, manual.* Stockholm: Psykologiförlaget.

Smith, G.J.W. & Westerlundh, B. (1980) Perceptgenesis: A process perspective on perception-personality. In L. Wheeler (Ed.), *Review of personality and social psychology: Vol. 1* (pp. 94–124). Beverly Hill, CA: Sage.

Sours, J.A. (1974) The anorexia nervosa syndrome. *International Journal of Psychoanalysis, 55,* 567–576.

Sours, J.A. (1981) Depression and the anorexia nervosa syndrome. *Psychiatric Clinics of North America, 4,* 145–157.

Stonehill, E. & Crisp, A. (1977) Psychoneurotic characteristics of patients with anorexia nervosa before and after treatment and a follow-up 4–7 years later. *Journal of Psychosomatic Research, 24,* 353–359.

Strober, M. (1981) The significance of bulimia in juvenile anorexia nervosa: An exploration of possible etiologic factors. *International Journal of Eating Disorders*, *1*, 28–43.

Sugarman, A. & Kurash, C. (1982) The body as a transitional object in bulimia. *International Journal of Eating Disorders*, *4*, 57–67.

Sugarman, A. & Quinlan, D.M. (1981) Anorexia nervosa as a defense against anaclitic depression. *International Journal of Eating Disorders*, *1*, 44–61.

Swift, W. & Letven, R. (1984) Bulimia and the basic fault: A psychoanalytic interpretation of the binge-vomiting syndrome. *Journal of American Academic Child Psychiatry*, *23*, 489–497.

Westerlundh, B. & Smith, G.J.W. (1983) Perceptgenesis and the psychodynamics of perception. *Psychoanalysis and Contemporary Thought*, *6*, 597–640.

Williamson, D.A., Kelley, M.L., Davis, C.J., Ruggiero, L., & Blouin, D.C. (1985) Psychopathology of eating disorders: A controlled comparison of bulimic, obese, and normal subjects. *Journal of Consulting and Clinical Psychology*, *2*, 161–166.

Winnicott, D.W. (1971) *Playing and reality*. London: Pelican Books.

27
Defense Styles in Eating Disorders

Inez Gitzinger

Why Is It Important To Look at Defense and Coping?

Defense and coping are important for the perception of reality and for dealing with internal conflicts and with everyday problems. How do we react to unwanted events, to unacceptable wishes, to threatening situations and feelings, and how can we deal with problems without an explicit system of coping and defense mechanisms? Defensive operations are—first of all —protective processes that exert control over the interaction between the internal and external world. Social and cultural effects are always intertwined with incompatible ideas. Whether we consider defense mechanisms to be functions of the mind (like memory or consciousness) or adopt a dynamic energy concept of defense or conceive of it as part of the ego organization, socialization constitutes one of the most import determinants for the development of defense mechanisms and defense organization. Specifically, defenses have been accorded a central role in the currently prominent and intrinsically important category of eating disorders.

Eating disorders occur at the rate of 1000:1 in women and men, respectively. Consequently, we have to look at gender issues. In the literature, defense and coping are typically discussed without reference to gender. In the classical description of defense mechanisms (Freud, 1936), they are viewed as "an attempt to repress an incompatible idea..." which has come into distressing opposition with one's ego. Haan (1963) described coping processes as actions by the ego that serve to coordinate the person's social, moral, and cognitive structures depending on the situation (cf. Gitzinger, 1988). Gender issues, however, were not explicitly taken into account by Haan either.

Differences in Defense Styles in Eating Disorders: How Can They Be Studied?

In empirical research on defense, there are major problems that must be solved: how to measure the unconscious, how to differentiate the defense mechanisms, and how to evaluate the adaptiveness of these mechanisms. Differences between men and women can be expected. Their nature, however, remains to be ascertained. The history of determining defense mechanisms has been long and frustrating. Methodological problems have proved to be intractable, and the results have been disappointing. The validity of questionnaires proved to be limited, interviews were not free of a taint of subjectivity, ratings were often not reliable enough, and clinical judgments did not correspond to the other results. Nonetheless, the concept of defense has exercised an abiding fascination on theorists and clinicians alike. In psychoanalytic treatment, the construct of defense is a key piece of the puzzle for understanding the nature of the disorder. The following research questions were posed in this study:

1. Defenses and reality perception:
1.1. Are there empirical differences between male and female patients in the type of defense and/or in defense organization?
1.2. Are the defenses of female patients with eating disorders different from the defenses of neurotic female patients?
2. Conflicts:
2.1. Do men and women differ in the conflict themes reported in association with the various defenses?
2.2. Do eating disorders differ from other disorders of female patients in reported conflicts?

Before the details of the study, are presented, some general problems associated with clinical samples must be addressed. Sufficiently large and homogeneous groups are essential. With studies based on clinical settings, it is very hard to define homogeneous groups as well as to obtain enough subjects within a diagnostic category. Another problem is inherent in the task of the psychoanalytic researcher who, in contrast to behaviorists, is dealing with theories of mental representation and with internal and private phenomena that can be known directly only through the analyst's experiences and are often unconscious and inaccessible. Thus, the observer has to provide a "third eye" (Bucci, 1988) on the psychoanalytic dialogue.

Participants

Seventy neurotic inpatients from a psychoanalytic hospital in Stuttgart, Germany, participated in this study. There were 49 women and 21 men (Gitzinger, 1990a). The diagnoses from the hospital's documentation center as well as the results of a German personality inventory, the FPI (Freiburger Persönlichkeitsinventar: Fahrenberg, Hampel, & Selg, 1984) were used in deriving clinical diagnostic criteria on the basis of which patient groups were defined.

The Instrument for Studying Defenses

Preconscious defense mechanisms must be distinguished from the precursors and the early mechanisms of defense. The problem of an adequate operationalization of variables representing these theoretical constructs must be tackled by finding instruments that can help translate defenses, feelings, and wishes dealing with the interrelationship of the unconscious, reality, perception, and words into an empirical measure. The DCT (Defense Mechanisms Computer Test: Gitzinger, 1993) appears to be an adequate instrument for perceptually coded defenses. The DCT is a computerized presentation and rating procedure with its roots in the DMT (Defense Mechanism Test: Kragh, 1960). The DMT is a tachistoscopic instrument based on subliminal perception and on the percept-genetic model (Kragh, 1960). It uses the subliminal presentation of stimuli to extend the process of perceptual development as understood in the percept-genetic model.

DCT Presentation

One screen picture with 20 trials per session is presented to the participant in the DCT. While reporting verbally immediately thereafter what she or he has seen, the patient is asked to draw a picture of each presentation. During the session, the picture is presented at exposures from 14 to 2000 ms; that is, the participant is shown the picture 20 times while exposure time is progressively increased. Presentation is by means of a personal computer, which is very reliable and easy to handle. The format (vertical or horizontal) and the gender of the person in the picture are varied as well as the brightness and the motivational valence or the stimulus. Presentation times were adapted for the computer version (Gitzinger, 1990b).

DCT Rating

The procedure above generated a verbal protocol for each exposure as well as 20 drawings in one series. In this verbal report the conflict themes are recorded, which are then rated, together with the drawings for 10 possible defense mechanisms on an interactive computer rating program. The defense mechanisms rated are as follows:

1. Repression.
2. Isolation.
3. Denial.
4. Reaction formation.
5. Identification with the aggressor.
6. Turning against self.
7. Introjection—identification with the opposite sex.

8. Multiple introjection.
9. Projection.
10. Regression.

The controlled computer rating is based on subliminal perception theory, Freudian defense theory, and the original operational definitions of defenses devised for scoring the DMT (Kragh, 1985). This procedure was modified to increase standardization and to require less time-consuming ratings. With the DCT rating, the rater only needs 10 to 15 minutes at the interactive program to produce a standardized defense result for one patient on:

The total percentage for each mechanism.
Ipsative percentage (one person's relative percentage of one defense in total).
Phases (and reality perception).
Frequencies of defenses and presentation number.
Unconscious, conscious, and preconscious defenses.

The new instrument is more reliable in its presentation and especially in its ratings than are the usual projective techniques. Within the psychoanalytic framework, this procedure makes possible the observation of the developmental process in perception whereby its relationship to personality problems can be investigated on the conscious and preconscious planes or in terms of the primary and secondary processes in the psychodynamic sense.

Questions Addressed in This Study

Do Female and Male Patients Differ in Defense Mechanisms?

A random sample of 70 neurotic inpatients in a German hospital were diagnosed as suffering from severe neurotic disorders. These patients were administered the DCT, not in its computerized version but by means of presenting slides tachistoscopically. The DCT interactive computer rating was then obtained and compared to the old version of ratings. The results reported below were found to be very reliable. There were several statistically significant differences between men and women in defense mechanisms. The results of these analyses are presented in Table 27.1.

Do Men and Women Differ in Reality Perception?

There was also a significant difference between men and women in reaching the "reality phase". Women attained the so-called C-phase in

TABLE 27.1. Defenses of female (f) and male f(m) patients ($N = 70$): B = bulimic, A = anorectic, h = high.

Defense	F	p	f	m	B	A
Repression	2.27	.04*	h		Sig.	
Isolation	1.44	.30	hs			
Denial	2.28	.00**	h			
Reaction formation	3.55	.00**		h	h	
Identification with aggressor	n.s.					
Turning against self	31.22	.00**		h		
Introjection	3.87	.00**	h			
Multiple introjection	2.01	.09				
Projection	5.01	.00*	h			Sig.
Regression	1.69	.14				

NOTES: Neurotics are known to display little regression (REG); it was therefore expected that as a group, neurotic patients would obtain high scores in isolation and in multiple introjection as well as low scores in regression. In this sample, both men and women were found to have high scores in isolation and multiple introjection and low scores in regression.

Isolation, multiple introjection, and regression were not significantly different for male and female patients. On a descriptive level there was a difference between women and men in the following six mechanisms: repression, denial, reaction formation, turning against self (TURN), introjection, and projection. Women tend more toward repression and denial of threatening conflicts than men do. Ratings of introjection and projection are also higher for women. Men in this sample tended to turn against self and to rely on reaction formation.

$^*p = .01$, $^{**}p = .001$, n.s. = not sign., Sig. = significant.

the DCT earlier than men. They perceived the threatening person in the picture earlier without showing any sign of defense. These results might be connected to the tendency of men to seek therapy at a rather late stage of their disturbance and to make such decisions with great reluctance. Women are used to assimilating and to accepting conflicts with greater ease. The women in this sample have a greater awareness of their conflicts even though they do not resolve them, while men have learned either to accept their conflicts totally or to reject them entirely. The defense styles mirror this contrast: masking, slighting, changing, or putting the threat outside themselves underlie women's defenses. Male patients' defenses demonstrate a more black-and-white tendency: that is, a conflict is fitted into a person's self-concept and is therefore accepted because the conflict is not perceived at all.

Do Men and Women Differ in the Kinds of Conflict Reported?

The conflicts analyzed are not necessarily connected to the defense mechanisms rated, but they are reported during testing. We looked at every story told by the patient and at every picture. On the basis of this information, we produced a category system based on the following themes: sexual abuse, fear of being abused physically (and robbed), fear of having illicit sexual fantasies, mother/daughter or father/son conflicts, religious transgressions, other cultural and social problems. An independent rater saw the results for the women as follows: most of the women talked about the fear of being physically abused, of being robbed, and of being sexually abused. Several of them talked about mother/daughter conflicts related to their wish for identity with and self–others differentiation from other against the mother's opposition to such striving. Men never reported anxieties of being abused sexually or physically. They reported father/son themes connected to achievement and intense fear of failure.

Do Female Patients with Eating Disorders (Bulimic and Anorectic) Differ in Defense from Other Neurotic Female Patients?

Women with eating disorders (anorectic and bulimic) differ negatively from other female patients: turning against self and reaction formation are entirely absent among them. They do not show denial in the DCT. Our explanation of these results is as follows. Anorectic and bulimic patients, in contrast to other neurotic patients, do not need the kinds of defense because of their acting out these conflicts against their own bodies.

Do Anorectic and Bulimic Patients Differ in Their Defense Mechanisms?

Anorectic patients were found to display more projection, while bulimic patients tended toward repression. Bulimic patients reacted with repression as did other female patients, but they resembled male patients in relying on introjection, perhaps because of their ambivalent sex role identity. This finding also supports the theory that views bulimia as a compromise in social conflict. Although anorectic patients react with introjection as other female patients do, they have a very high score in projection. This finding supports the explanation that anorexics believe that they are not ill at all and yet they are convinced that they cannot do anything on their own. It also supports the view that anorectic patients experience what is called an "early disease"; projection is a more psychotic defense mechanism. Thus bulimics tend to identify with the opposite sex and to avoid conflicts by means of repression, while anorexics tend not to identify with the opposite sex and attempt to solve their conflicts by externalizing their problems by means of projection. The common tendency for problem solving in eating disorders is not to face the problem. Bulimics express this tendency through a more internal and anorexics through a more external style of defense. If we posit that the perceived reality of the patient is reflected through the method of analyzing and interpreting defense mechanisms and that the basis of bulimia is the difficulty in separating from mother, the bulimics' ambivalence over having "female and male" defense styles offers support of this view. Keeping in mind the strong repressive tendencies of such patients might be very important in psychotherapy. The conflicts of anorexics are those typically found in "early disease," and their defenses are more psychotic.

Neither anorectic nor bulimic patients characteristically resort to turning against themselves. Neither group exhibits reaction formation or denial. In the DCT classification, the latter two defense mechanisms are very similar: they concern the possibility to turn something threatening into its opposite (i.e., into something "beautiful"). There may be several reasons for the failure of patients to show turning against self when bulimic and anorectic diagnoses are done by the DCT. For example, this result may be traced to socialization and education, and the impact of these variables may explain why there is so much total repression and introjection. Because neurotic male patients are used to turning conflicts into "black and white" feelings, they tend more toward reaction formation and turning against self than neurotic female patients do. The prominence of sex role identity problems and conflicts over self–other differentiation in bulimic patients is supported by their resort to defensive ambivalence in reacting both like other female patients and like male patients and in repressing every thought and feeling connected with this ambivalence. This study provides a basis for further research on defense styles to help therapists understand resistance and conflicts in eating disorders and to help patients analyze sex role conflicts from another point of view.

References

Bucci, W. (1988) Converging evidence for emotional structures: Theory and method. In H. Dahl, H. Kächele, & H. Thomae (Eds.), *Psychoanalytic process research*. New York: Springer.

Fahrenberg, J., Hampel, R., & Selg, H. (1984) *Das Freiburger Persönlichkeitsinventar. Handbuch zum FPI-R*. Göttingen: Verlag für Psychologie.

Freud, A. (1936) *Das Ich und die Abwehrmechanismen* [The ego and the mechanisms of defense]. Vienna: Internationaler Psychoanalytischer Verlag.

Gitzinger, I. (1988) *Operatonalisierung von Abwehrmechanismen*. Unpublished thesis, University of Freiburg.

Gitzinger, I. (1990a) Perceptual and linguistic coding of defense mechanisms in a clinical setting. *Psychotherapie, Psychosomatik, medizinische Psychologie, 40* [Disk Journal, Vol. 1, No. 1].

Gitzinger, I. (1990b) *Operationalization of defense mechanisms*. Paper read at the "Werkstatt für Empirische Forschung in der Psychoanalyse," University of Ulm, Germany, June.

Gitzinger, I. (1993) Mehrebenendiagnostik von Abwehrprozessen als eine Strategie der Psychotherapieforschung [Multilevel diagnostics of defense processes as a strategy for psychotherapy research]. Frankfurt: Peter Lang.

Haan, N. (1963) Proposed model of ego functioning: Coping and defense mechanisms in relationship to IQ change. *Psychological Monographs*, 77, No. 571.

Kragh, U. (1960) The Defense Mechanism Test. *Journal of Applied Psychology*, 40, 303–309.

Kragh, U. (1985) *DMT-Manual*. Stockholm: Persona.

28
Defense Mechanisms and Defense Organizations: Their Role in the Adaptation to the Acute Stage of Crohn's Disease

JOACHIM KÜCHENHOFF

Acute and severe somatic illnesses inflict severe psychological stress for the patient. The disturbance of bodily well-being has a serious impact on the narcissistic investment in the body. Thus a vital dimension of self-coherence is called into question. Being confronted with the diagnosis of a chronic illness implies that future life perspectives have become insecure, since the patient must live with the danger of possible relapse. He or she faces unusual dependencies on medical professionals and medical treatment. Therefore confrontation with an acute or chronic disease constitutes a challenge to the personality and its adaptive resources. From the psychoanalytic perspective, there is a special challenge to the defensive repertoire. The aim of defense, as Hoffmann (1987) has pointed out, is to regulate the individual narcissistic balance that is endangered by disease. It is therefore important to study the relationship of defense to the course of and adaptation to a disease. The relevant research issues that have increasingly become influential in present day psychosomatic research as a whole and in our Heidelberg research project on Crohn's disease can be summarized as follows:

1. What is the impact of the preexisting chronic course of a disease on the defense organization during an acute illness?
2. What are the adaptive values of the various defense mechanisms in the different phases of the disease?
3. What is the impact of the personality on the defense organization during the several phases of the disease?

The Heidelberg Research Project on Crohn's Disease

The Heidelberg research project (Küchenhoff, 1993) is a longitudinal study that analyzes the interrelations of personality, defense, coping, and course of the disease in patients suffering from Crohn's Disease (CD). CD is a severe and chronic relapsing illness mainly of the gastrointestinal tract, with abdominal pain, bloody diarrhea, fistula formation, and severe impairment of general health. Various extraintestinal symptoms may complicate the clinical picture.

Personality, disease process, and adaptation to the disease are interrelated in a complex manner. However, there are numerous empirical reports on the personality of Crohn's disease patients that do not take into account the course of the disease (e.g. Cohn et al., 1970); recent work done by the Lübeck research team (Leibig, Wilke, & Feiereis, 1985) has demonstrated that some psychological factors that had been assumed to be traits are clearly dependent on the somatic state. Therefore the course of the disease has to be taken into account in research. In the Heidelberg project, we see CD patients three times; in the acute phase, during remission, and 3 years after the first interview (cf. Table 28.1).

This chapter presents data on defense mechanisms from phase 1 of our project. At that time all patients were acutely ill. They were referred by the medical departments that cooperate with the project. Acuteness in generally approved medical terms means that the patients have surpassed 150 on a disease activity scale especially designed for CD patients, the so-Called Best Index or CDAI. Preexisting experience with the disease varied across patients, some of whom were confronted with CD for the first time ("new patients"), whereas others had experienced a relapse of a chronically recurring disease, the criterion for chronicity being a duration of CD exceeding 3 years (Ford, Glober, & Castelnuovo-Tedesco, 1970).

The comparison of both groups permits the investigation of the first of the three research issues: What impact does the long-lasting adaptation to a chronic disease have on the defense mechanisms in the acute phase? Is there a difference between new and chronic CD patients in the defense mechanisms employed during the acute phase?

The defense mechanisms were registered by the Clinical Assessment of Defense Mechanisms (CADM), an instrument for the clinical rating of defense mechanisms designed by Ehlers (1983) (cf. Chapter 17). The psychoanalytic interview was tape recorded and was played for three or four psychoanalytically trained raters, who listened to three 10-minute periods of the interview. Three individual ratings at the end of each interval were compared and discussed afterward; each of the 26 defense

TABLE 28.1. The Heidelberg study on Crohn's disease.

	First exploration: acute illness	Second exploration: first remission phase	
	Crohn's Disease Activity Index > 150	Crohn's Disease Activity Index < 100	Controls: 3 years later
New patients	N = 60	N = 60	N = 60
Chronic patients	N = 60	N = 60	N = 60

mechanisms was considered, and a generally agreed-upon result was recorded upon discussion (Küchenhoff, 1991).

Here we discuss ratings of 53 patients: the 27 chronic patients are about 2 years older (28 years vs. 25.9 years); the CDAI is comparable in both groups (274 vs. 245). In both groups there is a female predominance (17 vs. 10 in chronic patients, 19 vs. 7 in new patients).

Results

We begin with discrete defense mechanisms, as summarized in Fig. 28.1. The defense mechanisms are ranked according to their importance. We have defined as important defense mechanisms that have been rated 4 or 5 on the CADM rating scale with a range from 1 to 5 for at least 50% of the subsample. Three defense mechanisms are characteristic of both the chronic and the new patients: denial, rationalization, and isolation. Isolation exceeds 50% only in the chronic patients' group. Denial has a special importance in both groups: about three-quarters of the patients show strong denial. The very high incidence of denial is probably due to the acute stage of the illness. Of the several mechanisms, denial has been most thoroughly studied in psychoanalytic research on adaptation to illness (Beutel, 1985). As Gaus and Köhle (1986) have pointed out, it functions as an emergency mechanism ("Notfallmechanismus") that seems to be independent of personality and disease, but is peculiar to the situation. By preventing a complete perception of the disease reality, it cushions the person from the impact of traumatizing experiences and sustains his or her ego functioning at the expense of a restriction in ego functions (Freud, 1938/1964). Denial may be helpful during the acute phase by maintaining ego functioning that is needed for taking necessary steps toward treatment. Persistent denial might be maladaptive because it precludes working through of the disease reality in the long run. It is worth noting that chronic patients also show denial well. Living with the disease for a long time does not lessen denial at the acute stage. Assuming that denial is specific only to the situation, we expect that it does not play a major role in the state of remission.

Rationalization and isolation come next. Both defense mechanisms help repress the affective responses and serve to replace them by rational controls. There are two possible interpretations of these mechanisms:

1. Like denial, rationalization can be regarded as an answer to the situation; it may simply support denial. Laplanche and Pontalis (1972) argue that rationalization is a secondary defense mechanism that makes the more basic defenses acceptable to consciousness. Acute illness then might have a strong homogenizing effect on defense.

2. Since rationalization and isolation are defense mechanisms most often seen in obsessive–compulsive personalities, and since obsessive–

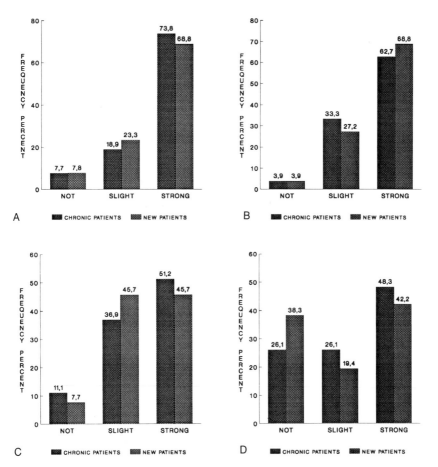

FIGURE 28.1. Group differences in discrete defenses. A. CADM 15 denial. B. CADM 11 rationalization. C. CADM 10 isolation. D. CADM 14 reaction formation.

compulsive traits have been found most often in other research studies on Crohn's disease, rationalization and isolation may in part constitute personality factors. We then would expect little change in phases 2 and 3 of our longitudinal study.

Up to now, we have studied discrete defense mechanisms. However, it should be kept in mind that defenses do not work in isolation, but form patterns or defensive organizations as Lichtenberg and Slap (1971) have pointed out. Evaluation of complex defense organizations allows a description that is closer to clinical reality. We have defined five defense organizations on a theoretical basis, proceeding from the model of defense proposed by Moser (1964). He differentiated between countercathectic defenses such as repression and regressive defense mechanisms, which

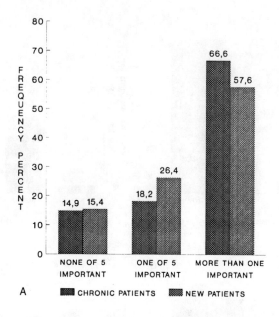

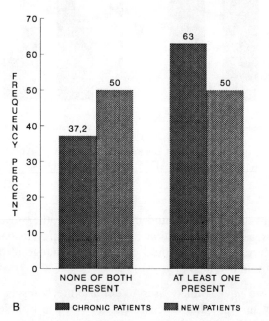

FIGURE 28.2. Group differences in neurotic defense organisations. A. Obsessive–compulsive defense. B. Depressive defense.

bring about alterations in self- and object representation, exemplified by projection. The former can be designated as neurotic defenses, the latter can be termed the early defense mechanisms. Let us consider the neurotic defense organizations first.

We have classified defense mechanisms 10–14 as an obsessive–compulsive defense and defense mechanisms 2 and 6 as depressive defenses. *Obsessive–compulsive defenses* are an arbitrary defensive organization consisting of isolation, rationalization, compulsive thinking, undoing, and reaction formation. In about two-thirds of the patients, high ratings were assigned for more than one of these mechanisms. Obsessive–compulsive defense is important for both groups.

Depressive defense is made up of a combination of depressive reaction and turning against the self; it is similar to the "self-sacrificing style" described by Bond (1986). Depressive defense is slightly less prominent in both groups, and again there is little difference between them (cf. Fig. 28.2).

Let me briefly return to Moser's (1964) theory. Whenever the ego cannot overcome anxiety by a neurotic defense, an additional defense is activated by alteration of self- and object representation. If the assumption is correct that acute and severe somatic illness can be traumatic (i.e., an experience that overwhelms neurotic defense), then early defense mechanisms might be additionally employed as a result of ego regression. The defensive repertoire then regresses to genetically early stages. We have distinguished three subgroups within the group of early defense mechanisms: borderline, narcissistic, and alexithymic (cf. Fig. 28.3).

1. Devaluation of objects and fantasies of omnipotent control are defense mechanisms that stabilize the ego through *narcissistic defense*. This objective is accomplished by activating a grandiose self as described by Kohut (1973). It is important to note that this combined occurrence of both defense mechanisms is given high ratings considerably more often in the group of the new patients.

2. Introjection, projection, splitting, projective identification, and primitive idealization are projective–introjective mechanisms that loom large in the defensive organization of borderline patients. We therefore apply the label of *borderline defense* for this cluster of mechanisms. For about half the patients, at least one of these mechanisms is important, but the conjunction at two or more mechanisms that received high ratings did not occur frequently in either group.

3. We grouped predominance of affective equivalents and primitive denial under the heading of *alexithymic defense*. This category requires a short explanation. Primitive denial, often termed psychotic denial in the literature, is defined as a radical exclusion of unbearable thoughts and affects from the intrapsychic experience. It seems to be equivalent to the defense mechanism of foreclosure (*Verwerfung*). Foreclosure has recently

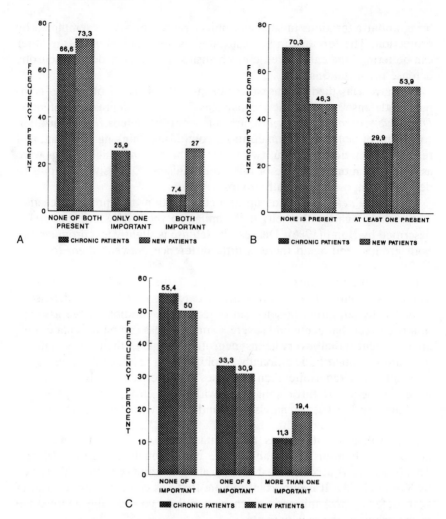

FIGURE 28.3. Group differences in early defense mechanisms. A. Narcissistic defense. B. Alexithymia-like defense. C. Borderline-like defense.

been described as the defense mechanism characteristic of alexithymic patients (McDougall, 1985). Such an exclusion of psychic representation brings about psychic stress that cannot be symbolized. It is then discharged by the body by forming affective equivalents. The presence of at least one of these mechanisms is noted in more than half the new patients as compared to only 30% of the chronic patients.

To summarize these results: for one-third to one-half of the new patients, early defense organizations play an important role; there is a clear difference between new and chronic patients with regard to narcissistic and alexithymic defense. This result is in harmony with Moser's (1964) theory: within the group of the new patients, the sudden onset of the unexpected acute disease may be more traumatic than for the chronic patients; thus the maintenance of ego activity for neurotic defense will be more often endangered, with the consequence of ego regression and additional regressive defense.

Let us return to the second of the three main research issues: What is the adaptive value of defense? Very little is known about possible factors that influence the disease process in CD (Farmer, Whelan, & Fazio, 1985). So far we have investigated the relationship between the defensive organization and the duration of the bowel inflammation in a subsample of our patients. Duration of the disease seems to be a sufficiently important parameter to serve as a preliminary criterion for adaptivity. In accordance with medical criteria, we have defined the duration of more than 34 weeks as a long inflammatory period (Summers et al., 1979). Remission has been defined by the normal medical standards, namely a CDAI lower than 100 for 4 weeks and no drugs or only maintenance pharmacotherapy. For the present preliminary evaluation, we used the data on 42 patients; 25 of them had remission within 34 weeks after the onset of the disease while in 17 cases acute inflammation lasted longer.

A relationship was found between the duration of the acute phase and two defensive organizations, alexithymic and obsessive–compulsive (cf. Figs. 28.4 and 28.5). More than half the long-term patients show an alexithymic defense organization, whereas the patients with a short disease duration show this pattern in only 20% of the cases. An inverse relationship can be found in obsessive–compulsive defensive organization. It is rated as important more frequently in patients who recover quickly. If we agree that a short duration of inflammation can be judged to be the better result, one can assume that the obsessive–compulsive defensive organization may be favorable in the acute phase, whereas the alexithymic pattern may be more adaptive in the chronic phase.

Summary and Conclusion

Patients suffering from CD do not constitute a homogeneous group. Their course of the disease is variable, as is their level of stress as well as their individual adaptations to the disease. The present study has inquired into a small portion of the various factors that influence the disease process, specifically the impact of the long-term experience with a chronic disease on the defensive mechanisms during the acute phase of the illness.

Evaluation of CADM ratings at the level of individual mechanisms has produced a surprising result: confrontation with an acute somatic crisis exerts a homogenizing influence on the defense. Denial and rational-

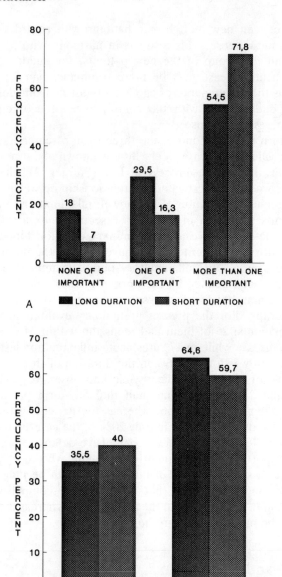

FIGURE 28.4. Duration of illness and neurotic defense organisations. A. Obsessive–compulsive defense. B. Depressive defense.

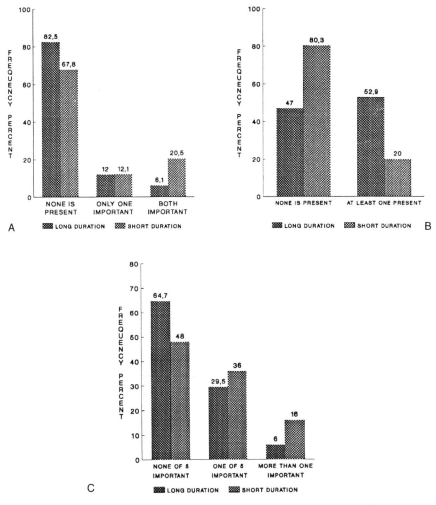

FIGURE 28.5. Duration of illness and early defense mechanisms. A. Narcissistic defense. B. Alexithymia-like defense. C. Borderline-like defense.

ization have been found in the great majority of the new as well as in the chronic patients. Chronicity has no moderating influence on the defense during the acute stage. Evaluation of phase 2 of our research project will help us to decide what defense mechanisms are stable and what defense mechanisms are activated during the acute phase only.

Evaluation of the CADM ratings at the level of defense organizations has provided data for further differentiation of the subgroups. Various defensive organizations play an important role; most important is an obsessive–compulsive defensive organization, but depressive defense is recognizable in about 50% of the patients. For a considerable number of the new patients, early defense mechanisms are important (i.e., alexithymic and narcissistic defenses that are of minor relevance for the chronic patients). A possible interpretation of this finding would focus on the traumatic impact of the disease, which can overwhelm the ego's capacity for integration and can mobilize regressive defense mechanisms.

In the course of our longitudinal study we hope to be able to elucidate more thoroughly the impact of defense mechanisms and defense organizations on adaptiveness. Preliminary results suggest that the study of defense organization can be useful for prognostic purposes. During the acute phase of the disease, obsessive–compulsive defenses seem to predict a favorable course, whereas the occurrence of early defense organizations suggests a poor prognosis. During the acute phase, the opportunity of minimizing the affective response to the disease by compulsive mechanisms can affect the course of the disease positively, whereas the overwhelming of ego functions that leads to the mobilization of early defense repertoires represents an unfavorable precondition for the disease process.

The CADM is a time-consuming rating method that is not very easy to handle because it requires prolonged training if it is to be used realistically. Sharp differentiation of the defense mechanisms must be accomplished by the rating team. Despite these disadvantages, it appears that the CADM can be very useful as a research tool for the study of adaptation to chronic diseases. With the help of the CADM, stability or variability of defense processes in the course of chronic diseases can be investigated. Furthermore, the adaptiveness of defense processes can be analyzed with the help of the CADM.

References

Beutel, M. (1985) Zur Erforschung der Verarbeitung chronischer Krankheit: Konzeptualisierung, Operationalisierung und Adaptivität von Abwehrprozessen am Beispiel von Verleugnung [Research into coping with chronic disease: Conceptual approach, operationalization and adaptivity of defense processes shown by the example of denial]. *Psychotherapie, Psychosomatik, medizinische Psychologie, 35*, 295–302.

Bond, M. (1986) An empirical study of defense styles. In G.D. Vaillant (Ed.), *Empirical studies of ego mechanisms of defense* (pp. 1–29). Washington, DC: American Psychiatric Press.

Cohen, E., Lederman, I., & Shore, E. (1970) Regional enteritis and its relation to emotional disorders. *American Journal of Gastroenterology, 54*, 378–387.

Ehlers, W. (1983) Dimensionen der klinischen Beurteilung von Abwehrmechanismen [Dimensions of clinical ratings of defense mechanisms]. *Praxis der Psychotherapie und Psychosomatik, 28*, 1–10.

Farmer, R.G., Whelan, G., & Fazio, V.W. (1985) Long-term follow-up of patients with Crohn's disease. *Gastroenterology, 88*, 1818–1825.

Ford, C.V., Glober, G.A., & Castelnuovo-Tedesco, P. (1969) A psychiatric study of patients with regional enteritis. *Journal of the American Medical Association, 208*, 311–315.

Freud, S. (1964) Splitting of the ego in the process of defense. In J. Strachey (Ed. and Trans.), *The standard edition of the complete psychological works of Sigmund Freud: Vol. 23* (pp. 230–233). London: Hogarth Press. (Original work published 1938)

Gaus, E. & Köhle, K. (1986) Psychische Anpassungs- und Abwehrvorgänge bei körperlichen Erkrankungen [Psychic processes of adaptation and defense in somatic illnesses]. In T. von Uexküll (Ed.), *Psychosomatische Medizin* [Psychosomatic medicin] (pp. 1127–1145). Munich: Urban & Schwarzenberg.

Hoffmann, S.O. (1987) Die psychoanalytische Abwehrlehre—Aktuell, antiquiert oder obsolet? [The psychoanalytic theory of defense: Up-to-date, antiquated or obsolete?]. *Forum der Psychoanalyse, 3*, 20–39.

Kohut, H. (1973) *Narzißmus* [Narcissism]. Frankfurt: Suhrkamp.

Küchenhoff, J. (1991) Zur Theorie und Methodik der Fremdeinschätzung von Abwehrprozessen [Clinical rating of defense processes: Theory and methodology]. *Psychotherapie, Psychosomatik, medizinische Psychologie, 41*, 216–223.

Küchenhoff, J. (1993) *Psychosomatik des Morbus Crohn. Zur Wechselwirkung seelischer und körperlicher Faktoren im Krankheitsverlauf* [Psychosomatics of Crohn's Disease. The interaction of psychological and somatic factors during the course of the disease]. Stuttgart: Enke.

Laplanche, J. & Pontalis, J.B. (1972) *Das Vokabular der Psychoanalyse* [The vocabulary of psychoanalysis]. Frankfurt: Suhrkamp.

Leibig, T., Wilke, E., & Feiereis, H. (1985) Zur Persönlichkeitsstruktur von Patienten mit Colitis ulcerosa und Morbus Crohn [On the personality structure in patients with ulcerative colitis and Crohn's disease]. *Zeitschrift für psychosomatische Medizin und Psychoanalyse, 31*, 380–392.

Lichtenberg, J.D. & Slap, J.W. (1971) On the defensive organization. *International Journal of Psychoanalysis, 52*, 451–457.

McDougall, J. (1985) *Plädoyer für eine gewisse Anormalität* [Plea for a measure of abnormality]. Frankfurt: Suhrkamp.

Moser, U. (1964) Zur Abwehrlehre: Das Verhältnis von Verdrängung und Projektion [On the theory of defense: The relationship of repression and projection]. *Jahrbuch der Psychoanalyse, 3*, 56–85.

Summers, R.W., Switz, D.M., Sessions, J.T., Becktel, J.M., & Best, W.R. (1979) National Cooperative Crohn's Disease Study: Result of drug treatment. *Gastroenterology, 77*, 847–869.

Index